ASPECTS OF PACEMAKERS – FUNCTIONS AND INTERACTIONS IN CARDIAC AND NON-CARDIAC INDICATIONS

Edited by **Oliver Vonend** and **Siegfried Eckert**

Aspects of Pacemakers – Functions and Interactions in Cardiac and Non-Cardiac Indications
Edited by Oliver Vonend and Siegfried Eckert

Published by InTech
Janeza Trdine 9, 51000 Rijeka, Croatia

Publishing Process Manager Dragana Manestar

Technical Editor Teodora Smiljanic

Cover Designer InTech Design Team

Additional hard copies can be obtained from orders@intechopen.com

Aspects of Pacemakers – Functions and Interactions in Cardiac and Non-Cardiac Indications, Edited by Oliver Vonend and Siegfried Eckert
p. cm.
ISBN 978-953-307-616-4

For EU product safety concerns:
IN TECH d.o.o., Prolaz Marije Krucifikse Kozulić 3, 51000 Rijeka, Croatia,
info@intechopen.com or visit our website at intechopen.com.

Meet the editors

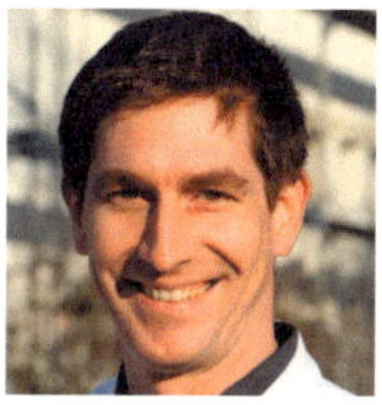

Dr. Oliver Vonend is born in Germany, he is currently an assistant professor of the department of Nephrology of the Heinrich-Heine-University Duesseldorf. Oliver Vonend was working in London, Baltimore and Boston concentrating on neuroscience and the sympathetic nervous system before he moved to the Ruhr-University Bochum. As a Junior-Professor he directed many doctoral theses in the he field of experimental nephrology. In 2008 he started his actual position in Duesseldorf. One of his major clinical fields of interest is the workup and treatment of resistant hypertension. He has various national and international publications in the areas of experimental and clinical hypertension. Besides the evaluation of secondary causes for hypertension he analyzes the efficiency of electrical baroreceptor stimulation and high frequency renal nerve ablation as new options for resistant hypertension.

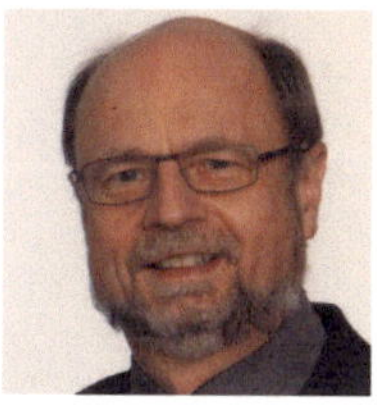

Dr. Siegfried Eckert is a senior assistant at The Clinic of Cardiology, Heart and Diabetes Center North Rhine-Westphalia, Ruhr University of Bochum in Bad Oeynhausen, Germany. He received his medical degree from the Westfälische Wilhelm-University Münster. Dr. Eckert is board certified in internal medicine, angiology, cadiology and diabetology. He is an active member of the German Society of Angiology, German Cardiac Society, Diabetes DE, International Neuromodulation Society, European Society of hypertension and board member of the German Hypertension League. Dr. Eckert research interests include therapy of arterial hypertension and other cardiovascular diseases, resistant angina pectoris and peripheral arterial diseases. He is a national coordinator of the DEBuT-HT and EXPAND-D studies and served on the editorial board for Diabetes, Metabolism, and the Heart.

Contents

Preface

Pacemakers play an important role in our body homeostasis. The identification of endogenous pacemakers and the exploration of their controllability lead to a remarkable progress in human medicine. On cellular basis proliferation and orientation are regulated, and contraction and organ interactions were modulated by pacemaking cells. Dysfunctions lead to acute and chronic organ damage and can be life-threatening. In this respect, overactive as well as underactive pacemaking can bring a person in a very dangerous situation.

In the last decades, "artificial" pacemakers made outstanding steps forward, in particular in cardiovascular science. The devices are now able to do much more than solely pacemaking of the heart. Sensing, pacing, resynchronization, overstimulation and defibrillation are just some of the functions that actual devices can cover. And not only is the heart dependant on pacemaking cells; the urinary tract, the central nervous system and the blood pressure is controlled to a certain extent by endogenous pacemakers.

However, one has to be careful to find the correct indication before device implantation. In addition, complications such as infections need to be minimised. It should be noted that some diagnostic or therapeutic procedures cannot be performed when a person carries an electrical device. Taken together, a correctly functioning device can improve the quality of life substantially.

New devices, beside cardiac pacemakers, are currently under investigation. In order to treat arterial hypertension various strategies were developed. Besides renal nerve ablation, baroreceptor stimulation is one approach to reduce the sympathetic nerve activity. Similar to a cardiac pacemaker, an electrical device stimulates the glomus caroticus to feed back to the central nervous system in order to re-adjust the elevated blood pressure.

In this book, through eleven chapters different aspects of pacemakers –functions and interactions were reviewed. In addition, various areas of application and the potential side effects and complications of the devices were discussed.

Dr. med. Oliver Vonend
Department of Nephrology, Medical Faculty,
Heinrich Heine University, Duesseldorf,
Germany

Dr. med. Siegfried Eckert
Department of Cardiology,
Heart and Diabetes Center North Rhine-Westphalia,
Ruhr-University Bochum, Bad Oeynhausen,
Germany

Part 1

Devices in Hypertension

1

Novel Approaches in Hypertension Treatment - Modulation of the Sympathetic Overactivity

Sebastian A. Potthoff, Lars-Christian Rump and Oliver Vonend
*Department of Internal Medicine / Nephrology, Medical Faculty,
Heinrich-Heine-University Duesseldorf,
Germany*

1. Introduction

Arterial hypertension is the leading cause of mortality in the world [1]. It is estimated that 25 to 35 % of modern populations suffer from this condition [2-4]. Hypertension is the major risk factor for the most common cardio vascular diseases which are a major cause for morbidity and mortality. Depending on the stage of hypertension, it dramatically increases the individual risk for heart failure, heart attack, stroke or chronic kidney failure if not treated adequately [5]. Since hypertension is usually not directly linked to specific symptoms, it is one of the most insufficiently treated diseases in the population with only 10-20 % of patients with controlled blood pressure levels [4]. It is estimated that the prevalence of hypertension is going to increase within the next decades. Aging populations contribute significantly to this trend [6]. Due to its impact on public health, it already is a major burden for modern societies [7].

New strategies and treatment options have to be evaluated in order to slow or prevent the rise in hypertension related morbidity and mortality. This chapter focuses on the role of the sympathetic nervous system in the pathogenesis of hypertension. After almost half a decade with only minor advancements in this field, sympathetic overactivity has been recognized as a major contributor to hypertension [8]. Many secondary causes can increase sympathetic activity which can lead to hypertension. Beyond the initial contribution, sympathetic overactivity can sustain hypertension. Therefore the sympathetic nervous system plays a role in the acute and chronic pathogenesis of hypertension. Understanding the mechanisms involved in the regulation of the sympathetic nervous system is currently leading to novel approaches in hypertension treatment.

2. Anatomy of the sympathetic nervous system

2.1 Efferent sympathetic neurons

Sympathetic innervation origins from the intermediolateral cell column of the spinal cord. Preganglionic neurons range from the thoracic to the lumbar parts (T1-L2). These short neurons usually travel to the paravertebral ganglia where they connect to the postganglionic neurons. Those postganglionic neurons sympathetically innervate most organs such as heart, kidney and blood vessels (Fig. 1). Sympathetic nerve endings release a variety of neurotransmitters notably norepinephrine, neuropeptide Y (NPY) and adenosine triphosphate (ATP) [9, 10].

Sympathetic overactivity is a major contributor to arterial hypertension which is one of the leading causes of stroke, chronic kidney failure, left ventricular hypertrophy and sudden cardiac death.

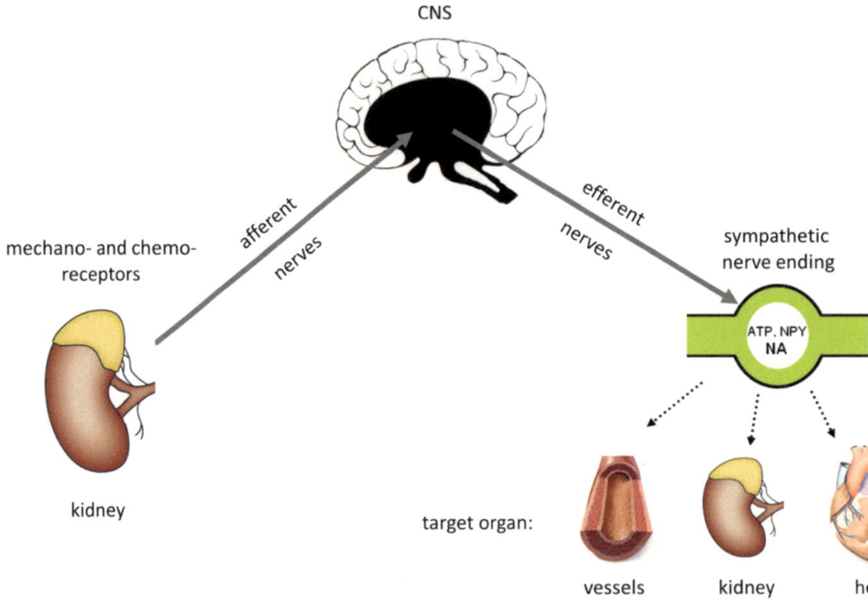

Fig. 1. Schematic of sensory, afferent and sympathetic efferent neurons and target organ innervation.

One of the distinct features of the sympathetic nervous system is the immediate regulation of peripheral vascular resistance through adaptation of the vascular tone. Besides this immediate action on blood pressure control through vasoconstriction, release of sympathetic neurotransmitters contribute to adaptive mechanisms through regulation of cell proliferation, transformation and apoptosis which are blood pressure independent [11-14].

2.2 Afferent sympathetic nerve activity

Besides the efferent innervation, sensory afferent neurons travel from target organs to the sympathetic nuclei of the central nervous system (CNS). These afferent nerves have been extensively described for the kidney but can also be found in the heart [15]. The pathogenesis of this sympathetic activation was elucidated in several animal models [16]. Afferent nerves are activated by baro- or chemoreceptors in ischemia or inflammation [17]. They travel along the renal artery and insert the posterior horn of the spinal cord at the level of TH6-L3 from where they travel to the sympathetic nuclei of the CNS (Fig.1). Neurotransmitters of these afferent neurons are ATP, substance P and calcitonin-gene related peptide (CGRP)[18].

The renin-angiotensin-aldosterone system (RAAS) contributes to the central nervous feedback in sympathetic activation. Especially angiotensin II and nitric oxide (NO) are important effectors of this system [19]. Inhibition of the RAAS leads to a decrease in efferent sympathetic activity in chronic kidney disease patients [18]. Not all inhibitors of the RAAS can penetrate through the blood-brain barrier, therefore peripheral actions of angiotensin II are likely to affect afferent signal transduction.

Renal ischemia leads to a release of adenosine as a paracrine transmitter. This leads to a potent activation of afferent neurons [17]. Interestingly, in an animal model, already minor kidney injury through local injection of phenol leads to a permanent neurogenic hypertension [20]. Severing afferent and efferent sympathetic nerve fibers prevents hypertension in an animal model of chronic kidney injury [21]. Independent from CNS-effects, chronic kidney injury leads to an increase of presynaptic norepinephrine release in the heart and kidney. This might be due to an increase in angiotensin II through RAAS activation [22-24]. However, it is still unclear which renal mechanisms contribute to a sustained activation of renal afferent neurons.

3. Detection of increased neuronal activity

3.1 Microneurography

Microneurography has been established at the university of Uppsala (Sweden) by Karl-Erik Habbarth und Åke Vallbo [25]. The sympathetic nerve activity can be measured by insertion of a micro electrode into a peripheral nerve (mostly peroneal nerve) [26].

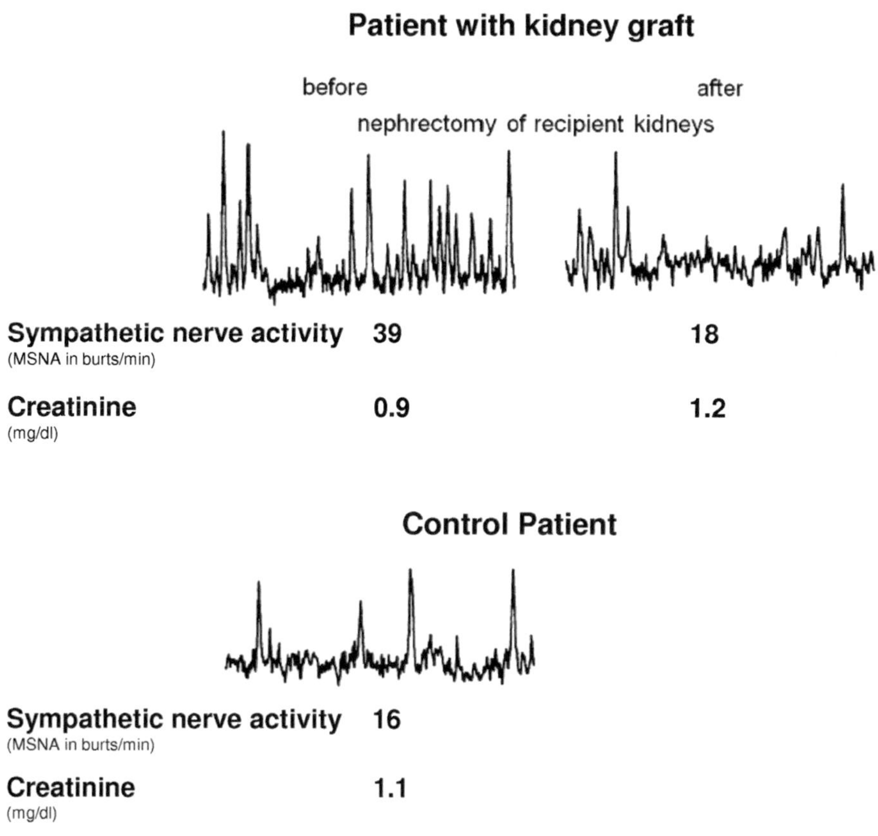

Fig. 2. Multiunit activity sympathetic nerve activity (MSNA) of the sural nerve. Kidney transplant patients show an increased sympathetic nerve activity despite normal serum creatinine levels. Only nephrectomy of the native kidneys is able to normalize the activity compared to healthy controls (modified from [28]).

Multiunit activity sympathic nerve activity (MSNA) is equivalent to the sympathetic activity. This activity is measured as "bursts" per minute. Using this method, the concept of the kidney as a pacemaker of sympathetic activity could be very well established. Converse et al. analyzed the sympathetic activity in dialysis patients vs. healthy controls [27]. Interestingly, in kidney transplant patients with normal serum levels of creatinine and urea, the sympathetic overactivity persisted. Only bilateral nephrectomy was able to abolish the pathologic sympathetic overactivity (Fig. 2) [28].

3.2 Norepinephrine release

Besides microneurography, norepinephrine release can be used to estimate the activity of the sympathetic nervous system. This concept has been established by Murray Esler from Melbourne, Australia [29]. Norepinephrine can be measured in blood samples. Also local norepinephrine release can be quantified in tissue samples from kidney and heart.
The heart is an important target organ of sympathetic activity. Especially patients with end stage renal disease show a dramatic and early increase of cardiovascular events. Zocalli et al. could demonstrate that norepinephrine and NPY serum levels correlate with the patient mortality (Fig. 3) [30, 31].

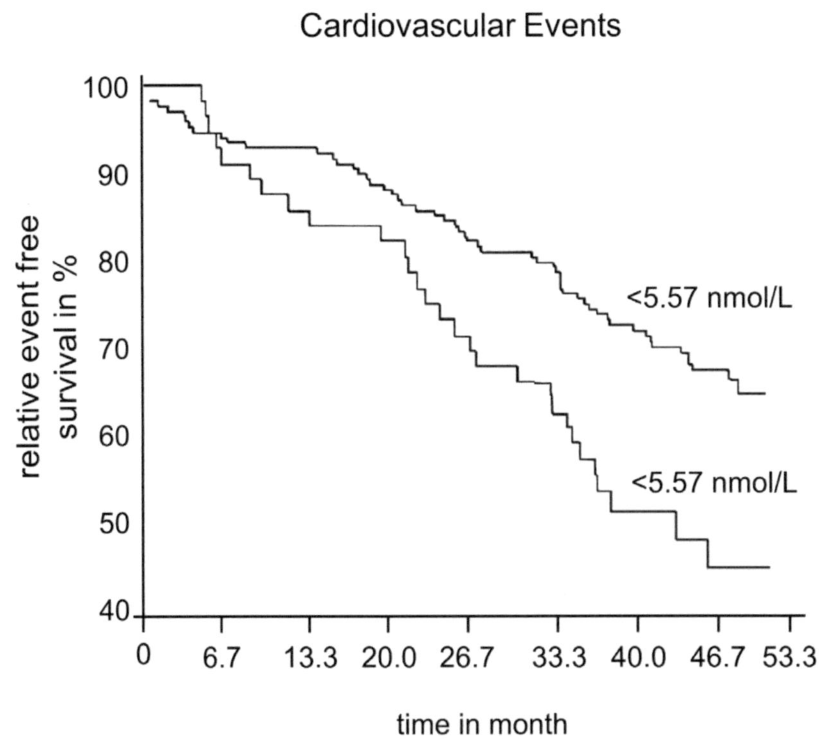

Fig. 3. Serum norepinephrine levels correlate well with the incidence of cardiovascular events in end stage renal disease patients (n = 228 patients on haemodialysis). Kaplan-Meier survival curves for cardiovascular events (fatal and nonfatal) in patients below and above 75th percentile of serum norepinephrine (5.57 nmol/L) (from [30]).

3.3 Modulation of sympathetic activity

The sympathetic nervous system allows for rapid adaptation of the body to current events. Orthostatic reaction is a well examined example of immediate activation of the sympathetic nervous system [32]. Besides pain, stress and urgency, changes in temperature, blood oxygenation and ambient sound level lead to a change in sympathetic activity [15, 32].
Instead of immediate alterations of sympathetic activity, it appears feasible that long-term change in sympathetic activity is the underlying mechanism which contributes to the development of hypertension. Aging people show an increase in sympathetic activity with an increase of MSNA of 1 burst/min per year [33]. Although female subjects are characterized by a lower MSNA, they exhibit a more significant annual increase [34]. It is likely that the increase in MSNA contributes to the development of hypertension in the aging population, since the prevalence of hypertension increases with age. There is a tight correlation between blood pressure and MSNA in subjects older than 40 which does not occur in younger patients (Fig. 4.) [34]. This might be due to diminished compensatory mechanisms in the elderly population (endothelial dysfunction, diminished baroreflex, etc.).
Sympathetic overactivity is the pathogenic link between hear failure, sleep apnea, metabolic syndrome and hypertension.

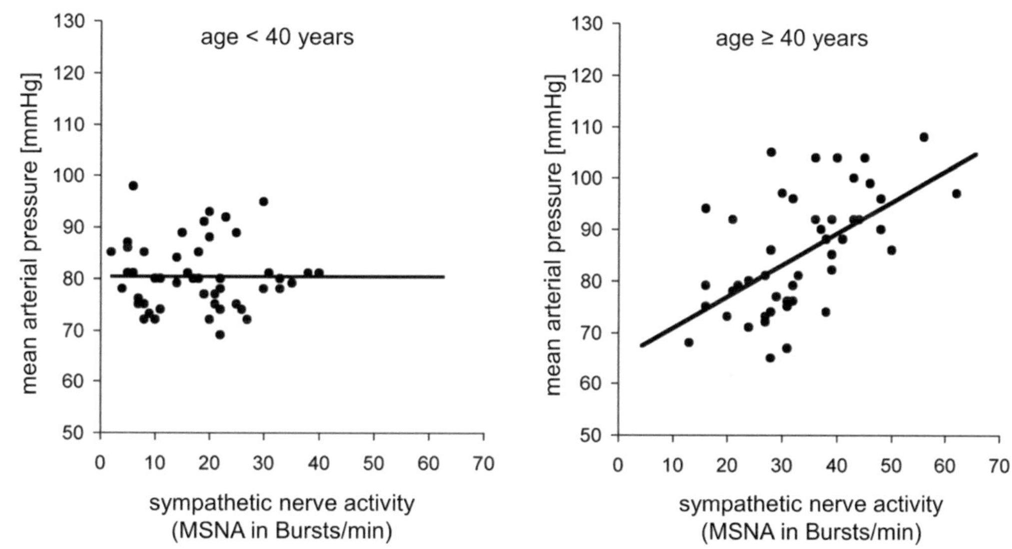

Fig. 4. Correlation between MSNA and mean arterial blood pressure in female subjects <40 and ≥ 40 years of age. A correlation between blood pressure and MSNA cannot be found until the age of 40 (modified from [34]).

3.4 Sympathic overactivity in chronic heart failure

Chronic heart failure is associated with an increased sympathetic activity [35]. There is a tight correlation between severity of heart failure and MSNA. However, MSNA does not allow direct conclusion on the degree of heart failure. Due to different mechanisms of sympathetic activation, high MSNA can also be found in patients with only mild to moderate heart failure [36].

The rise in MSNA causes an increase of norepinephrine release in the myocardium. The increased release of norepinephrine contributes to the increased risk of arrhythmogenic cardiac events and left ventricular hypertrophy.
In an animal model with genetically determined sympathetic overactivity (α2-adrenoceptor knockout - decreased adrenergic auto inhibition), increase of left ventricular mass and heart failure can be observed [37].
Hypernatremia is a common finding in severe chronic heart failure. This leads to an activation of the RAAS and sympathetic nervous system. However, the increase in sympathetic activity can already be observed in mild to moderate chronic heart failure. The underlying cause is not well understood. This might be linked to a change in baroreflex sensitivity or a maladaptation of the cardiopulmonary reflex [35].
A left ventricular systolic dysfunction with an increase of cardiopulmonary filling pressure can trigger sympathetic activity. Obesity and sleep apnea add to this condition.
Therefore, a goal in chronic heart failure has to be the inhibition of the self-sustaining pacing of sympathetic activity, in order to reduce the cardiovascular mortality.

3.5 Sympathetic overactivity in sleep apnea

Sleep related respiratory dysfunction is much more common in patients with hypertension compared to the common population [18]. Some authors estimate that every second patient with hypertension is prone to sleep related respiratory dysfunction [38]. An increase in blood pressure is almost always observable in sleep apnea patients. Apnea causes an immediate increase in sympathetic activity which is the underlying cause of the increase in blood pressure [39]. Chemo-receptors within the carotid body (glomus caroticum) are activated due to hypoxia. Those chemo-receptors can directly activate the sympathetic nervous system. [18].
In chronic sleep apnea, this activation of the sympathetic nervous system persists during daytime which results in increased MSNA and norepinephrine release [40]. Intermittent hypoxia leads to a sustained increase in blood pressure in an animal model. Denervation of the carotid body abolishes the blood pressure increase after hypoxia [41]. Desensitizing chemo-receptors through respiration of 100 % oxygen leads to a decrease in sympathetic activity, heart rate and blood pressure in wake sleep apnea patients but not in healthy controls [42]. Apparently, a sustained activity of chemo receptors contributes to the stimulation of the sympathetic nervous system while awake which is leading to hypertension.
Despite chemoreceptors, baroreceptors play a central role in regulation of the cardiovascular system. A dysfunction of baroreceptors can be observed in sleep apnea patients similar to chronic heart failure patients. In a canine animal model of sleep apnea, the baroreflex is adjusted to higher blood pressure levels [43]. Obstruction of the respiration at night leads to a sustained hypertension at daytime [44]. Continuous Positive Airway Pressure (CPAP) therapy is able to abolish or reduce sleep apnea. Night- and day-time sympathetic overactivity can be significantly reduced through this therapy [40].

3.6 Sympathic overactivity in metabolic syndrome

The increased sympathetic activity in metabolic syndrome patients contributes to the increased cardiovascular risk in this patient group [45]. In overweight patients, sympathetic overactivity appears to be linked to a dysfunction of the baroreflex [46]. This is also linked to the distribution of body fat mass. Accumulation of visceral fat is characterized by an increase in MSNA and cardiovascular risk [45].

Compared to healthy individuals, overweight people suffer significantly more often from hypertension and show an increased risk for the development of type 2 diabetes. An increased MSNA can also be observed in patients with type II diabetes [47].
The underlying cause for this interacting pathogenesis is unknown. Hyperinsulinemia appears to play an important role. For instance, administration of insulin in an increasing dose was able to increase MSNA in euglycemic individuals [48].

3.7 Sympathic overactivity in hypertension

Almost all studies measuring microneurographic sympathetic nerve activity in hypertensive patients could demonstrate the central role of sympathetic overactivity [49]. Smith et al. was able to show that especially in patients with observable target organ damage MSNA increase is more pronounced [50] (Fig. 5).

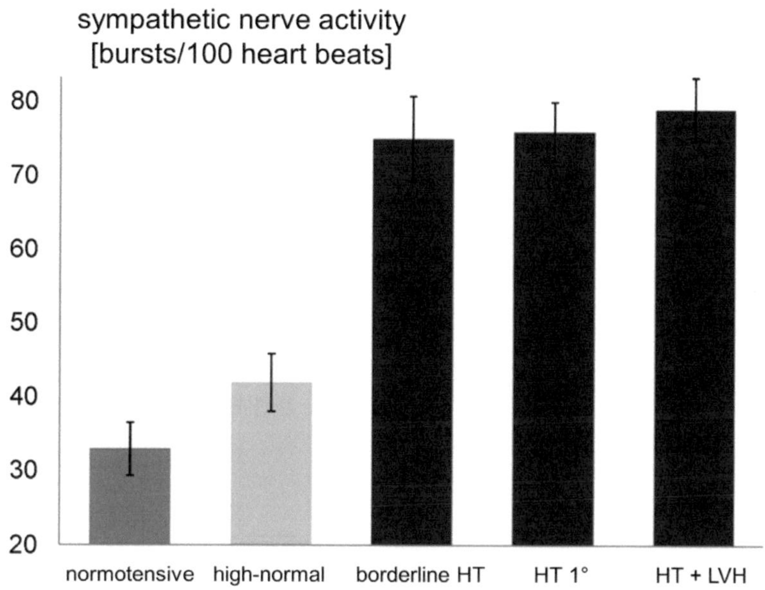

Fig. 5. Microneurographic measurements confirm a significant increase in sympathetic nerve activity (MSNA) in patients with hypertension (HT) compared to healthy individuals. An increased MSNA can already be found in high-normal blood pressure patients (130-139/85-89 mmHg) (modified from [50]).

The underlying conditions of sympathetic overactivity in hypertension are often linked and cannot be distinguished from each other. These conditions among others include chronic kidney disease, heart failure, obesity and sleep apnea. However, there is evidence that sympathetic reactivity might be genetically determined. Children of hypertensive individuals show normal MSNA-levels. When subjected to mental stress these children show a significantly increased MSNA if compared to children of non-affected parents [51].
Other hypertensive conditions such as preeclampsia [52] or pulmonary arterial hypertension [52] show an increased burst activity in microneurography.
Today, we have a distinct understanding of the pathogenesis of hypertension induced by chronic kidney injury. As seen in figure 1, activation of afferent neurons in the injured kidney leads to an increased sympathetic activity through central nervous mechanisms. It is

well established that increase of serum norepinephrine levels can indicate chronic kidney failure [53]. However, this finding is mostly based on reduced norepinephrine clearance in the kidney. Recently, it has been discovered that the kidney also releases a soluble monoamine-oxidase (Renalse) which degrades circulating catecholamines and thereby might regulate blood pressure [54]. Renalase serum levels are significantly decreased in chronic kidney failure. If Renalase actually plays a significant role in hypertension in chronic kidney failure patients has not been proven yet.
As stated above, bilateral nephrectomy is able to normalize MSNA. This can be reproduced in an animal model by renal denervation or selective dorsal rhizotomy [55]. Beside increased catecholamine levels, increased MSNA is an additional finding in renovascular hypertension [56]. The underlying mechanism for renovascular hypertension in renal artery stenosis is increased renin release which is dependent on renal innervation. Increase in blood pressure can be abolished in a Goldblatt-hypertension animal model ("2 kidney 1 clip") if the affected kidney is denervated [57]. Interestingly, denervation of the non-affected contralateral kidney also abolishes hypertension in this model [58].

4. Therapeutic approach in sympathetic overactivity

4.1 Pharmaceutical approach

In patients with chronic renal failure, the degree of the disease correlates very well with the sympathetic activity [59]. An increase of MSNA of 10 burts/min increases the event rate by 60 %. Concordantly, adverse cardiovascular events are also increased in these patients (Fig. 6.).

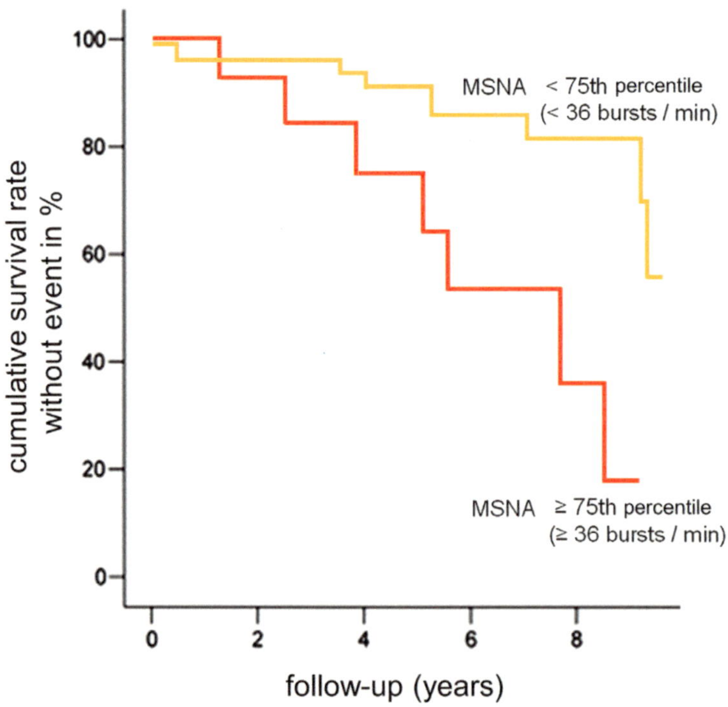

Fig. 6. Kaplan-Meier curve for adverse cardiovascular events in dependence of MSNA above (≥ 36 bursts/min) and below (< 36 bursts/min) the 75th percentile (modified from [59]).

RAAS blockade, through ACE-inhibitors or AT1-blockers, leads to a reduction in the efferent sympathetic activity [60, 61]. However, normalization of sympathetic activity can only be achieved if a central sympatholytic drug (moxonidine) is added to this treatment [62]. Moxonidine has been shown to have renoprotective properties in chronic renal failure and to reduce MSNA [63, 64]. This effect was independent from blood pressure reduction. In an animal model of chronic kidney failure, monoxidine is able to significantly improve histomorphologic and functional renal outcome. It is able to reduce albuminuria and the degree of glomerulosclerosis [65]. This might be dependent on an alteration of gene expression [14]. Adrenergic receptor activation (α- and β-receptors) is involved in this pathogenesis [66]. Therefore it appears feasible that adrenergic receptor inhibitors might be beneficial.

In patients with resistant hypertension, the suggested blood pressure goal of below 140/90 mmHg cannot always be achieved using oral antihypertensive medication. Therefore, there has been extensive research on alternative approaches for blood pressure control. Due to the pivotal role of sympathetic activity in the pathogenesis of hypertension, novel treatment strategies have focused on the alteration of sympathetic overactivity in order to control blood pressure and reduce overall cardiovascular risk.

There have been two major advancements in the field of non-pharmaceutical intervention: baroreflex activation therapy at the caroid body and catheter-based renal denervation. Each of these strategies significantly reduces sympathetic activity and controls blood pressure beyond pharmaceutical intervention.

4.2 Baroreflex activation therapy

As described above, dysfunction of the baroreceptor reflex causes an increase in sympathetic activity in a variety of diseases such as sleep apnea and chronic heart failure. In a canine animal model, Lohmeier et al. could demonstrate that activation of the baroreflex at the carotid artery by implanted pacemaker was able to reduce blood pressure as well as serum catecholamine levels [67, 68]. This approach is currently in clinical evaluation for resistant hypertension [69]. Promising data from a clinical trial for baroreflex activation therapy has been published recently. In this study, baseline mean blood pressure was 179/105 mmHg and heart rate was 80 beats/min, with a median of 5 antihypertensive drugs. After 3 months of device therapy, mean blood pressure was reduced by 21/12 mmHg. This result was sustained in 17 subjects who completed 2 years of follow-up, with a mean reduction of 33/22 mm Hg. The device exhibited a favorable safety profile [70].

In the Rheos Pivotal Trial, preliminary results (2010) also show similar results in blood pressure control [71]. In this study, subjects were enrolled if systolic blood pressure (SBP) was > 160 mmHg, 24-hour ambulatory SBP > 135 mmHg and they were on at least 3 antihypertensive drugs at maximum doses including a diuretic. 2010, 45 of 55 roll-in subjects have reached 6 months follow-up: Prior to baroreflex activation therapy mean blood pressure was 178/102 mmHg and post baroreflex activation therapy mean blood pressure was 144/87 ($p<0.001$). A reduction of > 20 mmHg was achieved in 69 % and > 30 mmHg in 58 % of subjects. In this study, antihypertensive medication remained unchanged during the follow-up period.

There are some issues of concern regarding this intervention. Previously, baroreflex activation therapy required bilateral carotid preparation and implantation of electrodes and the corresponding pacemaker aggregate. Due to the approach of bilateral activation, battery power of pacemakers lasts only for two years with the need of replacement after this period. However, advancements regarding baroreflex activation therapy are made. Recently, a single side baroreflex activation device has been introduced which is currently investigated in clinical trials.

4.3 Renal denervation therapy

As stated above, renal denervation in animals leads to a reduction of MSNA and blood pressure. In 1923, sympathectomy was performed for the first time in order to treat hypertension with stenocardia [72]. In 1935, Page and Heuer at the Rockefeller institute published data on surgical sympathectomy on blood pressure and renal function [73].

In 1953, a large study of 1266 cases was published on lumbal sympathectomy. However, this procedure was linked with severe side effects such as voiding dysfunction, intestinal dysfunction, impotence and orthostatic dysregulation [74]. Due to pharmaceutical alternatives, surgical sympathicolysis was replaced by antihypertensive drugs.

Recently, a novel, minimal-invasive, catheter-based approach is available which selectively severs renal nerve fibers at the site of the renal artery [75]. This renal denervation strategy can significantly reduce blood pressure in resistant hypertension (Fig. 7) [76]. In a multicentre, prospective, randomized trial, patients who had a baseline systolic blood pressure of 160 mmHg or more (≥150 mmHg for patients with type 2 diabetes) and were treated with at least 3 antihypertensive drugs were enrolled. After a 6-month follow-up period after renal denervation, office-based blood pressure measurements in the renal denervation group reduced by 32/12 mmHg (SD 23/11, baseline of 178/96 mmHg, $p<0.0001$) without significant side effects. Patients with a glomerular filtration rate of < 45 ml/Min/1.73 m^2 (MDRD) or renal artery abnormalities were excluded from the study.

Due to the pathogenesis of sympathetic overactivity in chronic kidney failure, it is feasible that this novel approach might also be beneficial in this patient group.

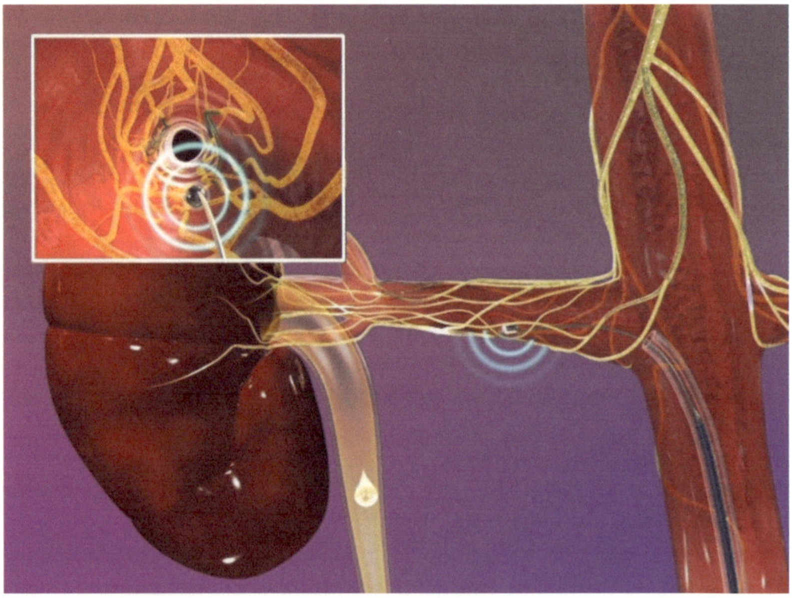

Fig. 7. Schematic of renal nerve fibres along the renal artery. Renal denervation is achieved by ablation using a catheter which is connected to a radiofrequency generator (picture by Ardian/Medtronic).

In a preliminary study, renal norepinephrine release was measured. There was a significant mean reduction of 47 %. Exemplary, MSNA was measured in a patient before and after renal denervation. A marked reduction in nerve activity could be demonstrated (Fig. 8) [77].

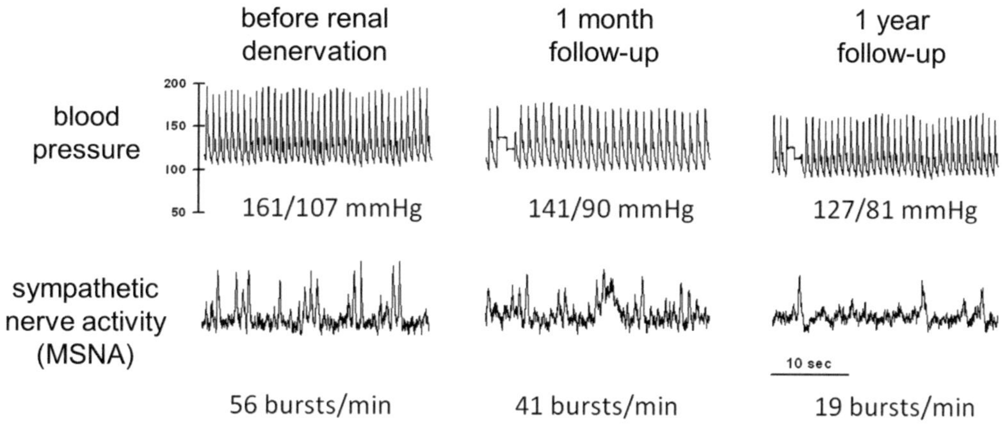

Fig. 8. Exemplary blood pressure and MSNA in a patient before and after renal denervation. There is a significant reduction in blood pressure and burst activity (modified from [77]).

5. Summary

Hypertension is the most significant health burden in modern societies. 25 to 35 % of the population suffers from this condition. Due to increasing age, the incidence of hypertension will increase in the future.

Overactivity of the sympathetic nervous system is a striking feature of a variety of cardiovascular and renal diseases. There is a distinct correlation between sympathetic activity, stage of disease and hypertension. Almost every hypertensive subject shows sympathetic overactivity. It correlates well with the cardiovascular event rate (heart failure, myocardial infarction, and stroke).

The kidney plays a pivotal role in the control of sympathetic nerve activity. Baro- and chemoreceptors which activate afferent sensory nerves travel from the kidney to the sympathetic nuclei of the central nervous system. This can lead to an increase in sympathetic activity which leads to an increase of neurotransmitter release in the target organs. This axis is especially pronounced in patients with chronic kidney disease. But also chronic heart failure, sleep apnea and obesity increase sympathetic nerve activity which can be measured by microneurography.

Pharmaceutical intervention can be achieved with RAAS-blockade (Renin- or ACE-inhibitors, or AT1-blockers) and peripheral adrenergic receptor antagonists and centrally acting sympatholytic drugs.

If pharmaceutical therapy fails in achieving target blood pressure levels, novel approaches in hypertension treatment such as baroreflex activation or renal denervation therapy are promising strategies for future treatment which directly inhibit the pacing of sympathetic activity.

6. References

[1] Lopez, A.D., et al., *Global and regional burden of disease and risk factors, 2001: systematic analysis of population health data.* Lancet, 2006. 367(9524): p. 1747-57.

[2] Hajjar, I. and T.A. Kotchen, *Trends in prevalence, awareness, treatment, and control of hypertension in the United States, 1988-2000.* JAMA, 2003. 290(2): p. 199-206.

[3] Yusuf, S., et al., *Effect of potentially modifiable risk factors associated with myocardial infarction in 52 countries (the INTERHEART study): case-control study.* Lancet, 2004. 364(9438): p. 937-52.

[4] Meisinger, C., et al., *Regional disparities of hypertension prevalence and management within Germany.* J Hypertens, 2006. 24(2): p. 293-9.

[5] Mancia, G., et al., *2007 ESH-ESC Practice Guidelines for the Management of Arterial Hypertension: ESH-ESC Task Force on the Management of Arterial Hypertension.* J Hypertens, 2007. 25(9): p. 1751-62.

[6] Ostchega, Y., et al., *Trends in hypertension prevalence, awareness, treatment, and control in older U.S. adults: data from the National Health and Nutrition Examination Survey 1988 to 2004.* J Am Geriatr Soc, 2007. 55(7): p. 1056-65.

[7] Heidenreich, P.A., et al., *Forecasting the future of cardiovascular disease in the United States: a policy statement from the American Heart Association.* Circulation, 2011. 123(8): p. 933-44.

[8] Hart, E.C. and N. Charkoudian, *Sympathetic neural mechanisms in human blood pressure regulation.* Curr Hypertens Rep, 2011. 13(3): p. 237-43.

[9] Vonend, O., et al., *Alpha(2A)-adrenoceptors regulate sympathetic transmitter release in mice kidneys.* Br J Pharmacol, 2007. 150(1): p. 121-7.

[10] Vonend, O., et al., *Renovascular effects of sympathetic cotransmitters ATP and NPY are age-dependent in spontaneously hypertensive rats.* Cardiovasc Res, 2005. 66(2): p. 345-52.

[11] Oberhauser, V., O. Vonend, and L.C. Rump, *Neuropeptide Y and ATP interact to control renovascular resistance in the rat.* J Am Soc Nephrol, 1999. 10(6): p. 1179-85.

[12] Vonend, O., et al., *P2Y-receptors stimulating the proliferation of human mesangial cells through the MAPK42/44 pathway.* Br J Pharmacol, 2003. 139(6): p. 1119-26.

[13] Vonend, O., et al., *ATP release in human kidney cortex and its mitogenic effects in visceral glomerular epithelial cells.* Kidney Int, 2002. 61(5): p. 1617-26.

[14] Vonend, O., et al., *Glomerular expression of the ATP-sensitive P2X receptor in diabetic and hypertensive rat models.* Kidney Int, 2004. 66(1): p. 157-66.

[15] Wallin, B.G. and N. Charkoudian, *Sympathetic neural control of integrated cardiovascular function: insights from measurement of human sympathetic nerve activity.* Muscle Nerve, 2007. 36(5): p. 595-614.

[16] Rump, L.C., K. Amann, and E. Ritz, *In: Bolis C, Licinio J, Govoni S (eds) Handbook of the Autonomic Nervous System in Health and Diesease.* New York - Basel: Marcel Dekker Verlag, 2002: p. 561-587.

[17] Siddiqi, L., et al., *Is kidney ischemia the central mechanism in parallel activation of the renin and sympathetic system?* J Hypertens, 2009. 27(7): p. 1341-9.

[18] Buchner, N., O. Vonend, and L.C. Rump, *[Pathophysiology of hypertension: what's new?].* Herz, 2006. 31(4): p. 294-302.

[19] Carlson, S.H. and J.M. Wyss, *Neurohormonal regulation of the sympathetic nervous system: new insights into central mechanisms of action.* Curr Hypertens Rep, 2008. 10(3): p. 233-40.

[20] Ye, S., et al., *A limited renal injury may cause a permanent form of neurogenic hypertension.* Am J Hypertens, 1998. 11(6 Pt 1): p. 723-8.

[21] Campese, V.M. and E. Kogosov, *Renal afferent denervation prevents hypertension in rats with chronic renal failure.* Hypertension, 1995. 25(4 Pt 2): p. 878-82.

[22] Rump, L.C., et al., *Beta 2-adrenergic receptor and angiotensin II receptor modulation of sympathetic neurotransmission in human atria.* Circ Res, 1994. 74(3): p. 434-40.

[23] Stegbauer, J., et al., *Angiotensin II modulates renal sympathetic neurotransmission through nitric oxide in AT2 receptor knockout mice.* J Hypertens, 2005. 23(9): p. 1691-8.

[24] Hoch, H., et al., *Regulation of renal sympathetic neurotransmission by renal alpha(2A) - adrenoceptors is impaired in chronic renal failure.* Br J Pharmacol, 2011. 163(2): p. 438-46.

[25] Vallbo, A.B., K.E. Hagbarth, and B.G. Wallin, *Microneurography: how the technique developed and its role in the investigation of the sympathetic nervous system.* J Appl Physiol, 2004. 96(4): p. 1262-9.

[26] Gandevia, S.C. and J.P. Hales, *The methodology and scope of human microneurography.* J Neurosci Methods, 1997. 74(2): p. 123-36.

[27] Converse, R.L., Jr., et al., *Sympathetic overactivity in patients with chronic renal failure.* N Engl J Med, 1992. 327(27): p. 1912-8.

[28] Hausberg, M., et al., *Sympathetic nerve activity in end-stage renal disease.* Circulation, 2002. 106(15): p. 1974-9.

[29] Esler, M., *The sympathetic system and hypertension.* Am J Hypertens, 2000. 13: p. 99S-105S.

[30] Zoccali, C., et al., *Plasma norepinephrine predicts survival and incident cardiovascular events in patients with end-stage renal disease.* Circulation, 2002. 105(11): p. 1354-9.

[31] Zoccali, C., et al., *Prospective study of neuropeptide y as an adverse cardiovascular risk factor in end-stage renal disease.* J Am Soc Nephrol, 2003. 14(10): p. 2611-7.

[32] Mano, T., *Microneurographic research on sympathetic nerve responses to environmental stimuli in humans.* Jpn J Physiol, 1998. 48(2): p. 99-114.

[33] Fagius, J. and B.G. Wallin, *Long-term variability and reproducibility of resting human muscle nerve sympathetic activity at rest, as reassessed after a decade.* Clin Auton Res, 1993. 3: 201-5.

[34] Narkiewicz, K., et al., *Gender-selective interaction between aging, blood pressure, and sympathetic nerve activity.* Hypertension, 2005. 45(4): p. 522-5.

[35] Floras, J.S., *Sympathetic nervous system activation in human heart failure: clinical implications of an updated model.* J Am Coll Cardiol, 2009. 54(5): p. 375-85.

[36] Oda, Y., et al., *Pulse-synchronous sympathetic burst power as a new index of sympathoexcitation in patients with heart failure.* Am J Physiol Heart Circ Physiol, 2004. 287(4): p. H1821-7.

[37] Gilsbach, R., et al., *Heterozygous alpha 2C-adrenoceptor-deficient mice develop heart failure after transverse aortic constriction.* Cardiovasc Res, 2007. 75(4): p. 728-37.

[38] Silverberg, D.S., A. Oksenberg, and A. Iaina, *Sleep-related breathing disorders as a major cause of essential hypertension: fact or fiction?* Curr Opin Nephrol Hypertens, 1998. 7: 353-7.

[39] Monahan, K.D., U.A. Leuenberger, and C.A. Ray, *Effect of repetitive hypoxic apnoeas on baroreflex function in humans.* J Physiol, 2006. 574(Pt 2): p. 605-13.

[40] Narkiewicz, K. and V.K. Somers, *Sympathetic nerve activity in obstructive sleep apnoea.* Acta Physiol Scand, 2003. 177(3): p. 385-90.

[41] Lesske, J., et al., *Hypertension caused by chronic intermittent hypoxia--influence of chemoreceptors and sympathetic nervous system.* J Hypertens, 1997. 15: 1593-603.

[42] Loredo, J.S., et al., *Obstructive sleep apnea and hypertension: are peripheral chemoreceptors involved?* Med Hypotheses, 2001. 56(1): p. 17-9.

[43] Carlson, J.T., et al., *Depressed baroreflex sensitivity in patients with obstructive sleep apnea.* Am J Respir Crit Care Med, 1996. 154(5): p. 1490-6.

[44] Brooks, D., et al., *Obstructive sleep apnea as a cause of systemic hypertension. Evidence from a canine model.* J Clin Invest, 1997. 99(1): p. 106-9.

[45] Alvarez, G.E., et al., *Sympathetic neural activation in visceral obesity.* Circulation, 2002. 106(20): p. 2533-6.

[46] Grassi, G., et al., *Body weight reduction, sympathetic nerve traffic, and arterial baroreflex in obese normotensive humans.* Circulation, 1998. 97(20): p. 2037-42.

[47] Huggett, R.J., et al., *Impact of type 2 diabetes mellitus on sympathetic neural mechanisms in hypertension.* Circulation, 2003. 108(25): p. 3097-101.

[48] Berne, C., et al., *The sympathetic response to euglycaemic hyperinsulinaemia. Evidence from microelectrode nerve recordings in healthy subjects.* Diabetologia, 1992. 35(9): p. 873-9.

[49] Schlaich, M.P., et al., *Sympathetic augmentation in hypertension: role of nerve firing, norepinephrine reuptake, and Angiotensin neuromodulation.* Hypertension, 2004. 43: 169-75.

[50] Smith, P.A., et al., *Relationship between central sympathetic activity and stages of human hypertension.* Am J Hypertens, 2004. 17(3): p. 217-22.

[51] Noll, G., et al., *Increased activation of sympathetic nervous system and endothelin by mental stress in normotensive offspring of hypertensive parents.* Circulation, 1996. 93(5): p. 866-9.

[52] Greenwood, J.P., et al., *The magnitude of sympathetic hyperactivity in pregnancy-induced hypertension and preeclampsia.* Am J Hypertens, 2003. 16(3): p. 194-9.

[53] Brecht, H.M., W. Ernst, and K.M. Koch, *Plasma noradrenaline levels in regular haemodialysis patients.* Proc Eur Dial Transplant Assoc, 1976. 12: p. 281-90.

[54] Desir, G.V., *Regulation of blood pressure and cardiovascular function by renalase.* Kidney Int, 2009. 76(4): p. 366-70.

[55] Rump, L.C., et al., *Sympathetic overactivity in renal disease: a window to understand progression and cardiovascular complications of uraemia?* Nephrol Dial Transplant, 2000. 15(11): p. 1735-8.

[56] Johansson, M., et al., *Increased sympathetic nerve activity in renovascular hypertension.* Circulation, 1999. 99(19): p. 2537-42.

[57] Oparil, S., *The sympathetic nervous system in clinical and experimental hypertension.* Kidney Int, 1986. 30(3): p. 437-52.

[58] Kalaitzis, C., et al., *Effects of renal denervation of the contralateral kidney on blood pressure and sodium and eicosanoid excretion in the chronic phase of two-kidney, one-clip renovascular hypertension in rats.* Scand J Urol Nephrol, 2005. 39(1): p. 15-20.
[59] Penne, E.L., et al., *Sympathetic hyperactivity and clinical outcome in chronic kidney disease patients during standard treatment.* J Nephrol, 2009. 22(2): p. 208-15.
[60] Klein, I.H., et al., *Enalapril and losartan reduce sympathetic hyperactivity in patients with chronic renal failure.* J Am Soc Nephrol, 2003. 14(2): p. 425-30.
[61] Ligtenberg, G., et al., *Reduction of sympathetic hyperactivity by enalapril in patients with chronic renal failure.* N Engl J Med, 1999. 340(17): p. 1321-8.
[62] Neumann, J., et al., *Moxonidine normalizes sympathetic hyperactivity in patients with eprosartan-treated chronic renal failure.* J Am Soc Nephrol, 2004. 15(11): p. 2902-7.
[63] Hausberg, M., et al., *Effects of moxonidine on sympathetic nerve activity in patients with end-stage renal disease.* J Hypertens, 2010. 28(9): p. 1920-7.
[64] Vonend, O., et al., *Moxonidine treatment of hypertensive patients with advanced renal failure.* J Hypertens, 2003. 21(9): p. 1709-17.
[65] Amann, K., et al., *Effects of low dose sympathetic inhibition on glomerulosclerosis and albuminuria in subtotally nephrectomized rats.* J Am Soc Nephrol, 2000. 11(8): p. 1469-78.
[66] Amann, K., et al., *Glomerulosclerosis and progression: effect of subantihypertensive doses of alpha and beta blockers.* Kidney Int, 2001. 60(4): p. 1309-23.
[67] Lohmeier, T.E., et al., *Prolonged activation of the baroreflex produces sustained hypotension.* Hypertension, 2004. 43(2): p. 306-11.
[68] Schmidli, J., et al., *Acute device-based blood pressure reduction: electrical activation of the carotid baroreflex in patients undergoing elective carotid surgery.* Vascular, 2007. 15: 63-9.
[69] Wustmann, K., et al., *Effects of chronic baroreceptor stimulation on the autonomic cardiovascular regulation in patients with drug-resistant arterial hypertension.* Hypertension, 2009. 54(3): p. 530-6.
[70] Scheffers, I.J., et al., *Novel baroreflex activation therapy in resistant hypertension: results of a European multi-center feasibility study.* J Am Coll Cardiol, 2010. 56(15): p. 1254-8.
[71] G. Bakris , J.B., M. Nadim , L. Sanchez , D. Sica, Rheos Pivotal Trial Investigators, *Achievement of Blood Pressure Goal in Patients With Resistant Hypertension Treated With Baroreflex Activation Therapy*, in *Journal of Hypertension*. 2010.
[72] Bruening, F., *Die operative Behandlung des Halsbrustsympathukus und Bemerkungen ueber die operative Behandlung der abnormen Blutdrucksteigerung.* . Klin Wochenschr, 1923. 2: p. 777-780.
[73] Page, I.H. and G.J. Heuer, *The Effect of Renal Denervation on Patients Suffering from Nephritis.* J Clin Invest, 1935. 14(4): p. 443-58.
[74] Smithwick, R.H. and J.E. Thompson, *Splanchnicectomy for essential hypertension; results in 1,266 cases.* J Am Med Assoc, 1953. 152(16): p. 1501-4.
[75] Krum, H., et al., *Catheter-based renal sympathetic denervation for resistant hypertension: a multicentre safety and proof-of-principle cohort study.* Lancet, 2009. 373(9671): p. 1275-81.

[76] Esler, M.D., et al., *Renal sympathetic denervation in patients with treatment-resistant hypertension (The Symplicity HTN-2 Trial): a randomised controlled trial.* Lancet, 2010. 376(9756): p. 1903-9.
[77] Schlaich, M.P., et al., *Renal sympathetic-nerve ablation for uncontrolled hypertension.* N Engl J Med, 2009. 361(9): p. 932-4.

Part 2

Mechanisms of Pacemaking

2

MicroRNAs as Possible Molecular Pacemakers

Emanuela Boštjančič and Damjan Glavač
University of Ljubljana, Faculty of Medicine, Institute of Pathology, Department of Molecular Genetics, Slovenia

1. Introduction

MicroRNAs (miRNAs) are endogenously expressed, small (approx. 22 nucleotides long) non-coding RNA molecules that regulate gene expression at the post-transcriptional level. They are encoded in almost all organisms, from viruses to humans (Soifer et al., 2007). Bioinformatic studies of the genomes of multiple organisms suggest that this short length maximizes target-gene specificity and minimizes non-specific effects. Generally, by targeting the 3'-untranslated region (UTR) of mRNAs in a sequence specific manner, they influence the translation (protein synthesis repression) or stability of the transcripts (mRNA degradation) (Ying et al., 2008). The role of endogenously expressed miRNA (the first miRNA to be discovered was *lin-4*) in down-regulating gene expression was first described by Victor Ambros and his colleagues in 1993 for *C. Elegans,* although the term microRNA was only introduced in 2001 (Lagos-Quintana et al., 2001; Lau, et al., 2001; Lee et al., 2001; Ruvkun, 2001). In humans, approx. 1700 mature miRNA have been cloned and sequenced (miRBase v17.0 database, release April 2011, http://www.mirbase.org). It is estimated that there could be as many as thousands of miRNAs in humans, thought to regulate approx. 30 % of genes within the human genome (Pillai et al., 2007).

1.1 MicroRNA biology

MicroRNAs are genome encoded, derived from the intergenic regions, exon sequences of non-coding transcription units or intronic sequences of either protein coding or non-coding transcription units. They are encoded as a single gene or gene clusters. It has been predicted that miRNAs constitute more than 3 % of human genes (Pillai, 2005). Intergenic miRNAs are transcribed as an independent transcription unit, as a monocistronic, bicistronic or polycistronic primary transcript (Bartel, 2004). Intronic miRNA are usually part of introns of pre-mRNA, preferentially transcribed in the same orientation as the mRNA, probably not transcribed from their own promoters but instead processed from introns, as are many snoRNA. Intronic miRNAs and their host transcripts are co-regulated and co-transcribed from the same promoter (Kim & Kim, 2007). Within the genome, there might be more than one copy of particular miRNAs. The suggestion has been made that some miRNAs are also encoded in antisense DNA, which is not transcribed to the mRNA (Bartel, 2004).

1.1.1 MicroRNA processing

Regulation of miRNA expression depends on transcription factors and epigenetic mechanisms, such as DNA methylation and histone modification of the miRNA genomic region. Over the course of their lifecycle, miRNAs must undergo extensive post-transcriptional modifications. Genes encoding miRNAs are transcribed with RNA-polymerase II or RNA-polymerase III (Pol II or Pol III) into a primary transcript, 200 nucleotides (nt) to several kilobases (kb) long, known as a *pri-miRNA*. Mature miRNA sequences are usually localized to regions of imperfect stem-loop. The resulting *pri-miRNA* (with poly-A tail and 7-methylguanosine cap) is processed by an RNase III enzyme called Drosha and a double-stranded RNA-binding protein, DGCR8 (DiGeorge syndrome critical region) in the cell nucleus, into a 70-nt stem-loop structure called a *pre-miRNA*. The resulting stem-loop structure, with a monophosphate at the 5' terminus and a 2-nt overhang with a hydroxyl group at the 3' terminus, is imported into the cytoplasm by a transporter protein, Exportin 5. After GTP hydrolysis, with consequent release of the *pre-miRNA*, the double-stranded RNA portion of *pre-miRNA* is bound and cleaved by Dicer (RNase III enzyme) together with co-factor TRBP (transactivating region binding protein). The action of these proteins removes the terminal loop and produces a miRNA:miRNA* duplex, which is a transient intermediate in miRNA biogenesis (20–25 nt), with a 2-nt overhanging its 3' UTR. One of the two strands of each fragment, known as the *guide strand* (miRNA), together with proteins argonaute (Ago 1-4), helicases, nucleases and RNA binding proteins, is incorporated into a complex called the miRNA-containing ribonucleoprotein complex (miRNP) or RNA-induced silencing complex (RISC). The resulting complex is responsible for base-pairing with complementary mRNA sequences. The other strand, miRNA* or *passenger strand*, is presumably degraded, although there are increasing prospects that either or both strands may be functional. It is believed that the *guide strand* is determined on the basis of the less energetically stable 5' end (Bartel, 2004; Pillai, 2005; Pillai et al., 2007; Ying et al., 2008). Intronic miRNAs bypass Drosha cleavage and rely on the action of the *pre-mRNA* splicing/debranching machinery to produce an approx. 60 nt precursor miRNA hairpin (*pre-miRNA*) (Kim & Kim, 2007). The miRNA processing is summarized in Figure 1.

1.1.2 MicroRNAs mechanism

The functional role of miRNA varies, depending on the organism, but the primary mechanism of miRNA action in mammals is to inhibit mRNA translation. The catalytic components of miRNP/RISC complex are Ago proteins. After base pairing between the miRNA and target mRNA, degradation of the target mRNA results when complementarity is perfect, or suppression of the translation occurs when base pairing between these two molecules is incomplete. Especially in animals, each miRNA can inhibit the translation of many different mRNAs (as many as 200 predicted target genes) without degrading the target mRNA. In addition, mRNA can be regulated by more than one miRNA. The cooperative action of multiple identical or different miRNP/RISCs appears to provide the most efficient translational inhibition. This explains the presence of multiple miRNA complementary sites in most genetically identified targets, and the cooperative action of miRNA:UTR interactions would provide an additional mechanism to increase the specificity of miRNAs. Proteins or mRNA secondary structures could restrict miRNP/RISC accessibility to the UTRs, or may facilitate recognition of the authentic mRNA targets (Bartel, 2004; Pillai, 2005; Pillai et al., 2007; Ying et al., 2008). It has been suggested that miRNAs may also be involved in regulation by binding to the 5' UTR of the target genes (Liu z. Et al, 2008). There is still the prospect that some miRNA might specify more than just post-transcriptional repression; some might in addition target DNA for transcriptional silencing. Each of the examples (DNA methylation and silencing in plants, heterochromatin formation in fungi, DNA rearrangements in ciliates) suggests the existence of a nuclear RISC-like complex (Bartel, 2004).

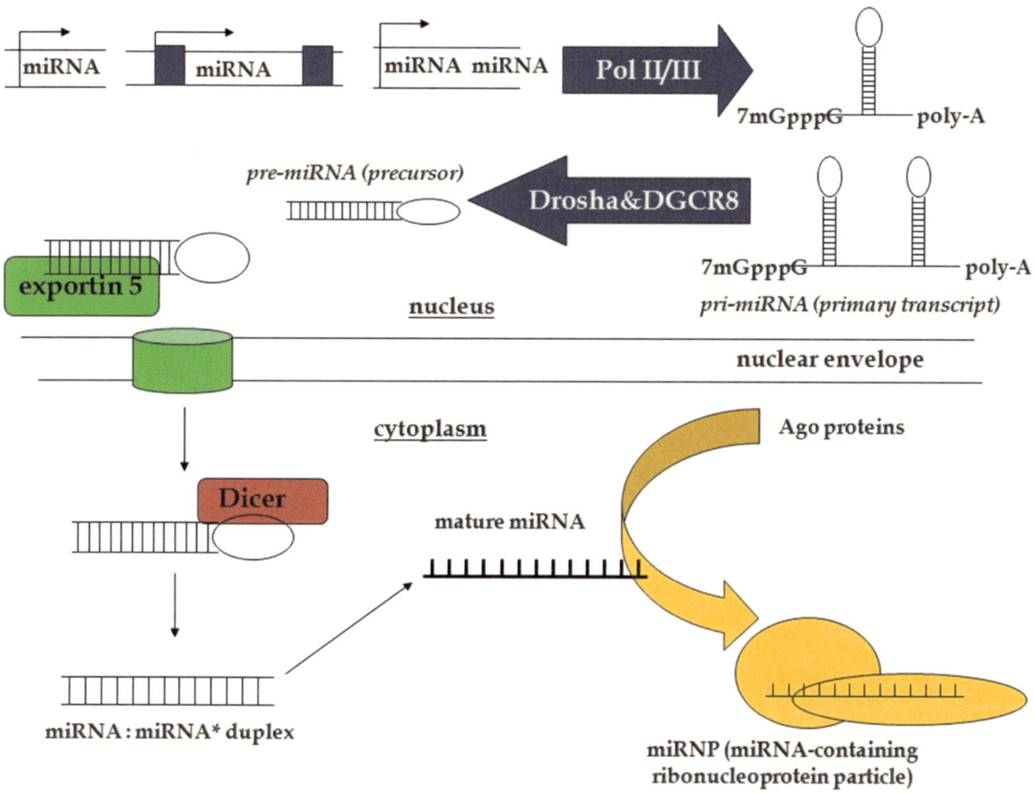

Legend: Pol II/PolIII, RNA-polymerase II and III; poly-A, poly-A tail; 7mGpppG, 7-methylguanosine cap; Drosha, RNase III enzyme; DGCR8, double stranded RNA-binding protein; Exportin 5, transporter protein; Dicer, RNase III enzyme.

Fig. 1. Schematic overview of the miRNA biogenesis pathway

1.2 MicroRNA annotation in humans

After the small isolated RNAs are annotated as miRNAs, based on expression and biogenesis criteria, they need to be named (Ambros et al., 2003; Berezikov et al., 2006). Perhaps the best examples of naming annotated miRNA in this context are those of muscle-specific *hsa-miR-133a-1, hsa-miR-133a-2* and *hsa-miR-133b,* and heart associated *hsa-miR-199a-3p* and *hsa-miR-199a-5p.* The prefix *hsa* is designated for human miRNA (Homo sapiens), the term *miR* is designated for miRNA gene; the numbers *133* and *199* are unique identifying numbers that characterize the exact miRNA sequence; the letters *a* and *b* are used for paralogous miRNAs; numbers after the miRNA gene name, e.g., *hsa-miR-133a* numbers *1* and *2,* are used for one copy of genes encoded within the genome; *3p* or *5p,* in this case for *hsa-miR-199a,* is used when none of the miRNA duplex is degraded, or it has not yet been determined from which *pre-miRNA* arm the miRNA is degraded and from which *pre-miRNA* arm the miRNA is incorporated in the miRNP/RISC (Griffiths-Jones et al., 2008).

1.3 Target prediction and bioinformatics

MicroRNAs are generally conserved in evolution, some quite broadly, others only in more closely related species (Bartel, 2004). Many computational methods have recently been developed for identifying potential miRNA targets (Ioshikes et al., 2007). Most of these methods search for multiple conserved regions of miRNA complementarities within 3' UTR; the most important parameters are therefore evolutionary conservation with regard to the quality and stability of base pairing. The interaction between seven consecutive nucleotides in the target mRNAs 3' UTR and the 2-8 nt ("seed sequence") at the 5' miRNA end is believed to be important for base pairing. The majority of prediction programmes use pairing with the seed sequence as one of the major criteria. There are several available programs for predicting mRNA targets for specific miRNA or for predicting possible miRNA binding sites for specific mRNA, but none of these programs can be used as a means of independently validating the targets, and all predicted targets must be validated *in vitro* and *in vivo* (Kuhn et al., 2008). Further complicating target site prediction in mammals is the fact that not all 3' UTR sites with perfect complementarities to the miRNA seed nucleotides are functional. Moreover, mRNAs sites with imperfect seed complementarities can themselves be very good miRNA targets. In animals, there are far fewer mRNAs with near perfect complementarities to miRNAs. Bioinformatic analysis is therefore much noisier and more prone to false positives (Barnes et al., 2007). The most often used target prediction programs are perhaps TargetScan and PicTar, although others are often used, such as miRanda, microrna.org, miRBase etc. There is also a database available containing dysregulated miRNAs in different diseases or their profiling in various tissues (HMDD, Human MicroRNA Disease Database; Lu et al., 2008). Another useful database is Tarbase, in which all experimentally validated targets for all organisms and miRNAs are incorporated (Sethupathy et al., 2006).

2. MicroRNA in regulating physiological functions

Importance of miRNA processing pathway components. MicroRNAs and their associated proteins appear to be one of the more abundant ribonucleoprotein complexes within cells. Perhaps the best evidence of miRNAs being important for normal physiological functions is provided by experiments in which the components of the miRNA biogenesis pathway are depleted or over-expressed. Biochemical experiments in several eukaryotes have shown that DGCR8 is an essential co-factor of the RNAse II enzyme Drosha. In addition, the reduced enzymes Dicer and Drosha have been demonstrated in several diseases, as well as over-expression of Dicer, Ago 2 and exportin-5 (Soifer et al., 2007).

Outcomes of translational repression. By translational repression, miRNAs, in normal cell conditions can function in different ways. Firstly, for mRNAs that should not be expressed in a particular cell type, miRNAs reduce protein production to inconsequential levels (switch off the targets). Secondly, miRNAs can adjust protein output in a manner that allows for customized expression in different cell types but a more uniform level within each cell type (fine-tuning target expression). Thirdly, some miRNAs act as bystanders, for which down-regulation by miRNAs is tolerated or is negated by feedback processes (neutral target expression). MicroRNA functions have mainly been determined by *in vivo* experiments, by the phenotypic consequences of a mutated miRNA or an altered mRNA complementarity site, either of which can disrupt miRNA regulation. In some cases, function has been inferred from the effects of transgenic constructs that lead to ectopic expression of the miRNA (Bartel, 2004).

Physiological functions. Many miRNAs are expressed in a tissue-specific manner, e.g., *miR-208* is cardiac specific (van Rooij et al., 2007), *miR-122* is liver specific (Girard et al., 2008), and/or cell-type specific manner (e.g. *miR-223* is primarily expressed in granulocytes); they are important at distinct stages of development and have been found to regulate a variety of developmental and physiological processes (Williams, 2008). In terms of development, miRNAs are important in regulating morphogenesis and the maintenance of undifferentiated or incompletely differentiated cell types, such as stem cell differentiation, cardiac and skeletal muscle development, neurogenesis, hematopoiesis etc. Recently discovered miRNA functions include control of cell-fate decision, cell proliferation, cell death, neuronal patterning, modulation of hematopoietic lineage differentiation and controlling the timing of developmental transitions (Callis et al., 2007; Fazi & Nervi, 2008; Li & Gregory, 2008). In physiological conditions, miRNAs are involved in metabolism, regulation of insulin secretion, cholesterol metabolism, resistance to viral infection and oxidative stress, immune response etc (Lodish et al., 2007; Williams, 2008). With all different genes and expression patterns, it is reasonable to propose that every cell type at each developmental stage might have a distinct miRNA expression profile. MicroRNA biogenesis and activity is now regarded as a key regulatory mechanism in maintenance tissue identity during embryogenesis and adult life.

3. MicroRNAs and disease

Presence of SNPs. Disruption of miRNA target interaction in the form of single-nucleotide polymorphisms (SNPs), either in the miRNA gene or its target site (3' UTR mRNA), can lead to complete gain or loss of the miRNA function and thus account for a diseased state (e.g. *AT_1R* and *miR-155*, Martin et al., 2007). In contrast to the miRNA target sites in mRNA transcripts, in which the potential of variation is huge, variants identified in miRNA precursor sequences tend to be extremely rare, usually restricted to one individual. The presence of SNPs in *pri-miRNA* or *pre-miRNA* can also affect the processing of miRNAs and their expression, which can also result in different disease outcomes (Barnes et al., 2007).
Aberrant expression of miRNAs. Recent advances in miRNA research have provided evidence of an miRNA association with various pathological conditions. These can be due to abnormal miRNA expression profiles, genomic rearrangements or epigenetic mechanisms activated in diseased human tissues. Aberrant miRNAs expression and processing is associated with genetic disorders, cancer, autoimmune and inflammatory diseases, and neurodegenerative and cardiovascular disorders (Perera & Ray, 2007). It is estimated that 50 % of miRNA genes are located at fragile chromosome sites and associated with the development of cancer. MicroRNAs can in addition act as tumour suppressors or proto-oncogens during the course of carcinogenesis (Cho, 2009).

4. MicroRNAs in heart physiology and disease

Cardiac specific Dicer deletion. One of the most important studies showing that miRNAs are important in heart physiology, as well as in heart disease, concerned the cardiac specific knockout of Dicer in prenatal mice. Dicer deletion resulted in rapidly progressive dilated cardiomyopathy, heart failure and postnatal mortality; early mortality was due to heart defects, such as pericardial edema and underdevelopment of the ventricular myocardium. Dicer mutant mice showed a severe decrease in heart contractile function, due to aberrant expression and loss of cardiac contractile proteins, and profound sarcomere disarray, resulting in reduced heart rates. Decreased Dicer expression has consistently been detected in end-stage human cardiomyopathy and heart failure. In contrast, increased expression has been observed after left ventricular assist device support in humans, which is used to improve cardiac function (Chen et al., 2008). Furthermore, postnatal experiments of Dicer loss in cardiomyocytes of young mice resulted in sudden cardiac death, probably due to arrhythmias. Loss of Dicer in adult myocardium induces rapid and dramatic biventricular enlargement, accompanied by myocyte hypertrophy, myofiber disarray, ventricular fibrosis and strong induction of foetal gene transcripts (da Costa Martins et al, 2008). These results clearly demonstrated that components of miRNA processing are important for cardiac contractility, suggesting one of the crucial roles of miRNAs in normal and pathological functions of the heart. Changes in miRNA biogenesis affect both juvenile and adult myocardial morphology, suggesting a huge biological impact of miRNAs in the postnatal heart. It can therefore be concluded that Dicer down-regulation probably affects the expression of hundreds of miRNAs, which results in a severe disease outcome.

Heart disease. MicroRNA research in cardiovascular diseases has only just started. There is growing evidence to suggest that miRNAs are involved in the regulation of developmental, physiologic and pathologic conditions of the heart. Cardiac diseases, including those with progressive degeneration, might involve abnormal miRNA regulation leading to loss of renewal of the cardiac muscle cells. The majority of studies have been concerned with development, conduct and pathology, focusing on hypertrophy, end-stage heart failure, cardiomyopathy and myocardial infarction (Schipper et al., 2008; Thum et al., 2007; Xiao et al., 2008; Yin et al, 2008). Stress, associated with cardiac diseases, contributes to miRNA expression patterns in the heart, suggesting that miRNAs might function in stress-related factors affecting cardiac structure and function. Previous studies of cardiac disease have focused on miRNAs that are primarily expressed in cardiomyocytes; however, there is mounting evidence that other miRNAs expressed in the human heart have an impact on cardiovascular disease (Cordes et al., 2009; Rane et al., 2009; Roy et al., 2009; Song et al., 2010). In several studies, miRNA microarray analysis has been performed using cell lines and an animal model of hypertrophy (Cheng et al., 2007; Sayed et al., 2007; van Rooij et al., 2006; Tatsuguchi et al., 2007; Thum et al., 2008), human cardiomyopathies and aortic stenosis (Ikeda et al., 2007; Sucharov et al., 2008), end-stage heart failure (Matkovich et al., 2009; Thum et al., 2007), fibrosis (van Rooij et al., 2008), myocardial infarction (Roy et al., 2009) and development (Niu et al., 2008) and animal model of remodelling and reverse remodelling of the heart (Wang et al., 2009) and all other forms of myocardial ischemia. Among the genes activated by oxidative stress are the transcription factors that orchestrate the expression of a wide variety of responses affecting metabolism, angiogenesis, cell survival and oxygen delivery and, in addition, miRNA expression, thought to be critical for adaptation to low oxygen. In response to low oxygen, a number of miRNAs are up- or down-regulated, with several of these dependent on hypoxia-inducible-factor, a transcription factor that plays essential role in the homeostatic response to hypoxia (Kulshreshtha et al., 2007; Kulshreshtha et al., 2008).

Heart development. The heart is the first organ to form and to function during development. It has been established that miRNAs represent developmental expression patterns, important for timing developmental decisions and pattern formation (Morton et al., 2008). In addition, it has been shown that some miRNA patterns are similar in diseased and foetal hearts, supporting the concept of reactivation of the foetal gene program in cardiovascular diseases.

MicroRNA expression in failing hearts has an increased similarity to that of foetal cardiac tissue, suggesting that foetal gene expression in diseased hearts is a hallmark of cardiac stress (Thum et al., 2007).

4.1 Cardiac and muscle specific microRNAs in heart

MicroRNAs *miR-1, miR-133, miR-206* and *miR-208,* are considered to be muscle and/or cardiac specific because they are preferentially but not exclusively expressed in muscle and/or cardiac tissue. Among mammalian miRNAs identified so far, *miR-1* and *miR-133* are believed to have a muscle specific expression pattern, with an impact on the regulation of heart development. Cardiac expression of *miR-1* is controlled by *SRF* (serum response factor) and myocardin; similar to *miR-1, miR-133* expression in the heart is controlled by *SRF* (Niu et al., 2008). Currently, a number of miRNAs have been described as enriched or muscle specific, but, to the best of our knowledge, only *miR-208* has been described as cardiac specific.

4.1.1 Cardiac specific *miR-208*

As an identified cardiac specific miRNA, *miR-208* is believed to play an important role in response to stress, such as pressure overload, activated calcineurin or hypothyroidism. MicroRNA *miR-208* is encoded by an intron of *Myh6,* a gene encoding human and mouse α-cardiac muscle myosin heavy chain (*aMHC*). By targeting *THRAP1,* a co-factor of the thyroid hormone nuclear receptor, it mediates down-regulation of *aMHC* and up-regulation of β-cardiac muscle myosin heavy chain (*βMHC*) in mice, the primary contractile proteins of the heart. Changes in contractile proteins are accompanied by hypertrophy and fibrosis, resulting eventually in the diminution of contractility; these changes are also referred to as remodelling. Experimental models of *miR-208* null animals (mice), which failed to undergo stress-induced remodelling and hypertrophic growth in response to activated calcineurin signalling or pressure-overload-induced stress, and failed to induce *βMHC* up-regulation in response to hypothyroidism, support the suggested role of *miR-208* in remodelling (van Rooij et al, 2007). It was recently determined that this *miR-208* gene corresponds to *miR-208a* and that it is a member of a family that also includes *miR-208b,* which is encoded within an intron of *Myh7* (gene coding *βMHC*). These two miRNAs (*miR-208a* and *miR-208b*) are differentially expressed in mice heart during development, paralleling the expression of their host genes (Callis et al., 2009).

4.1.2 Muscle specific *miR-1* and *miR-133*

Development. Muscle miRNAs are mainly controlled by myogenic transcription factors; through cardiac development they fine-tune regulatory protein levels in a spatiotemporal manner. MicroRNAs *miR-1* and *miR-133* are clustered on the same chromosome loci (*miR-1-1* and *miR-133a-2* on chromosome 20, and *miR-1-2* and *miR-133a-1* on chromosome 18) and are transcribed together in a tissue specific manner. Using cell culture and animal model experiments, it has recently been shown that *miR-1* and *miR-133* have opposite roles in muscle development, with *miR-1* promoting myoblast differentiation and *miR-133* promoting myoblast proliferation; both *miR-1* and *miR-133* target *SRF,* with *miR-1* also targeting transcription repressor, histone deacteylase *HDAC4* thus promoting myogenesis (Chen et al., 2006; Niu et al., 2008). Over-expression of *miR-1* in developing mouse hearts results in decreased cardiomyocyte proliferation and premature differentiation through down-regulation of transcription factor *Hand2*. Target deletion of *miR-1* causes death *in utero* of the majority of offspring, due to defects in cardiac morphogenesis. The surviving ones die later due to conductivity problems. It is suggested that a precise dosage of *Hand2* is essential for normal cardiomyocyte development and morphogenesis (Zhao et al., 2005). Experiments using mouse models of an *miR-1-2* null animal suggest that *miR-1-2* has a non-redundant role with *miR-1-1* in the heart, despite their apparent overlapping expression patterns. Half of the *miR-1-2* null animals died, others suffered from incomplete ventricular septation, indicating abnormal cardiogenesis. It would be useful to know whether deletion of *miR-1-1* invokes a similar phenotype, and whether deletion of both copies causes a more severe phenotype (Zhao et al., 2007). Finally, it has been shown that, during development, *miR-133* regulates cardiogenesis by targeting nuclear factor *Nelf-A/Whsc2* (Care et al., 2007).

Apoptosis. Loss of cardiac muscle cells due to apoptotic cell death is a common process in heart development, as well as in myocardial ischemia, cardiac hypertrophy and heart failure. MicroRNAs are also implicated in cardiovascular disease as regulators of apoptosis. Opposite effects of *miR-1* and *miR-133* regulating cardiomyocyte apoptosis induced by oxidative stress have been described, with a pro-apoptotic role of *miR-1* (targeting *HSP60* and *HSP70,* heat-shock proteins) and anti-apoptotic role of *miR-133* (targeting caspase-9) (Xu et al., 2007).

Hypertrophy. Both *miR-1* and *miR-133* have been demonstrated to be dysregulated in hypertrophic and failing hearts and in myocardial infarction in both animals and humans. MicroRNA *miR-133* showed down-regulation in patients with hypertrophic cardiomyopathy and in mouse models of cardiac hypertrophy. The predicted targets for *miR-133* are *Rhoa,* a GDP-GTP exchange protein regulating cardiac hypertrophy, and *Cdc42,* a signal transduction kinase implicated in hypertrophy; both miRNAs are involved in cell growth, myofibrillar rearrangements and regulation of contractility. Another target was determined, *Nelf-A/Whsc2,* a nuclear factor involved in cardiogenesis but the role of *Nelf-A/Whsc2* in cardiac hypertrophy has not yet been defined (Care et al., 2007). Although it is also believed that *miR-1* expression is down-regulated during cardiac hypertrophy, results are somewhat controversial; additional genetic studies are therefore needed to demonstrate clearly a direct role of *miR-1* in the regulation of cardiac hypertrophy. However, *miR-1* targets in the context of cell growth, contractility and extracellular matrix have been determined, including *RasGAP, Cdk9, Rheb* and fibronectin (Care et al., 2007).

4.2 MicroRNAs controlling cardiac excitability

The electrical-conduction system, which maintains proper heart rhythmicity, has been shown to be regulated by miRNAs that regulate the expression of its components and therefore possess the potential to induce arrhythmia. Dysregulated miRNA expression might affect the expression of ion channel genes, leading to arrhythmogenesis; it has been postulated that miRNAs control cardiac excitability through this regulation. Using bioinformatics and experimental approaches, a number of miRNAs have recently been proposed as having the potential to regulate human ion channel genes. The matrix of miRNAs that are expressed in cardiac myocytes has been established, with the potential to regulate genes encoding cardiac ion channels and transporters. The author proposed that multiple miRNAs might be critically involved in the electrical/ionic remodelling process in heart disease through altering the expression of the genes in cardiac myocytes (Luo et al., 2010). MicroRNAs known up to date to target cardiac excitability are listet in Table 1 with corresponding target genes and their functions.

4.2.1 Cardiac specific *miR-208*

As previously reported, the expression of *miR-208a* and *miR-208b* is not just developmentally regulated in the heart, but also pathologically. In a recent study, it was postulated that *miR-208a* expression was sufficient to induce arrhythmias; furthermore, experiments on genetic deletion of *miR-208a* in mice revealed that *miR-208a* is required for proper cardiac conduction and expression of the transcription factor *GATA4* and gap junction protein connexin 40 (*Cx 40*). MicroRNA *miR-208* is therefore required for maintaining the expression of cardiac transcription factors known to be important for the development of the conduction system. Over-expression of *miR-208a* results in cardiac conduction abnormalities and suggests that *miR-208a* regulates cardiac conduction system components. Studies on mice lacking *miR-208a* suggest that these mice suffer atrial fibrillation. Furthermore, *Cx 40* expression is restricted to the atria, more precisely in the His bundle and Purkinje fibres. Consistent with the phenotype of mice lacking *miR-208a*, mice lacking *Cx 40* also suffer from first-degree AV block. It can be concluded, therefore, that *miR-208a* gain- and lost-of-function are associated with arrhythmias (Callis et al., 2009).

4.2.2. Muscle specific *miR-1* and *miR-133*

MicroRNAs miR-1 and miR-133. The slow delayed rectifier current I_{ks}, is constituted of channel complex, which is formed from *KCNQI* and *KCNEI*. Their expression is regionally heterogeneous; it is also changed by the pathological state of the heart. It has been experimentally established that the two genes, *KCNQI* and *KCNEI*, are targets for *miR-133* and *miR-1*, respectively. It was shown that expressions of *miR-1* and *miR-133* in the heart are spatially heterogeneous and that this may contribute to regional differences in the distribution of *KCNQI* and *KCNE1*. To confirm the hypothesis, it was shown that *KCNQI* has the opposite patterns of transmural and apical-basal gradients to those of *miR-133*, whereas the characteristic regional distribution of *miR-1* may be one of the causal factors for the converse transmural and apical-base gradients of *KCNEI*. Thus, in areas in which *miR-1* and *miR-133* are less abundant, I_{ks} are more densely expressed (Luo et al., 2007). In one of the first studies of miRNA influence on the cardiac conduction system, it was suggested that down-regulation of *miR-1* and *miR-133* contributes to arrhythmogenesis in hypertrophic and failing hearts, and that *miR-1* and *miR-133* play an important role in determining cardiac automaticity, possibly by re-expression of the pacemaker channel genes *HCN2* and *HCN4*. Both miRNAs are involved in hypertrophy, with *miR-133* believed to be a negative regulator of hypertrophic growth of heart muscle. By undergoing a remodelling process and hypertrophic growth, the heart adapts to impaired cardiac function. The remodelling process in the heart also includes electrical remodelling, which increases the risk of arrhythmogenesis by re-expression of the pacemaker channel *HCN* genes (hyperpolarization–activated cyclic-nucleotide-gated channels). The *HCN2* gene has been shown to be a target of *miR-133*. In addition, pacemaker channels *HCN2* and *HCN4* have both been shown to be targets for *miR-1*, so its down-regulation may also lead to re-expression of these pacemaker channels in a diseased heart. To date, these two miRNAs have a postulated role in regulating automaticity in the functioning of the I_f current. This is a mixed Na^+K^+ inward current, which is activated by hyperpolarization and is the main current of pacemaker activity in the sinoatrial node. I_f may therefore be controlled by *miR-1* and *miR-133* through the regulation of *HCN* density (Luo et al., 2008).

MicroRNA miR-1. Up-regulation of *miR-1* has been reported in patients with coronary artery disease and in animal models in the border zone of myocardial infarction. Over-expression of *miR-1* in the hearts of adult rats leads to widened QRS complex, indicative of intraventricule conduction delay and the development of severe cardiac arrhythmia. Target mRNAs for *miR-1* have been predicted as ion channel genes *GJA1,* which encodes gap-junction protein connexin 43, and *KCNJ2,* which encodes the K^+ channel subunit Kir2.1. Knockdown of endogenous *miR-1* can inhibit ischemic arrhythmias. Therefore, *miR-1* might contribute to re-entry through decreased intracellular coupling via the repression of *GJA1* (Yang et al., 2007). In contrast to this research, it was shown that *miR-1* levels are greatly reduced in the left atrium of patients with persistent atrial fibrillation (AF), possibly resulting in up-regulation of Kir2.1 subunits, which leads to increased I_{k1}. Up-regulation of this inward-rectifier current is important for AF maintenance (Girmatsion et al., 2009). A further *miR-1* target involved in regulation of cardiac conductance is *Irx5,* a transcription factor that regulates cardiac repolarization by repressing *Kcnd2.* This gene encodes for potassium channel Kv4.2, which is responsible for transient outward K^+ current. Normal expression of all three components, *miR-1, Irx5* and *Kcnd2,* is required for maintaining the ventricular repolarisation gradient. Evidence was provided by deletion of the *miR-1-2* gene, which resulted in the death of half of the mice at birth, and those surviving to adulthood showed an aberrant heart rate and repolarization (Zhao et al., 2007). Calcium channels account for excitation-contraction coupling and also contribute to pacemaker activities. The effect of increased expression of *miR-1* on excitation-contraction coupling and Ca^{2+} cycling has been investigated in rat ventricular myocytes. It was shown that *miR-1* over-expression increased phosphorylation of the ryanodine receptor (*RyR2*) by selective decrease in expression of protein phosphatase *PP2A*. *RyR* channels on the sarcoplasmic reticulum (SR) are essential for activation of contractile filaments during myocardial contraction; *RyR2* is regulated by kinases and phosphathases, its activity depends on the phosphorylation state. Through translational inhibition, *miR-1* causes hyperphosphorylation of *RyR2* thus enhancing *RyR2* activity and promoting arhythmogenic SR Ca^{2+} release. The author concluded that *miR-1* enhances cardiac excitation-contraction coupling by selectively increasing phosphorylation of the L-type and *RyR2* channels via disrupting localization of *PP2A* activity to these channels (Terenteyev et al., 2009).

MicroRNA miR-133. In vitro studies have identified ERG (ether-a-go-go related gene) as an *miR-133* target, K^+ channel (I_{Kr}), in cardiomyocytes; its repression may contribute to depression and subsequent QT prolongation in diabetic hearts. ERG protein level was decreased in the ventricle of diabetic hearts; in contrast, increased expression of *miR-133* and SRF was detected in the same diabetic subjects. Down-regulation of *ERG* is responsible for arrhythmias in diabetic hearts caused by QT prolongation (Xiao et al., 2006).

4.2.3 Other miRNAs regulating cardiac excitability

Another possible mechanism of miRNA regulating the L-type Ca^{2+} current, reduction of which is associated with atrial electrical remodelling and atrial fibrillation, has recently been suggested. In particular, *miR-328* level was approx. 4-fold up-regulated, targeting the L-type Ca^{2+} channel genes, *CACNA1C* and *CACNB1.* The author therefore concluded that *miR-328* contributes to adverse atrial electric remodelling in AF and was postulated as a novel molecular mechanism for AF (Lu et al., 2010). Furthermore, it has been shown that nicotine-induced atrial remodelling, which represents an increased risk for atrial fibrillation, results in significant up-regulation of *TGF-ß1* and *TGF-ßRII* and, remarkably, a decrease in the levels of *miR-133* and *miR-590,* which at least partly accounts for *TGF-ß1* and *TGF-ßRII* up-regulation. It is suggested that the antifibrotic effect of both *miR-133* and *miR-590* are implicated in AF (Shan et al., 2009).

miRNA	Target gene	Target gene description	Regulating process	Reference
miR-1	*Hand2*	transcription factor, heart- and neural crest derivatives-expressed protein 2	developing ventricular chambers, cardiac morphogenesis	Zhao et al., 2005
	Irx5	iroquois homeobox 5	pattern formation of vertebrate embryos, heart development	Zhao et al., 2007
	GJA1	gap junction protein, alpha 1, connexin 43	conduction between cells and within a cell	Yang et al., 2007
	KCNJ2	potassium inwardly-rectifying channel, subfamily J, member 2		
	KCNEI	potassium voltage-gated channel, I_{ks}-related family, member 1	regional heterogeneity of expression	Luo et al., 2007
	HCN2, HCN4	hyperpolarization activated cyclic nucleotide-gated potassium channel	pacemaker channels	Luo et al., 2007
	PP2A	protein phosphatase 2A	regulating RyR2 phosphorylation	Terenteyev et al., 2009
miR-133	*ERG*	ether-a-go-go-like gene	long QT sindrom, diabetes mellitus	Xiao et al., 2007
	KCNQI	potassium voltage-gated channel, KQT-like subfamily, member 1	regional heterogeneity of expression	Luo et al., 2007
	HCN2	hyperpolarization activated cyclic nucleotide-gated potassium channel 2	pacemaker channels	Luo et al., 2007
	TGFB1, TGFBRII	transforming growth factor, beta 1 and its receptor	nicotin-induced atrial remodelling	Shan et al., 2009
miR-208	*GATA4, Cx 40*	GATA binding protein 4 and connexin 40	heart conduction and arrhythmia	Callis et al., 2009
miR-590	*TGFB1, TGFBRII*	transforming growth factor, beta 1 and its receptor	nicotin-induced atrial remodelling	Shan et al., 2009
miR-328	*CACNA1/ CACNB1*	voltage-dependent calcium channel	calcium transport	Lu et al., 2010

Table 1. MicroRNAs regulating cardiac excitation, its target genes and function.

5. Therapeutic potentials of microRNAs

MicroRNA expression patterns are dynamically regulated during various diseases, thus providing an opportunity to use them as biomarkers or diagnosis indicators and for prognosis. MicroRNAs are small molecules, making their *in vivo* delivery feasible. The use of chemically modified oligonucleotides either to target a specific miRNA or disrupt miRNA-mRNA binding may lead to inactivation of pathological miRNA. MicroRNAs may therefore serve as therapeutic targets in the future (Liu Z. et al, 2008; Soifer et al., 2008).

5.1 Replenishing small RNAs

For an miRNA that is under-expressed, re-introduction of the mature miRNA into the affected tissue would restore regulation of the target gene. For this purpose, artificial miRNA have been developed (miRNA mimic) to enhance the expression of beneficial miRNAs or the introduction of short hairpin duplex, similar to *pre-miRNA,* into the cell. These findings raise the hope that re-introduction of certain miRNAs (e.g., *miR-1, miR-133* or *miR-208),* depending on the disease outcome, might reduce life threatening arrhythmias, a frequent cause of death in patients with cardiovascular disease, or heart remodelling associated with prolonged ischemia, which often results in end-stage heart failure and poor prognosis (Liu Z. et al, 2008; Soifer et al., 2008). *In vivo* over-expression of *miR-133* protected animals from agonist induced cardiac hypertrophy, whereas reduction in wild-type mice (anti-miRNA antisense antagomir molecules secreted by implanted osmotic pumps) caused an increase in hypertrophic markers. This suggests that individual miRNAs are potential therapeutic agents, provided that their expression or delivery can be targeted to appropriate tissue. However, care should be taken, since over-production of *miR-133* induces arrhythmias (Care et al., 2007). Most of the developed protocols have used local administration in easily accessible tissue; systemic delivery has also some promising results; the major challenge remains tissue and cell-type specific targeting (Liu Z. et al, 2008; Soifer et al., 2008).

5.2 Inhibiting small RNAs

ASOs are short and single-stranded antisense oligonucleotides and, in the context of miRNA inhibition, are called AMOs, anti-miRNA oligonucleotides. Over-expressed miRNA can be down-regulated by reducing the mature miRNA level through direct targeting (mature miRNA, *pri-miRNA* or *pre-miRNA*) or by reducing the components of miRNA biogenesis. Chemically engineered oligonucleotides, termed "antagomirs", have been developed and proven to be efficient and specific silencers of endogenous miRNAs in mice. Chemical modifications and cholesterol conjugations stabilize and facilitate intravenous delivery of antagomirs. They interact with miRNAs in the cytoplasm and lead to specific miRNA down-regulation when injected systemically or locally (Liu Z. et al, 2008; Soifer et al., 2008). Direct injection of lipid-complexed antagomir oligonucleotides against *miR-1* into rat hearts protected the animals from induced arrhythmias, suggesting that transient down-regulation of *miR-1* could provide therapeutic benefits to those suffering from acute myocardial infarctions (Yang et al., 2007). In another approach, miRNA sponges have been developed to inhibit several miRNAs; miRNA sponges possess multiple binding sites and could be useful for sequestering an miRNA family. Furthermore, miR-masks and miR-erasers have also been developed; an miR-mask has been designed for masking the miRNA binding site on target mRNA, whereas an miR-eraser is similar to miR-sponges, except that the miR-eraser

uses only two copies of the antisense sequence. Gene-specific miRNA mimic and miRNA-masking antisense approaches have been used to test the possibility of using miRNAs and their corresponding targets as therapeutic targets. The expression of the cardiac pacemaker channel genes, *HCN2* and *HCN4*, has been manipulated via the mentioned approaches. MicroRNA mimics repressed protein levels, whereas miRNA masking markedly enhanced *HCN2/HCN4* expression and function (Xiao et al., 2007). In a recent study, the authors proposed that arhhythomgenesis after intracardiac skeletal myoblast (SKM) transplantation, a promising therapy for myocardial infarct repair, may be related to the differentiation state of (SKM). It was shown that *miR-181a* plays an important role in myobast differentiation, so using lentivirus mediated oligonucleotides against *miR-181a,* the authors demonstrated reduced arrhythmias post SKM transplantation (Li et al., 2009).
We need more knowledge concerning which miRNAs to target, how to produce and stabilize them, how to direct them to the heart and not systemically. The specificity of drug-like oligonucleotides is important, because of the off-target effect. The off-target effect is also a significant challenge, especially considering that miRNA-mediated repression often requires a homology of only six to seven nucleotides in the seed region of the miRNA and mRNA target site. Toxicity due to chemical modifications, which is used to facilitate cellular uptake and prevent degradation, should be take into account (Liu Z. et al, 2008; Soifer et al., 2008).

6. Conclusions

The field of miRNA is largely undiscovered territory, a young, emerging field of research, and we are just beginning to understand the role of miRNAs in the cardiovascular context. Recent advances in the research of miRNAs suggest that miRNAs modulate a wide variety of cardiac functions with developmental, (patho)physiological and clinical implications. The miRNA level in the myocardium must be kept within a proper concentration range to maintain normal cardiac conduction; excessive either decrease or increase in the level of some miRNAs can induce arrhythmia, which supports the central role of some miRNAs in fine-tuning the regulation of cardiac electrophysiology in pathological and normal conditions. The role of miRNAs in the pathogenesis of the heart and vessels points to the possibility of miRNA targets for the treatment of cardiovascular disease in previously unconsidered medical therapies.

7. References

Ambros, V., Bartel, B., Bartel, D.P., Burge, C.B., Carrington, J.C., Chen, X., Dreyfuss, G., Eddy, S.R., Griffiths-Jones, S., Marshall, M., Matzke, M., Ruvkun, G. & Tuschl, T. (2003) A uniform system for microRNA annotation. *RNA*, Vol. 9, No. 3, (Mar 2003), pp. 277-9, ISSN 1355-8382

Barnes, M.R., Deharo, S., Grocock, R.J., Brown, J.R. & Sanseau, P. (2007) The micro RNA target paradigm: a fundamental and polymorphic control layer of cellular expression. *Expert Opin Biol Ther*, Vol. 7, No. 9, (Sep 2007), pp. 1387-1399, ISSN 1471-2598

Bartel, D.P. (2004) MicroRNAs: genomics, biogenesis, mechanism, and function. *Cell*, Vol. 116, No.2 (Jan 2004), pp. 281-297, ISSN 0092-8674

Berezikov, E., Cuppen, E. & Plasterk, R.H. (2006) Approaches to microRNA discovery. *Nat Genet,* Vol. 38, Suppl, (Jun 2006), pp. S2-7, ISSN 1061-4036

Callis, T.E., Pandya, K., Seok, H.Y., Tang, R.H., Tatsuguchi, M., Huang, Z.P., Chen, J.F., Deng, Z., Gunn, B., Shumate, J., Willis, M.S., Selzman, C.H. & Wang, D.Z. (2009) MicroRNA-208a is a regulator of cardiac hypertrophy and conduction in mice. *J Clin Invest*, Vol. 119, No. 9, (Sep 2009), pp. 2772-2786, ISSN 0021-9738

Callis, T.E., Chen, J.F. & Wang, D.Z. (2007) MicroRNAs in skeletal and cardiac muscle development. *DNA Cell Biol*, Vol. 26, No. 4, (Apr 2007), pp. 219-225, ISSN 1044-5498

Carè, A., Catalucci, D., Felicetti, F., Bonci, D., Addario, A., Gallo, P., Bang, M.L., Segnalini, P., Gu, Y., Dalton, N.D., Elia, L., Latronico, M.V., Høydal, M., Autore, C., Russo, M.A., Dorn, G.W. 2nd, Ellingsen, O., Ruiz-Lozano, P., Peterson, K.L., Croce, C.M., Peschle, C. & Condorelli, G. (2007) MicroRNA-133 controls cardiac hypertrophy. *Nat Med*, Vol. 13, No. 5, (May 2007), pp. 613-618, ISSN 1078-8956

Chen, J.F., Mandel, E.M., Thomson, J.M., Wu, Q., Callis, T.E., Hammond, S.M., Conlon, F.L. & Wang, D.Z. (2006) The role of microRNA-1 and microRNA-133 in skeletal muscle proliferation and differentiation. *Nat Genet*, Vol. 38, No. 2, (Feb 2006), 228-233, ISSN 1061-4036

Chen, J.F., Murchison, E.P., Tang, R., Callis, T.E., Tatsuguchi, M., Deng, Z., Rojas, M., Hammond, S.M., Schneider, M.D., Selzman, C.H., Meissner, G., Patterson, C., Hannon, G.J. & Wang, D.Z. (2008) Targeted deletion of Dicer in the heart leads to dilated cardiomyopathy and heart failure. *Proc Natl Acad Sci U S A*, Vol. 105, No. 6, (Feb 2008), pp. 2111-2116, ISSN 0027-8424

Cheng, Y., Ji, R., Yue, J., Yang, J., Liu, X., Chen, H., Dean, D.B. & Zhang, C. (2007) MicroRNAs are aberrantly expressed in hypertrophic heart: do they play a role in cardiac hypertrophy? *Am J Pathol*, Vol. 170, No. 6, (Jun 2007), 1831-1840, ISSN 0002-9440

Cho, W.C. (2010) MicroRNAs: potential biomarkers for cancer diagnosis, prognosis and targets for therapy. *Int J Biochem Cell Biol*,Vol. 42, No. 8, (Aug 2010), pp. 1273-1281, ISSN 1357-2725

Cordes, K.R., Sheehy, N.T., White, M.P., Berry, E.C., Morton, S.U., Muth, A.N., Lee, T.H., Miano, J.M., Ivey, K.N. & Srivastava, D. (2009) miR-145 and miR-143 regulate smooth muscle cell fate and plasticity. *Nature*, Vol. 460, No. 7256, (Aug 2009), pp. 705-710, ISSN 0028-0836

da Costa Martins, P.A., Bourajjaj, M., Gladka, M., Kortland, M., van Oort, R.J., Pinto, Y.M., Molkentin, J.D. & De Windt, L.J. (2008) Conditional dicer gene deletion in the postnatal myocardium provokes spontaneous cardiac remodeling. *Circulation*, Vol. 118, No. 15, (Oct 2008), pp. 1567-1576, ISSN 0009-7322

Fazi, F. & Nervi, C. (2008) MicroRNA: basic mechanisms and transcriptional regulatory networks for cell fate determination. *Cardiovasc Res*, Vol. 79, No. 4, (Sep 2008), pp. 553-561, ISSN 0008-6363

Girard, M., Jacquemin, E., Munnich, A., Lyonnet, S. & Henrion-Caude, A. (2008) miR-122, a paradigm for the role of microRNAs in the liver. *J Hepatol*, Vol. 48, No. 4, (Apr 2008), pp. 648-656, ISSN 0168-8278

Girmatsion, Z., Biliczki, P., Bonauer, A., Wimmer-Greinecker, G., Scherer, M., Moritz, A., Bukowska, A., Goette, A., Nattel, S., Hohnloser, S.H. & Ehrlich, J.R. (2009) Changes in microRNA-1 expression and IK1 up-regulation in human atrial fibrillation. *Heart Rhythm*, Vol. 6, No. 12, (Dec 2009), pp. 1802-1809, ISSN 1547-5271

Griffiths-Jones, S., Saini, H.K., van Dongen, S. & Enright, A.J. (2008) miRBase: tools for microRNA genomics. *Nucleic Acids Res*, Vol. 36, Database issue, (Jan 2008), pp. D154-D158, ISSN 0079-6603

Ikeda, S., Kong, S.W., Lu, J., Bisping, E., Zhang, H., Allen, P.D., Golub, T.R., Pieske, B. & Pu, W.T. (2007) Altered microRNA expression in human heart disease. *Physiol Genomics*, Vol. 31, No. 3, (Nov 2007), pp. 367-373, ISSN 1094-8341

Ioshikhes, I., Roy, S. & Sen, C.K. (2007) Algorithms for mapping of mRNA targets for microRNA. *DNA Cell Biol*, Vol. 26, No. 4, (Apr 2007), pp. 265-272. ISSN 1044-5498

Kim, Y.K. & Kim, V.N. (2007) Processing of intronic microRNAs. *EMBO J*, Vol. 26, No. 3, (Feb 2007), pp. 775-783, ISSN 0261-4189

Kuhn, D.E., Martin, M.M., Feldman, D.S., Terry, A.V. Jr, Nuovo, G.J. & Elton, T.S. (2008) Experimental validation of miRNA targets. *Methods*, Vol. 44, No. 1, (Jan 2008), pp. 47-54, ISSN 1046-2023

Kulshreshtha, R., Ferracin, M., Negrini, M., Calin, G.A., Davuluri, R.V. & Ivan, M. (2007) Regulation of microRNA expression: the hypoxic component. *Cell Cycle*, Vol. 6, No. 12, (Jun 2007), pp. 1426-1431, ISSN 1538-4101

Kulshreshtha R, Davuluri RV, Calin GA, Ivan M. (2008) A microRNA component of the hypoxic response. *Cell Death Differ*, Vol. 15, No. 4, (Apr 2008), pp. 667-671, ISSN 1350-9047

Lagos-Quintana, M., Rauhut, R., Lendeckel, W. & Tuschl, T. (2001) Identification of novel genes coding for small expressed RNAs. *Science*, Vol. 294, No. 5543, (Oct 2001), pp. 853-858, ISSN 0036-8075

Lau, N.C., Lim, L.P., Weinstein, E.G. & Bartel, D.P. (2001) An abundant class of tiny RNAs with probable regulatory roles in Caenorhabditis elegans. *Science*, Vol. 294, No. 5543, (Oct 2001), pp. 858-62, ISSN 0036-8075

Lee, R.C. & Ambros, V. (2001) An extensive class of small RNAs in Caenorhabditis elegans. *Science*, Vol. 294, No. 5543, (Oct 2001), pp. 862-4, ISSN 0036-8075

Li, Q. & Gregory, R.I. (2008) MicroRNA regulation of stem cell fate. *Cell Stem Cell*, Vol. 2, No. 3, (Mar 2008), pp. 195-196, ISSN 1934-5909

Li, Y.G., Zhang, P.P., Jiao, K.L. & Zou, Y.Z. (2009) Knockdown of microRNA-181 by lentivirus mediated siRNA expression vector decreases the arrhythmogenic effect of skeletal myoblast transplantation in rat with myocardial infarction. *Microvasc Res*, Vol. 78, No. 3, (Dec 2009), pp. 393-404, ISSN 0026-2862

Liu, N., Bezprozvannaya, S., Williams, A.H., Qi, X., Richardson, J.A., Bassel-Duby, R. & Olson, E.N. (2008) microRNA-133a regulates cardiomyocyte proliferation and suppresses smooth muscle gene expression in the heart. *Genes Dev*, Vol. 22, No. 23, (Dec 2008), pp. 3242-54, ISSN 0890-9369

Liu, Z., Sall, A. & Yang, D. (2008) MicroRNA: An emerging therapeutic target and intervention tool. *Int J Mol Sci*, Vol. 9, No. 6, (Jun 2008), pp. 978-99, ISSN 1422-0067

Lodish, H.F., Zhou, B., Liu, G. & Chen, C.Z. (2008) Micromanagement of the immune system by microRNAs. *Nat Rev Immunol*, Vol. 8, No. 2, (Feb 2008), pp. 120-130, ISSN 1474-1733

Lu, M., Zhang, Q., Deng, M., Miao, J., Guo, Y., Gao, W. & Cui, Q. (2008) An analysis of human microRNA and disease associations. *PLoS One*, Vol. 3, No. 10, (2008), pp. e3420, ISSN 1932-6203

Lu, Y., Zhang, Y., Wang, N., Pan, Z., Gao, X., Zhang, F., Zhang, Y., Shan, H., Luo, X., Bai, Y., Sun, L., Song, W., Xu, C., Wang, Z. & Yang B. (2010) MicroRNA-328 contributes to adverse electrical remodeling in atrial fibrillation. *Circulation*, Vol. 122, No. 23, (Dec 2010), pp. 2378-87, ISSN 0009-7322

Luo, X., Lin, H., Pan, Z., Xiao, J., Zhang, Y., Lu, Y., Yang, B. & Wang, Z. (2008) Down-regulation of miR-1/miR-133 contributes to re-expression of pacemaker channel genes HCN2 and HCN4 in hypertrophic heart. *J Biol Chem*, Vol. 283, No. 29, (Jul 2008), pp. 20045-52, ISSN 0021-9258

Luo, X., Xiao, J., Lin, H., Li, B., Lu, Y., Yang, B. & Wang, Z. (2007) Transcriptional activation by stimulating protein 1 and post-transcriptional repression by muscle-specific microRNAs of IKs-encoding genes and potential implications in regional heterogeneity of their expressions. *J Cell Physiol*, Vol. 212, No. 2, (Aug 2007), pp. 358-67, ISSN 0021-9541

Luo, X., Zhang, H., Xiao, J. & Wang, Z. (2010) Regulation of human cardiac ion channel genes by microRNAs: theoretical perspective and pathophysiological implications. *Cell Physiol Biochem*, Vol. 25, No. 6, (2010), pp. 571-86, ISSN 1015-8987

Matkovich, S.J., Van Booven, D.J., Youker, K.A., Torre-Amione, G., Diwan, A., Eschenbacher, W.H., Dorn, L.E., Watson, M.A., Margulies, K.B. & Dorn, G.W. 2nd. (2009) Reciprocal regulation of myocardial microRNAs and messenger RNA in human cardiomyopathy and reversal of the microRNA signature by biomechanical support. *Circulation*, Vol. 119, No. 9, (Mar 2009), pp. 1263-71, ISSN 0009-7322

Martin, M.M., Buckenberger, J.A., Jiang, J., Malana, G.E., Nuovo, G.J., Chotani, M., Feldman, D.S., Schmittgen, T.D. & Elton, T.S. (2007) The human Angiotensin II Type 1 Receptor +1166A/C Polymorphism Attenuates MicroRNA-155 Binding. *J Biol Chem*, Vol. 282, No. 33, (Avg 2007), pp. 24262-24269, ISSN 0021-9258

Morton, S.U., Scherz, P.J., Cordes, K.R., Ivey, K.N., Stainier, D.Y. & Srivastava, D. (2008) microRNA-138 modulates cardiac patterning during embryonic development. *Proc Natl Acad Sci U S A*, Vol. 105, No. 46, (Nov 2008), pp. 17830-5, ISSN 0027-8424

Niu, Z., Iyer, D., Conway, S.J., Martin, J.F., Ivey, K., Srivastava, D., Nordheim, A. & Schwartz, R.J. (2008) Serum response factor orchestrates nascent sarcomerogenesis and silences the biomineralization gene program in the heart. *Proc Natl Acad Sci USA*, Vol. 105, No. 46, (Nov 2008), pp. 17824-9, ISSN 0027-8424

Perera, R.J. & Ray A. (2007) MicroRNAs in the search for understanding human diseases. *BioDrugs*, Vol. 21, No. 2, (2007), pp. 97-104, ISSN 1173-8804

Pillai, R.S., Bhattacharyya, S.N. & Filipowicz, W. (2007) Repression of protein synthesis by miRNAs: how many mechanisms? *Trends Cell Biol*, Vol. 17, No. 3, (Mar 2007), pp. 118-126, ISSN 0962-8924

Pillai, R.S. (2005) MicroRNA function: multiple mechanisms for a tiny RNA? *RNA*, Vol. 11, No. 12, (Dec 2005), pp. 1753-1761, ISSN 1355-8382

Rane, S., He, M., Sayed, D., Vashistha, H., Malhotra, A., Sadoshima, J., Vatner, D.E., Vatner, S.F. & Abdellatif, M. (2009) Downregulation of miR-199a derepresses hypoxia-inducible factor-1alpha and Sirtuin 1 and recapitulates hypoxia preconditioning in cardiac myocytes. *Circ Res*, Vol. 104, No. 7, (Apr 2009), pp. 879-86, ISSN 0009-7330

Roy, S., Khanna, S., Hussain, S.R., Biswas, S., Azad, A., Rink, C., Gnyawali, S., Shilo, S., Nuovo, G.J. & Sen, C.K. (2009) MicroRNA expression in response to murine myocardial infarction: miR-21 regulates fibroblast metalloprotease-2 via phosphatase and tensin homologue. *Cardiovasc Res*, Vol. 82, No. 1, (Apr 2009), pp. 21-29, ISSN 0008-6363

Ruvkun, G. (2001) Molecular biology. Glimpses of a tiny RNA world. *Science*, Vol. 294, No. 5543, (Oct 2001), pp. 797-9, ISSN 0036-8075

Sayed, D., Hong, C., Chen, I.Y., Lypowy, J. & Abdellatif, M. (2007) MicroRNAs play an essential role in the development of cardiac hypertrophy. *Circ Res*, Vol. 100, No. 3, (Feb 2007), pp. 416-24, ISSN 0009-7330

Schipper, M.E., van Kuik, J., de Jonge, N., Dullens, H.F. & de Weger, R.A. (2008) Changes in regulatory microRNA expression in myocardium of heart failure patients on left

ventricular assist device support. *J Heart Lung Transplant,* Vol. 27, No. 12, (Dec 2008), pp. 1282-5, ISSN 1053-2498
Sethupathy, P., Corda, B., Hatzigeorgiou, A.G. (2006) TarBase: A comprehensive database of experimentally supported animal microRNA targets. *RNA,* Vol. 12, No. 2, (Feb 2006), pp. 192-197, ISSN 1355-8382
Shan, H., Zhang, Y., Lu, Y., Zhang, Y., Pan, Z., Cai, B., Wang, N., Li, X., Feng, T., Hong, Y. & Yang, B. (2009) Downregulation of miR-133 and miR-590 contributes to nicotine-induced atrial remodelling in canines. *Cardiovasc Res,* Vol. 83, No. 3, (Aug 2009), pp. 465-72, ISSN 0008-6363
Soifer, H.S., Rossi, J.J. & Saetrom, P. (2007) MicroRNAs in disease and potential therapeutic applications. *Mol Ther,* Vol. 15, No. 12, (Dec 2007), pp. 2070-9, ISSN 1525-0016
Song, X.W., Li, Q., Lin, L., Wang, X.C., Li, D.F., Wang, G.K., Ren, A.J., Wang, Y.R., Qin, Y.W., Yuan, W.J. & Jing, Q. (2010) MicroRNAs are dynamically regulated in hypertrophic hearts, and miR-199a is essential for the maintenance of cell size in cardiomyocytes. *J Cell Physiol,* Vol. 225, No. 2, (Nov 2010), pp. 437-43, ISSN 0021-9541
Sucharov, C., Bristow, M.R. & Port, J.D. (2008) miRNA expression in the failing human heart: functional correlates. *J Mol Cell Cardiol,* Vol. 45, No. 2, (Aug 2008), pp. 185-192, ISSN 0022-2828
Tatsuguchi, M., Seok, H.Y., Callis, T.E., Thomson, J.M., Chen, J.F., Newman, M., Rojas, M., Hammond, S.M. & Wang, D.Z. (2007) Expression of microRNAs is dynamically regulated during cardiomyocyte hypertrophy. *J Mol Cell Cardiol,* Vol. 42, No. 6, (Jun 2007), pp. 1137-41, ISSN 0022-2828
Terentyev, D., Belevych, A.E., Terentyeva, R., Martin, M.M., Malana, G.E., Kuhn, D.E., Abdellatif, M., Feldman, D.S., Elton, T.S. & Györke, S. (2009) miR-1 overexpression enhances Ca(2+) release and promotes cardiac arrhythmogenesis by targeting PP2A regulatory subunit B56alpha and causing CaMKII-dependent hyperphosphorylation of RyR2. *Circ Res,* Vol. 104, No. 4, (Feb 2009), pp. 514-521, ISSN 0009-7330
Thum, T., Galuppo, P., Wolf, C., Fiedler, J., Kneitz, S., van Laake, L.W., Doevendans, P.A., Mummery, C.L., Borlak, J., Haverich, A., Gross, C., Engelhardt, S., Ertl, G. & Bauersachs, J. (2007) MicroRNAs in the human heart: a clue to fetal gene reprogramming in heart failure. *Circulation,* Vol. 116, No. 3, (Jul 2007), pp. 258-67, ISSN 0009-7322
Thum, T., Gross, C., Fiedler, J., Fischer, T., Kissler, S., Bussen, M., Galuppo, P., Just, S., Rottbauer, W., Frantz, S., Castoldi, M., Soutschek, J., Koteliansky, V., Rosenwald, A., Basson, M.A., Licht, J.D., Pena, J.T., Rouhanifard, S.H., Muckenthaler, M.U., Tuschl, T., Martin, G.R., Bauersachs, J. & Engelhardt, S. (2008) MicroRNA-21 contributes to myocardial disease by stimulating MAP kinase signalling in fibroblasts. *Nature,* Vol. 456, No. 7224, (Dec 2008), pp. 980-4, ISSN 0028-0836
van Rooij, E., Sutherland, L.B., Liu, N., Williams, A.H., McAnally, J., Gerard, R.D., Richardson, J.A. & Olson, E.N. (2006) A signature pattern of stress-responsive microRNAs that can evoke cardiac hypertrophy and heart failure. *Proc Natl Acad Sci USA,* Vol. 103, No. 48, (Nov 2006), pp. 18255-60, ISSN 0027-8424
van Rooij, E., Sutherland, L.B., Qi, X., Richardson, J.A., Hill, J. & Olson, EN. (2007) Control of stress-dependent cardiac growth and gene expression by a microRNA. *Science,* Vol. 316, No. 5824, (Apr 2007), pp. 575-9, ISSN 0036-8075
van Rooij, E., Sutherland, L.B., Thatcher, J.E., DiMaio, J.M., Naseem, R.H., Marshall, W.S., Hill, J.A. & Olson, E.N. (2008) Dysregulation of microRNAs after myocardial

infarction reveals a role of miR-29 in cardiac fibrosis. *Proc Natl Acad Sci U S A,* Vol. 105, No. 35, (Sep 2008), pp. 13027-13032, ISSN 0027-8424

Wang, J., Xu, R., Lin, F., Zhang, S., Zhang, G., Hu, S. & Zheng, Z. (2009) MicroRNA: novel regulators involved in the remodeling and reverse remodeling of the heart. *Cardiology,* Vol. 113, No. 2, (2009), pp. 81-88, ISSN 0008-6312

Williams, A.E. (2008) Functional aspects of animal microRNAs. *Cell Mol Life Sci,* Vol. 65, No. 4, (Feb 2008), pp. 545-562, ISSN 1420-682X

Xiao, J., Luo, X., Lin, H., Zhang, Y., Lu, Y., Wang, N., Zhang, Y., Yang, B. & Wang, Z. (2007) MicroRNA miR-133 represses HERG K+ channel expression contributing to QT prolongation in diabetic hearts. *J Biol Chem,* Vol. 282, No. 17,(Apr 2007), pp. 12363-12367, ISSN 0021-9258

Xiao, J., Yang, B., Lin, H., Lu, Y., Luo, X. & Wang, Z. (2007) Novel approaches for gene-specific interference via manipulating actions of microRNAs: examination on the pacemaker channel genes HCN2 and HCN4. *J Cell Physiol,* Vol. 212, No. 2; (Aug 2007), pp. 285-292, ISSN 0021-9541

Xiao, L., Xiao, J., Luo, X., Lin, H., Wang, Z. & Nattel, S. (2008) Feedback remodeling of cardiac potassium current expression: a novel potential mechanism for control of repolarization reserve. *Circulation,* Vol. 118, No. 10, (Sep 2008), pp. 983-92, ISSN 0009-7322

Xu, C., Lu, Y., Pan, Z., Chu, W., Luo, X., Lin, H., Xiao, J., Shan, H., Wang, Z. & Yang, B. (2007) The muscle-specific microRNAs miR-1 and miR-133 produce opposing effects on apoptosis by targeting HSP60, HSP70 and caspase-9 in cardiomyocytes. *J Cell Sci* Vol. 120, No. Pt 17, (Sep 2007), pp. 3045-3052, ISSN 0021-9533

Yang, B., Lin, H., Xiao, J., Lu, Y., Luo, X., Li, B., Zhang, Y., Xu, C., Bai, Y., Wang, H., Chen, G. & Wang, Z. (2007) The muscle-specific microRNA miR-1 regulates cardiac arrhythmogenic potential by targeting GJA1 and KCNJ2. *Nat Med,* Vol. 13, No. 4, (Apr 2007), pp. 486-491, ISSN 1078-8956

Yin, C., Wang, X. & Kukreja, R.C. (2008) Endogenous microRNAs induced by heat-shock reduce myocardial infarction following ischemia-reperfusion in mice. *FEBS Lett,* Vol. 582, No. 30, (Dec 2008), pp. 4137-42, ISSN 0014-5793

Ying, S.Y., Chang, D.C. & Lin, S.L. (2008) The microRNA (miRNA): overview of the RNA genes that modulate gene function. *Mol Biotechnol,* Vol. 38, No. 3, (Mar 2008), pp. 257-68, ISSN 1073-6085

Zhao, Y., Ransom, J.F., Li, A., Vedantham, V., von Drehle, M., Muth, A.N., Tsuchihashi, T., McManus, M.T., Schwartz, R.J. & Srivastava, D. (2007) Dysregulation of cardiogenesis, cardiac conduction, and cell cycle in mice lacking miRNA-1-2. *Cell,* Vol. 129, No. 2 (Apr 2007), pp. 303-17, ISSN 0092-8674

Zhao, Y., Samal, E. & Srivastava, D. (2005) Serum response factor regulates a muscle-specific microRNA that targets Hand2 during cardiogenesis. *Nature,* Vol. 436, No. 7048, (Jul 2005), pp. 214-20, ISSN 0028-0836

3

Atrio-Ventricular Block-Induced Torsades de Pointes: An Update

Chevalier Philippe[1] and Scridon Alina[2]
[1]*Hôpital Louis Pradel, Lyon*
[2]*University of Medicine and Pharmacy, Targu Mures*
[1]*France*
[2]*Romania*

1. Introduction

Torsades de pointes is a potentially life threatening form of rapid, polymorphic ventricular tachycardia. Literally meaning "twisting of the points", torsades de pointes is electrocardiographically characterized by QRS axis undulations over runs of several beats, with a specific twist of the QRS complex around the isoelectric baseline. The definition also requires that an abnormal QT-prolongation be present (usually to 600 msec or greater) and / or abnormal TU complexes. The arrhythmia usually terminates spontaneously, with the exception of rare degeneration into ventricular fibrillation. The episodes are often repetitive and frequency dependent.

In 1966, Dessertenne first described torsades de pointes in a patient with atrio-ventricular block (Dessertenne, 1966). Ever since, several reports have associated torsades de pointes with bradycardia, especially with atrio-ventricular block (Viskin, 1999). From 5% to 30% of patients with atrio-ventricular block have been reported to develop torsades de pointes (Motté, 1970, Jensen, 1975, Guize, 1993) - an observation that suggests the participation of yet other intrinsic or extrinsic sensitising factors.

Most episodes of torsades de pointes are paroxystic, not longer than 5-20 beats, with a very elevated heart rate (160-300 bpm). The typical morphology of torsades de pointes includes a complete twist at 180° of QRS complexes and a progressive change of the surface ECG. A QT interval prolongation to 600 ms or longer is always evident. These episodes are often preceded by ventricular bigeminism with fixed and long coupling interval.

2. Risk factors

Several studies have proposed different risk factors for torsades de pointes. Among them, the most commonly encountered are female gender, advanced age, bradycardia, different metabolic disorders, and a number of therapeutic agents (Haverkamp, 2000). The gender-specific preponderance in females to develop drug-induced torsades de pointes when treated with antiarrhythmic drugs or during spontaneous bradyarrhythmias is also well documented. In the general population, women have a longer corrected QT interval than men.

Several endocrine disorders as well as a number of electrolytic imbalances have been incriminated as torsades de pointes facilitators (hypothyroidism, mental anorexia, hypokalaemia, hypomagnesaemia, hypocalcaemia, acidosis).

A great number of drugs are currently considered "torsadogenic". Almost all of these drugs have an IKr channel blocking effect, which explains QT interval prolongation. These agents belong to both "cardiotropic" and "non-cardiotropic" drugs (an exhaustive list is available on Internet at http://www.qtdrugs.org).

2.1 Atrio-ventricular block – a piece in the puzzle

The common element between atrio-ventricular block and torsades de pointes seems to be the presence of QT interval prolongation. Still, the association between atrio-ventricular block and QT interval prolongation is infrequent. Several studies have shown that this exact category of patients who present atrio-ventricular block induced - QT prolongation has the most elevated risk of developing torsades de pointes.

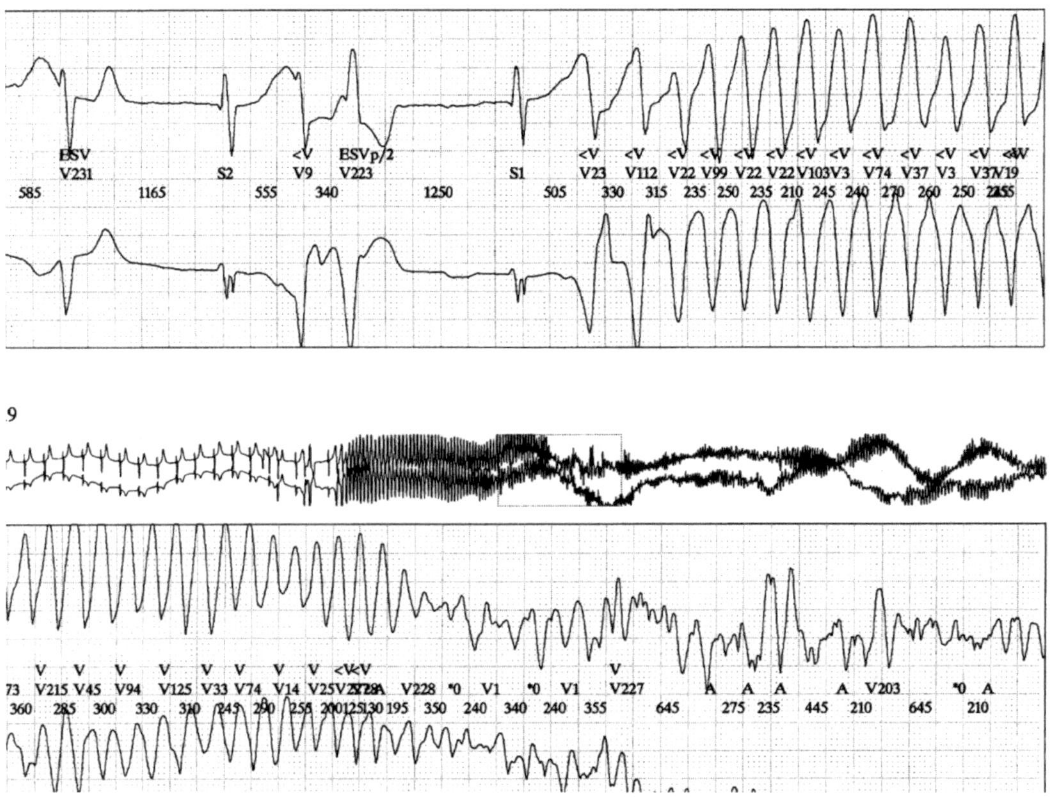

Fig. 1. Holter recording in a patient with post-operative atrio-ventricular block and typical torsades de pointes. Note the association of long QT interval, ventricular bigeminism, bradycardia, and bradycardia-dependant polymorphic ventricular tachycardia degenerating in ventricular fibrillation.

Kurita et al. have reported that patients with bradycardia-induced torsades de pointes have abnormally long QT intervals at slow heart rates, compared with patients with bradycardia but no tachyarrhythmia (Kurita, 1992). Strasberg et al. compared patients with atrio-ventricular block with torsades de pointes to those without torsades de pointes, and mentioned that the QT interval in patients with torsades de pointes was longer than in those without torsades de pointes, whereas heart rate and QRS interval during the escape rhythm were not significantly different (Strasberg, 1986). Moreover, they reported that QT interval above 600 ms and premature ventricular beats on electrocardiogram appear to indicate an increased risk for the development of polymorphic ventricular tachycardia in a patient with atrio-ventricular block.

In a retrospective review of 43 young patients with congenital atrio-ventricular block, Sholler et al. found QT interval prolongation to be an independent predictor of symptoms, including cardiac arrest and syncope. Overall, the outcome was poor with 21% of the atrio-ventricular block patients in their symptomatic group with rate-corrected QT intervals >0.45 seconds, in contrast with none in the asymptomatic group (Sholler, 1989). Marked QT interval prolongation complicated by torsades de pointes, as a sequela of acquired atrio-ventricular block, has been convincingly demonstrated in paediatric and adult patients. In each of these patients, who ranged in age from 18 months to 80 years on initial presentation with torsades de pointes, there was QT interval normalization and complete suppression of torsades de pointes after institution of ventricular pacing at age-appropriate rates.

Experimental data confirm these observations. In a dog model with chronic atrio-ventricular block, the QT interval was prolonged by 20%.

3. Genetic bases

3.1 Genetic bases of acquired long QT syndrome

In contrast to congenital long QT syndrome, the acquired form has been considered a non-familial disease, which is not transmitted in specific genetic patterns of inheritance. This does not automatically exclude genetic components from the pathogenesis of acquired long QT syndrome, but it implies that these are only cofactors in the pathogenesis.

The unpredictability of acquired long QT syndrome, its similarity to the congenital form and identification of manifest congenital long QT syndrome in patients with the drug-induced form, all suggest a genetic contribution to risk.

With the identification of mutations in ion channel genes underlying congenital long QT syndrome and the investigation of large families, a variable clinical expressivity and especially incomplete penetrance have become apparent (Raviña, 2000). In a given family, some individuals with a certain mutation have frank long QT intervals, while others with the same mutation have normal QT intervals at baseline. In some cases, the latter, who represent less than 10% of the patients with acquired long QT syndrome, experience torsades de pointes only after intervention of a QT-prolonging stressor. In autosomal dominant long QT syndrome (Romano-Ward syndrome), the aspect of incomplete penetrance was reported to be approximately 25% in a specific group of families. This raises the question of the frequency and importance of silent ion channel gene mutations that may become functionally significant in presence of coexisting factors.

Mutations in KCNE1 and KCNE2, KCNH2, HERG itself, and SCN5A have been identified in acquired forms of long QT syndrome (Abbott, 1999). However, the gene in which mutations are seen most commonly is KCNQ1, encoding for potassium channel IKs (Donger, 1997, Napolitano, 2000, Kubota, 2000).

Several frequently occurring polymorphisms have also been described in the long QT syndrome population, distributed in nearly all the genes associated with this condition. Although these changes are apparently not pathogenic, some can generate individual susceptibility to the development of arrhythmia. This is the case of the K897T polymorphism in KCNH2 (Crotti, 2005), which is present in up to 15% of the population and is linked with susceptibility to certain drugs. Another example is the R1047L polymorphism, the second most frequent polymorphism encountered in KCNH2, which has been associated with the development of torsades de pointes while using the drug dofetilide (Sun, 2004).

Polymorphisms that confer susceptibility to the development of ventricular arrhythmia have also been documented in sodium channel Na1.5. This is the case of the H558R polymorphism (Viswanathan, 2003), which is present in up to 30% of the population, or S1103Y, found mainly in blacks, with an incidence of nearly 13%, and associated with an increased risk of sudden death in childhood (Splawski, 2002, Paulussen, 2004). Most of these DNA polymorphisms do not occur in coding regions and may either have no functional significance, or modulate expression levels of functionally normal proteins. Other rare polymorphisms with minor allele frequencies (1-2%) that have been implicated in drug-induced torsades de pointes include D85N (KCNE1) (Paulussen, 2004) and T8A (KCNE2) (Sesti, 2000). I447 polymorphism in KCR1 was also proposed as potential modulator of the risk of drug-induced torsades de pointes (Roden, 2005). The valine variant was seen in 1.1% of patients, compared with 7% in controls, suggesting that the presence of valine in this position protects against drug-induced torsades de pointes.

It is not yet clear if all patients with acquired long QT syndrome have a genetic predisposition. Systematic evaluation of genes known to be involved in congenital long QT syndrome has therefore been recommended in patients with acquired long QT syndrome.

3.2 Genetic bases of atrio-ventricular block-induced torsades de pointes

A general observation is that only a minority of patients with atrio-ventricular block develop torsades de pointes. Moreover, in the early nineties, in patients with atrio-ventricular block and torsades de pointes compared with those without torsades de pointes, it was reported that the QT interval was longer than the bradycardia could account for. These observations suggested a genetic predisposition of the affected subjects. Furthermore, common clinical features and the presence of long QT intervals in patients with congenital long QT syndrome and in those with atrio-ventricular block–induced torsades de pointes suggested that patients with atrio-ventricular block-mediated QT-related arrhythmia could have latent congenital long QT syndrome or a vulnerable genetic polymorphism.

Moreover, several similarities have been found between experimental models of atrio-ventricular block–induced torsades de pointes and specific forms of human congenital long QT syndrome. Frequent episodes of spontaneous torsades de pointes during day and night, abnormal QTU complex, and reduction of both IKr and IKs in a rabbit atrio-ventricular block model (Tsuji , 2002) closely resemble the clinical characteristics of the malignant form of human congenital long QT syndrome caused by double mutation of HERG and KCNQ1. An enhanced susceptibility to acquired torsades de pointes, the adrenergic dependence of torsades de pointes, the typical T-wave patterns during prolonged QT intervals and the reduction of IKs in dog with chronic atrio-ventricular

block closely resemble the clinical characteristics of the LQT1 or LQT5 form of human congenital long QT syndrome.
Using recently introduced molecular biology techniques, these bradycardia-related repolarisation abnormalities appear to be allelic variants in the coding region of congenital long QT syndrome genes, variants that can be identified in 10–15% of affected subjects. A recent retrospective study showed that 14% to 18% of subjects with atrio-ventricular block-related QT-interval prolongation were carriers of a genetic mutation in genes coding for potassium channels. Another study showed that 36% of patients with complete atrio-ventricular block and torsades de pointes had a genetic mutation involving HERG and SCN5A (Yoshida, 2001). In fact, the most commonly encountered mutation in this setting is in HERG genes, coding for potassium channel IKr.
The scarcity of this association in the general population is directly responsible for the limited amount of information that we dispose of regarding this issue. Still, much is expected from future molecular testing in these patients.

4. Pathophysiology

4.1 Pathophysiology of torsades de pointes

The association between torsades de pointes and a prolonged QT interval has long been known, but the underlying mechanisms of torsades de pointes have yet to be satisfactorily elucidated. In general, alterations in cardiac ion currents which dictate the normal action potential play a major role in arrhythmogenesis. Both early afterdepolarisation - induced triggered activity (Cosio, 1991, Shimizu,1995, Burashnikov, 2002) and increased dispersion of repolarisation have been suggested as playing a role in the genesis of torsades de pointes. Significantly increased transmural dispersion of repolarisation favours re-entrant substrates that initiate and maintain torsades de pointes.
QT intervals in humans are very variable, being strongly influenced by age, sex, heart rate or heart diseases. It would appear that subjects with a propensity to develop the syndrome have a subclinical abnormality in some of the ion channels dictating repolarisation, and / or a reduced repolarisation reserve.
The latter hypothesis has been suggested by Roden et al (Roden, 1998). They hypothesized that the extent of QT lengthening in response to specific environmental triggers depends on the ventricular "repolarisation reserve". This concept proposes that loss of one component (e.g. IKs) ordinarily will not lead to failure of repolarisation since multiple other currents flow across the myocyte membrane (e.g. IKr) also act to maintain repolarisation in normal ranges. However, when a reduction or down regulation in any of the currents involved in the repolarisation phase is overlapped by a destabilizing factor, this "reserve" is overcome and acquired long QT syndrome may become clinically obvious (Roden, 1998). This issue may occur in the female gender, when a factor such as bradycardia or hypokalaemia is present, in conditions that predispose to electrical remodelling such as heart failure, myocardial ischemia, or ventricular hypertrophy.
It is well known that local action potential duration of myocardial cells displays considerable variability depending on many factors, including, in normal conditions, location in the ventricular wall (epicardium, mid-myocardium or endocardium) and rate of stimulation. These differences in action potential duration across the ventricular wall determine the transmural dispersion of repolarisation. When this transmural dispersion is exaggerated, opposite voltage gradients may occur and trigger oscillatory potentials,

namely phase 2 early afterdepolarisations and sustained abnormal electrical activity (Dangman, 1981, Brachmann, 1983, Levine, 1985, Roden, 1985, Davidenko, 1989).
Rarely, a single severe abnormality in a major repolarizing current can elicit an abnormal phenotype, as in congenital long QT syndrome (Roden, 1996). More commonly, one or more pre-existing minor abnormalities of repolarisation result in a subclinical phenotype. Following recent advances in molecular biology and genetics, it has become clear that in some clinical instances (e.g. congestive heart failure or cardiac hypertrophy) ion channel genes become down-regulated and the consequent reduced ion currents are likely to cause prolonged myocardial repolarisation. If, within this framework, an environmental stressor able to further destabilize the "repolarisation reserve" interferes, a long QT syndrome may be unburied and the arrhythmic consequences may appear.
Thus, a potentially dangerous stressor may appear completely safe when present in a large number of subjects. The risk may only be evident when the factor is present in a certain individual under certain circumstances.

4.2 Pathophysiology of atrio-ventricular block-induced torsades de pointes

Although a slow ventricular rate may be a major factor for inducing abnormal QT prolongation, the mechanism of QT prolongation in patients with bradycardia-related torsades de pointes is poorly understood.
Farkas et al. showed for the first time that bilateral vagotomy can prevent drug-induced torsades de pointes in an in vivo rabbit model, demonstrating that vagally-mediated reductions in heart rate are necessary for the development of torsades de pointes (Farkas, 2008). Torsades de pointes has been described in many conditions associated with bradycardia, such as atrio-ventricular block, drugs, vagotonia or hypothyroidism. Moreover, the occurrence of torsades de pointes in the presence of bradycardia is influenced by other factors such as gender, degree of QT prolongation or duration of bradycardia.
An interesting observation shows that arrhythmogenic bradycardias are most commonly chronic, with a slow ventricular escape rhythm – a profile corresponding to atrio-ventricular block. Studies have reported that patients with atrio-ventricular block have significantly longer QT intervals than those with sinus bradycardia, even at comparable heart rates. This relative QT prolongation may be one of the major reasons that torsades de pointes is more commonly observed in chronic atrio-ventricular block than in sinus bradycardia.
Clinical and experimental data show that the duration of atrio-ventricular block is an important determinant of the susceptibility to acquired torsades de pointes. Experimental studies show that torsades de pointes is rarely inducible at 0 weeks of atrio-ventricular block (acute atrio-ventricular block) but is inducible at 5 weeks (chronic atrio-ventricular block) in most animals (Vos, 1998). In a series of 64 patients with chronic atrio-ventricular block, Yiginer et al. reported a longer duration of bradycardia in the three patients who developed torsades de pointes (Yiginer, 2010). Concomitant to the duration of atrio-ventricular block, the likelihood of structural and electrical alterations in myocardial cells may increase.

4.2.1 Bradycardia-induced cardiac remodelling

Atrio-ventricular block-induced volume overload initiates a number of adaptative processes that are aimed to compensate the decreased cardiac output and the increased end-diastolic pressure. These remodelling processes offer both the "trigger" and "substrate" for the occurrence of torsades de pointes.

Bradycardia-induced volume overload causes the development of a biventricular eccentric hypertrophy and consequently a non-homogenous lengthening of the ventricular action potential duration. Exact information concerning the sequence and nature of the time-related electrophysiological process in hypertrophy are lacking, but there seems to be a parallelism between the evolutions of the two processes. These adaptations, alone or synergistically, increase the risk of early afterdepolarisations and / or delayed afterdepolarisation and therefore the risk of torsades de pointes.

4.2.2 Structural remodelling during atrio-ventricular block

Ventricular hypertrophy in this setting is a response of the heart to compensate the altered hemodynamic load induced by atrio-ventricular block (Vos, 1998). The process is initiated by mechanical factors and thereafter amplified by neurohumoral factors, such as adrenergic stimuli, the renin-angiotensin system, endothelin, or insulin-like growth factor.

Autopsy studies have demonstrated increased heart weight to body weight ratios, with significant contributions of both the right and left ventricular mass. Morphologically, biventricular hypertrophy is characterized by an eccentric expansion with increased right and left ventricular diameters, as seen during volume overload (Verduyn, 2001). Photo- and electron-micrograph analyses have shown myocardial cell hypertrophy together with the parallel increases of collagen fibbers and extracellular space.

Morphopathological studies have shown larger growth responses in the right than left ventricular myocytes, supporting the autopsy finding of a larger relative increase of the right than the left ventricular weight, as well as a more significant hypertrophy of right ventricular free wall and septal wall than of the left ventricular free wall (Verduyn, 2001, Sugiyama, 2002). The preponderance of right ventricular cell growth in atrio-ventricular block may reflect a greater impact on this chamber after the transition from sinus rhythm to idioventricular rhythm.

This structural adaptation process is accompanied by electrophysiological remodelling. Prolongation of the left ventricular action potential is a consistent observation in myocardial hypertrophy of different causes in several species. Many of the sarcolemmal ion channels, exchangers, and pumps, as well as intracellular ion transporters, can show functional defects leading to delayed repolarisation.

4.2.3 Electrical remodelling during atrio-ventricular block

While electrical and structural changes in chronic atrio-ventricular block are aimed to maintain cardiac function, they also predispose to QT prolongation, leading to the onset of torsades de pointes. This association has been extensively evaluated in animal studies.

Tsuji et al. reported the results obtained in a rabbit model with atrio-ventricular block induced by injection of formaldehyde into the atrio-ventricular node (Tsuji, 2002). These rabbits received ventricular pacing support after atrio-ventricular block induction. The authors demonstrated significant QT interval prolongation in the same day that they discontinued pacing, with further prolongation later on. Seventy % of the animals developed spontaneous torsades de pointes, with most episodes occurring during the first week of uncompensated bradycardia. Even more information has been offered by a rabbit model with atrio-ventricular block induced by transcatheter radiofrequency ablation of atrio-ventricular node. Chronic endocardial ventricular pacing at near-physiologic rate was installed immediately after the ablation procedure. The authors showed identical amplitudes of all repolarizing currents in atrio-ventricular block group and sham-operated group. Moreover, they showed a similar down-regulation in the affected currents regardless of ventricular cavity stimulation (left or right ventricle) and they concluded that secondary electrical remodelling is unrelated to the loss of atrio-ventricular synchrony, suggesting that bradycardia alone suffices to turn on the electrical remodelling process.

In vivo experiments in dogs indicate the importance of bradycardia-dependent early afterdepolarisations, increased regional dispersion of repolarisation and multiple ectopic beats for the initiation of torsades de pointes. Fast heart rates tend to oppose these actions, preventing torsades de pointes.

Several mechanisms have been proposed for early afterdepolarisations occurrence in this setting (Emori, 2001, Yan, 2001). These abnormalities appear to be secondary to both bradycardia-dependent depression of electrogenic Na^+ pumping and more complete inactivation of K^+ currents. Vos et al. showed a high incidence of early afterdepolarisations in dogs with chronic atrio-ventricular block after d-sotalol administration and proposed significant down-regulation of the slow component of the delayed rectifier K^+ current (IKs) and that of the rapid component (IKr) as potential mechanism (Vos, 1995, 1998).

Enhanced regional dispersion of repolarisation is considered to be the consequence of inhomogeneous prolongation of ventricular action potential (more in the left than the right ventricle), probably reflecting the existence of significant repolarisation gradients in closely adjacent areas, possibly the septum. Interventricular differences of the action potential are known to exist in the normal myocardium of dogs with sinus rhythm. In chronic atrio-ventricular block, larger action potential durations have been documented in left mid-myocardial compared with right ventricular myocytes, in contrast to the larger degree of hypertrophy in the latter. The observation that a down-regulation of IKs is present in both ventricles while IKr down-regulation is mainly expressed in the right ventricle could explain these abnormalities.

Other currents such as It0, ICaL or IK1 have been reported as unchanged in a number of studies.

However, the observations are contradictory. While some suggest that the role of It0 is unlikely given the fact that the spike-and-dome configuration of the action potential is preserved, others suggest that low ventricular rates are associated with submaximal activation of It0, which would shift the plateau phase of the action potential to voltage levels in which Ca^{2+} window current availability is increased, predisposing to torsades de pointes.

The fact that the action potential duration to 95% of complete repolarisation and action potential duration to 50% of complete repolarisation have been found to be increased to a similar extent indicates that the delay of repolarisation is most likely due to a disturbance at the plateau level, sustaining the central role of IKr and IKs in this setting.

Additional insights into the ionic mechanisms of action potential prolongation in chronic atrio-ventricular block come from experiments with almokalant. After block of IKr during almokalant treatment, the action potential duration was found much larger in chronic atrio-ventricular block myocytes than in sinus rhythm controls. This suggests that ionic currents other than IKr contribute to the abnormal repolarisation in chronic atrio-ventricular block, even though the role of IKr can not be excluded. These results have been confirmed by other similar studies, which show uniformly distributed IKs down-regulation by 50% in both

ventricles, while a similar degree of IKr inhibition was apparent only in the right but not in the left ventricle.
In vivo recordings in dog with chronic atrio-ventricular block demonstrate that another important factor involved in the occurrence of torsades de pointes is represented by ventricular ectopic beats. However, their origin and mechanisms remain obscure for the moment.

5. Conclusions

Investigations of the clinical aspects and molecular mechanisms of long QT syndrome have provided novel and important insights into the basis of ventricular arrhythmias and shown how small perturbations in ion flow can have important consequences in human health.
Even if molecular diagnosis appears to be an appealing way of integrating contemporary genomics with arrhythmia science, several obstacles limit its wide availability. Molecular diagnosis is restricted by the very large number of candidate genes and the correspondingly huge number of described polymorphisms. Moreover, most association studies have not proven to be reproducible, raising the problem of false positives. There is also the issue that, owing to its restrictive costs, mutation screening will be limited to a limited number of specialized centres for some time.
Though great progress has been made, many important issues require further clarification. A major challenge in the future will be to understand the complex mechanisms of repolarisation and to assess the individual risk of malignant arrhythmia more precisely. Moreover, mutations in other ion channel genes, still unrecognized, could be responsible for different variants of long QT syndrome.
We recommend systematically genotyping patients with acquired long QT syndrome and torsades de pointes. The next step could be represented by case-control studies of gene polymorphisms in pace-maker patients to find the possible markers of susceptibility to malignant arrhythmias during bradycardia.

6. References

Abbott GW, Sesti F, Splawski I, et al. (1999) MiRP1 Forms IKr Potassium Channels with HERG and Is Associated with Cardiac Arrhythmia. *Cell*. 97(2): 175-187.
Brachmann J, Scherlag BJ, Rosenshtraukb LV, et al. (1983) Bradycardia-dependent triggered activity: relevance to drug-induced multiform ventricular tachycardia. *Circulation*. 68: 846-85.
Burashnikov A, Antzelevitch C. (2002) Prominent IKs in epicardium and endocardium contributes to development of transmural dispersion of repolarization but protects against development of early afterdepolarizations. *J Cardiovasc Electrophysiol*. 13: 172–177.
Cosio FG, Goicolea A, López-Gil L, et al. (1991) Suppression of Torsades de Pointes with verapamil in patients with atrio-ventricular block. *Eur Heart J*. 12: 635–63 8.
Crotti L, Lundquist AL, Insolia R et al. (2005) Common KCNH2 polymorphism (K897T) as a genetic modifier of congenital long QT syndrome. *Circulation*. 112: 1251–1258.
Dangman KH, Hoffman BF. (1981) In vivo and in vitro antiarrhythmic and arrhythmogenic effects of N-acetyl procainamide. *J Pharmacol Exp Ther*. 217: 851-862.

Davidenko JM, Cohen L, Goodrow R, et al. (1989) Quinidine-induced action potential prolongation, early afterdepolarizations, and triggered activity in canine purkinje tibsrs: effects of stimulation rate, potassium, and magnesium. *Circulation.* 79: 674-686.

Dessertenne F. (1966) La tachycardie ventriculaire a deux foyers opposes variables. *Arch Mal Coeur Vaiss.* 59 (2): 263–272.

Donger C, Denjoy I, Berthet M, et al. (1997) KVLQT1 c-terminal missense mutation causes a forme fruste long-QT syndrome. *Circulation.* 96: 2778–2781.

Emori T, Antzelevitch C. (2001) Cellular basis for complex T wave and arrhythmic activity following combined IKr and IKs block. *J Cardiovasc Electrophysiol.* 12: 1369 –1378.

Farkas A, Dempster J, Coker SJ. (2008) Importance of vagally mediated bradycardia for the induction of torsade de pointes in an in vivo model. *British Journal of Pharmacology.* 154: 958–970.

Guize L, Iliou MC, Bayet G, et al. (1993) Les torsades de pointes. *Arch Mal Coeur Vaiss.* 86: 769 –776.

Haverkamp W, Breithard G, Camm AJ et al. (2000) The potential for QT prolongation and proarrhythmia by non-antiarrhythmic drugs: clinical and regulatory implications. Reports on a policy conference of the European Society of Cardiology. *Cardiovasc Res.* 47: 219-233.

Jensen G, Sigurd B, Sandoe E. (1975) Adams-Stokes seizures due to ventricular tachydysarrhythmias in patients with heart block: prevalence and problems of management. *Chest.* 67: 43-48.

Kubota T, Shimizu W, Kamakura S, et al. (2000) Hypokalemia-induced long QT syndrome with underlying novel missense mutation in S4-S5 linker of KCNQ1. *J Cardiovasc Electrophysiol.* 11: 1048 –1054.

Kurita T, Ohe T, Marui Aihara N, et al. (1992) Bradycardia-induced abnormal QT prolongation in patients with complete atrioventricular block with torsades de pointes. *Am J Cardiol.* 69: 628–633.

Levine JH, Spear JF, Guamieri T, et al. (1985) Cesium chlorideinduced long QT syndrome: demonstration of afterdepolarizations and triggered activity in vivo. *Circulation.* 72: 1092-110.

Motté G, Coumel P, Abitbol G, et al. (1970) Le syndrome du QT long et syncopes par torsades de pointes. *Arch Mal Coeur Vaiss.* 63: 831-853.

Napolitano C, Schwartz PJ, Brown AM, et al. (2000) Evidence for a cardiac ion channel mutation underlying drug-induced QT prolongation and life-threatening arrhythmias. *J Cardiovasc Electrophysiol.* 11: 691–696.

Paulussen AD, Gilissen RA, Armstrong M, et al. (2004) Genetic variations of KCNQ1, KCNH2, SCN5A, KCNE1, and KCNE2 in drug-induced long QT syndrome patients. *J Mol Med.* 82(3): 182-188.

Raviña T, Gutierrez J. (2000) Amiodarone-induced AV block an ventricular standstill. A forme fruste of an idiopathic long QT syndrome. *Int J Cardiol.* 75: 105-108.

Roden DM. (1998) Taking the "idio" out of "idiosyncratic": predicting Torsades de Pointes. *PACE.* 21: 1029–1034.

Roden DM, Hoffman BF. (1985) Action potential prolongation and induction of abnormal automaticity by low quinidine concentrations in canine purkinje fibers:relationship to potassium and cycle length. *Circ Res.* 56: 857-86.

Roden DM, Lazzara R, Rosen M, et al. (1996) Multiple mechanisms in the long-QT syndrome: current knowledge, gaps, and future directions. *Circulation.* 94: 1996–2012.

Roden DM, Viswanathan PC. (2005) Genetics of acquired long QT syndrome. *J Clin Invest.* 115: 2025–2032.

Sesti F, Abbott GW, Wei J, et al. (2000) A common polymorphism associated with antibiotic-induced cardiac arrhythmia. *Proc Natl Acad Sci U S A.* 97(19): 10613-10618.

Shimizu W, Ohe T, Kurita T, et al. (1995) Effects of verapamil and propranolol on early afterdepolarizations and ventricular arrhythmias induced by epinephrine in congenital long QT syndrome. *J Am Coll Cardiol.* 26: 1299 -1309.

Sholler GF, Walsh EP. (1989) Congenital complete heart block in patients without anatomic cardiac defects. *Am Heart J.* 118: 1193-1198.

Splawski I, Timothy KW, Tateyama M, et al. (2002) Variant of SCN5A sodium channel implicated in risk of cardiac arrhythmia. *Science.* 297: 1333–1336.

Strasberg B, Kusniec J, Erdman S, et al. (1986) Polymorphous ventricular tachycardia and atrioventricular block. *Pacing Clin Electrophysiol.* 9: 522-526.

Sugiyama A, Ishida Y, Satoh Y, et al. (2002) Electrophysiological, Anatomical and Histological Remodeling of the Heart to AV Block Enhances Susceptibility to Arrhythmogenic Effects of QT-Prolonging Drugs. *Jpn J Pharmacol.* 88: 341 - 350.

Sun Z, Milos PM, Thompson JF, et al. (2004) Role of a KCNH2 polymorphism (R1047 L) in dofetilide-induced torsades de pointes. *J Mol Cell Cardiol.* 37: 1031-1039.

Tsuji Y, Opthof T, Yasui K, et al. (2002) Ionic mechanisms of acquired QT prolongation and torsades de pointes in rabbits with chronic complete atrioventricular block. *Circulation.* 106: 2012–2018.

Verduyn SC, Ramakers C, Snoep G, et al. (2001) Time course of structural adaptations in chronic AV block dogs: evidence for differential ventricular remodeling. *Am J Physiol Heart Circ Physiol.* 280: H2882-H2890.

Viskin S. (1999) Long QT syndromes and torsades de pointes. *Lancet.* 354: 1625-1633.

Viswanathan PC, Benson DW, Balser JR. (2003) A common SCN5A polymorphism modulates the biophysical effects of an SCN5A mutation. *J Clin Invest.* 111: 341–346.

Vos MA, Groot SHM, Verduyn SC, et al. (1998) Enhanced susceptibility for acquired Torsade de Pointes arrhythmias in the dog with chronic, complete AV block is related to cardiac hypertrophy and electrical remodeling. *Circulation.* 98: 1125–1135.

Vos MA, Verduyn SC, Gorgels APM, et al. (1995) Reproducible induction of early afterdepolarizations and Torsade de Pointes arrhythmias by d-sotalol and pacing in dogs with chronic atrioventricular block. *Circulation.* 91: 864 -872.

Yan GX, Wu Y, Liu T, et al. (2001) Phase 2 early afterdepolarization as a trigger of polymorphic ventricular tachycardia in acquired long-QT syndrome, direct evidence from intracellular recordings in the intact syndrome, direct evidence from intracellular recordings in the intact. *Circulation.* 103: 2851- 2856.

Yiginer O, Kilicaslan F, Aparci M, et al. (2010) Bradycardia-induced Torsade de Pointes - An arrhythmia Less Understood." *Indian Pacing Electrophysiol J.* 10(10): 435-438.

Yoshida H, Horie M, Otani H, et al. (2001) Bradycardia-induced long QT syndrome caused by a de novo missense mutation in the S2-S3 inner loop of HERG. *Am J Med Genet.* 98: 348 –352.

4

Ultradian Rhythms Underlying the Dynamics of the Circadian Pacemaker

Carolina Barriga-Montoya, Pablo Padilla-Longoria,
Miguel Lara-Aparicio and Beatriz Fuentes-Pardo
Universidad Nacional Autónoma de México
México

1. Introduction

Before discussing rhythms and pacemakers, we would like to begin this chapter by quoting Albert Einstein (Einstein, 1934):

> "Our experience hitherto justifies us in trusting that nature is the realization of the simplest that is mathematically conceivable. I am convinced that purely mathematical construction enables us to find those concepts and those lawlike connections between them that provide the key to the understanding of natural phenomena".

Indeed, it seems that nature can be described and understood in mathematical terms. In the context of physical phenomena nobody can deny the usefulness, applicability and relevance of mathematical models. However, as strange and paradoxical as it might appear, the importance of mathematics in biology is still questioned.

In the case of biological systems it is particularly important to discuss whether this confidence is based on facts. Among life scientists it is a widespread opinion that mathematical models just put in very complicated terms what they already knew.

On the other hand this is in sharp contrast with what Darwin expresses in a letter, regretting not having deepened in some basic mathematical principles (Nowak, 2006).

Mathematical models incorporate experimental information, both, quantitative and qualitative. Models have to mimic the observed behavior, but this is not enough. They have to allow for the understanding of the mechanisms underlying the studied phenomenon and also have to be able to make predictions (again, both qualitative and quantitative).

The construction of a mathematical model is not an unidirectional process. The feedback at the different stages of the process is one of the most important and useful characteristics (see Figure 1). A mathematical model provides the necessary elements to compare and even discard different hypotheses, and, in many cases, to propose new experiments (Fuentes-Pardo et al., 2005).

Just to provide a few examples in which the construction of a mathematical model has been essential in the understanding of a biological process we mention the work by Hodgkin and Huxley in the early fifties, on the existence of selective ion channels on the membrane of a neuron. Their model not only enabled them to test this hypothesis, namely, but also to deduce qualitative properties of the transmission of electrical impulses, leading to the notion of action potential (Hodkgin et al., 1952a; Hodgkin & Huxley, 1952b, 1952c, 1952d, 1952e). In the past few years, important progress has been made in establishing mathematical models at the basis of the understanding of many biological systems: genetic regulatory networks, ecological dynamics, morphogenetic process and so on. At the same time, it is important to mention the fact that some of these models have been proven efficient tools in the design of new treatments or in implementing new therapies (Murray, 2003a, 2003b).

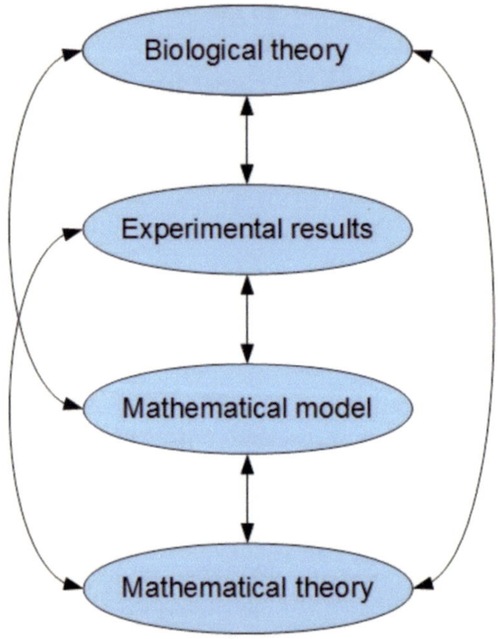

Fig. 1. Relationship among experiments, models, and theories.

As we hope we will make clear in what follows, it is absolutely necessary to incorporate modeling tools in the study of circadian rhythms and their pacemakers. We could use the title of the famous song by George Gershwin "I've got rhythm" to express our conviction that without a solid mathematical framework, we will never have rhythms or at least a good understanding of them.

In the rest of this chapter we are going to explain the main characteristics of a circadian rhythm and the possible organization of the structures in charge of generating the circadian oscillation, i.e. the pacemaker(s). Also we are going to expose the importance of high frequency oscillators (ultradian oscillators) in the generation of the circadian oscillation in the pacemaker and finally we are going to discuss the development of a mathematical model related to the emergence of an oscillation with a period of about 24 hours in a circadian pacemaker and the concomitant phenomenon of synchronization.

The story began a few years ago, when a biologist asked a mathematician to construct a mathematical model for the emergence of the crayfish circadian rhythm. The mathematician asked her what the goal was. The reply can be summarized as follows:

—To understand in depth the observed experimental phenomena in order to explain the mechanisms underlying to the emergence of circadian rhythms in the corresponding pacemaker.

What followed was a close collaboration which involved, among other things, a great deal of patience from both, in order to be able to establish a common language and the possibility of "translating" questions, problems and assertions phrased in a biological way in the mathematical jargon and the other way around. As a result of this collaboration (that still continues) an important point was made:
A focal point to the understanding the generation of the 24 hour oscillation in the circadian pacemaker is a more primeval time-base, one that encompasses both biophysics and biochemistry, both cellular biology and cell reproduction. This is a high frequency clock or ultradian clock (Lloyd et al., 2008).
Considering that the physiological basis for the pacemaker function has to be at the cellular level, it is a fundamental question how individual cells interact among themselves in order to produce a coherent collective behavior that exhibits periodic features. The study of how biological systems organize themselves in time (including the study of biological clocks and biological rhythms), how time and space-time structures and hierarchies arise in living organisms, what we might call space-time morphogenesis, is still far from satisfactory. In what follows we present a concrete attempt to provide a mathematical framework in a specific example.
The chapter is organized as follows. In section 2 we briefly discuss the basic features of circadian rhythms and the circadian pacemaker(s) organization. Section 3 is devoted to the molecular and cellular basis of the circadian pacemaker functioning. In section 4 we provide a short review of the presence of ultradian oscillators that are believed to be responsible for the emergence of oscillatory behavior in the circadian pacemaker. Section 5 deals with the specific case of the crayfish, presenting both experimental results as well as a mathematical model. We present in section 6 a very simple model that might account for the appearance of low frequency oscillations in the (circadian) pacemaker as a result of the coupling of ultradian (high frequency) nonlinear oscillators. We conclude with some general remarks and, more importantly, with open problems and further questions on the subject.

2. What are circadian rhythms?

Many physiological variables change according to some temporal signals like the hour of the day or the seasons during the year. The study of biological rhythms is centered on the understanding of the mechanisms underlying the periodical changes exhibited by the functions of the organisms, as well as the relationship they maintain with external signals.
Among the collection of biological rhythms it can be distinguished those belonging to the *circa* (*lit.* near) class. These rhythms are designed in that way because when periodical signals from the environment are eliminated, the oscillation persists with a period similar, but different from that of the external influence. For example, under constant environmental conditions, the circatidal, circadian, circalunar, and circannual rhythms show a period of approximately 12 hours, 24 hours, 28 days, and 365 days respectively. In natural conditions, however, the external perturbations are present, the period of these rhythms is exactly equal to the period of the external perturbation.
A common feature of *circa* rhythms is that are all the expression of endogenous oscillator networks. In *circa* rhythm there exists a structure, known as the pacemaker, which has the ability to oscillate even under constant environmental conditions. This is true under normal circumstances, when it is part of the organism and even when it has been removed from it.

This structure has also the ability to impose its rhythm to other related units within the organism called effectors.

In this presentation, we discuss circadian rhythms, which are based on a circadian biological clock or circadian pacemaker that has a free-running period of 20-28 hour. This clock is able to synchronize itself to 24-hour environmental cycles, namely the light-dark cycles from the Earth rotation.

Circadian rhythms are relevant to many processes and have received considerable attention. We mention the following two important facts:

1. Their universality. With the exception of bacteria and simpler organisms, all living organisms that have been studied exhibit some kind of rhythm.
2. Their fundamental role in the temporal organization of the physiological and behavioral functions of living organisms.

Although circadian rhythms have been well known since antiquity, the existence of the corresponding biological clocks has only been, relatively speaking, recently accepted (around the sixties). Since then, researchers have gathered evidence in favor of the existence of endogenous biological circadian oscillators or circadian pacemakers.

2.1 Organization of circadian pacemakers

In the early days of chronobiology the notion of circadian organization was quite simple: inside the organism there was a clock (pacemaker) able to be entrained by light via photoreceptors and to impose its rhythm to some structures in the body called effector organs (Zivkovic B., 2006).

This model became difficult to sustain because of new experimental evidence. For example, it was recognized that other signals as temperature, food, or social cues are able to synchronize the pacemaker (Zivkovic B., 2006).

Moreover, experimental results pointed out to the existence of more than one pacemaker inside the organism: in certain environmental conditions circadian rhythms would split into two or more components, each with a different endogenous period; every component observed corresponds to the dynamics of each pacemaker (Zivkovic B., 2006).

In some organisms it appeared that the organization between multiple pacemakers was hierarchical, i.e., there was a master or central pacemaker whose output affects the phase (synchronizes) of the group of peripheral or slaves pacemakers. However in other organisms it appeared that the organization was non-hierarchical, i.e., each pacemaker influences all the others, and as a group, generates an output that drive all the overt rhythms (Zivkovic B., 2006).

The next step was the recognition that the information does not necessarily flow in just one direction: from the environment, via sensory systems, to the pacemakers, to the effector organs. The pacemaker(s) also generate(s) a circadian rhythm in sensory sensitivity. For example the eye may be more sensitivity to light during the night than during the day. Other form of feedback was, for example, the effect of an hormone released from an effector organ over the pacemaker dynamics (Zivkovic B., 2006).

2.2 Synchronization

Other remarkable characteristic of the *circa* rhythms is that, although their oscillations are due to endogenous mechanisms, they have the ability "to follow" the rhythm coming from external signals. An alignment of the period and phase of the *circa* rhythms to the period

and phase of some external rhythms can be observed. This property is known as extrinsic synchronization or synchronization by external stimulus.
In contrast to extrinsic synchronization, in which, as we just mentioned, an external signal plays a fundamental role in inducing a coherent collective behavior, there is another kind of coordinated in time regime. We could call this intrinsic or spontaneous synchronization. In this, there is no distinguished agent.
In order to have this functionality of external synchronization, it has been postulated that the biochronometric system has to possess an internal synchronization system regulating the pacemaker functional units and their interactions with an external synchronization system.

3. How does the circadian pacemaker work?

In several organisms including fungi, plants, worms, crustaceans, insects, mollusca, birds and mammals, circadian pacemakers, centrals and peripherals, have been identified by performing lesion studies, *in vitro* and *in vivo* functional studies, as well as transplant studies. However the way the pacemakers work is far from being understood (Paranjpe & Sharma, 2005).
It is now common to begin from a general assertion the circadian oscillation exhibited by the pacemaker will be describable as a circular list of causes and effects that closes within the bounds of a single cell, even in the most complicated systems as in mammals (Dunlap, 1999).
In an attempt to understand the mechanisms underlying the dynamics of circadian pacemaker, molecular models have been proposed. As in any other self-sustaining oscillatory process, these molecular models are based on negative and positive feedback loops. Clock genes turn on and off because of the proteins they encode. It has been suggested that synchronization of the intracellular clock with the geophysical cycles is due to the degradation of a substance and formation of another, both induced by light (Harmer et al., 2001).
Now, assuming that there is (and that we reasonably understand) "an intracellular synchronizable clock" in each circadian pacemaker cells, it still remains to be elucidated how the molecular time arising from the molecular clock is transferred to the cell in order to promote changes in its excitability and modify the physiology and behavior of the organism. This is a very complicated problem for which, up to the present, there is no adequate model. Moreover, it was discovered that every cell in the body contain a molecular clock, i.e. every cell is a secondary or slave pacemaker with a molecular machinery very similar to one in the central or master pacemaker. However it is known that if we remove a central pacemaker all overt rhythms finished, while removal a peripheral pacemaker does not; that transplantation of a central pacemaker tissues also transplant the phase and the period of all overt rhythms of the donor to the host, while transplantation of peripheral pacemaker does not do, i.e., the observed period and phase were that of the host; that the central pacemakers cells kept in a dish cycling "indefinitely" while peripheral pacemaker damp into arrythmicity after just a few cycles (Zivkovic, 2006).
Recent results have made evident the important role of electrical signaling at the cellular level. It was shown that in order to maintain a robust circadian oscillation, the molecular feedback loops are necessary but not sufficient. The rhythmic nature of pacemaker cells was traditionally described considering the individual properties of the cells. Nitabatch and cols.

questioned this premise showing that interneuronal communication is necessary to sustain molecular, cellular and systemic rhythms (Nitabach et al., 2002, 2005, 2006).
So, as we can see, the panorama is very complicated.

4. The oscillation in the circadian pacemaker by coupling ultradian oscillations

Research on biological clocks has been centered in the circadian ones. That is why they were frequently employed as a reference point, in particular with respect to the value of its frequency: rhythms that have a frequency less than that of the circadian rhythms were called infradian and those having a bigger frequency were called ultradian rhythms.
As we previously noted, organisms possess a pacemaker that matches physiological functions to the 24 hour cycle of day and night on the Earth. Since 1971 when R. J. Konopka and S. Benzer (Konopka & Benzer, 1971) identified the first clock-gene up to date, there were many significant advances in the comprehension about the mechanisms underlying the generation of circadian rhythms. However the paradigm that mechanisms generating a period of about 24 hours also have a period of 24 hours (that is the fact that every cell in the pacemaker is capable of sustaining a 24 hour oscillation individually in its own activity), every time is less solid because of new experimental evidences that explore the possibility that the circadian pacemaker is an emergent property of circuit interactions. In this section we argue that ultradian oscillators are coupled to yield a composite circadian pacemaker.
As Paetkau and collaborators. pointed out (Paetkau et al., 2006), "the beats" mechanism has been largely ignored because of a number of critical arguments, but most of the criticisms predated gene regulatory model of circadian oscillation.
First of all, 24 hours is a long time in terms of the coherent intracellular dynamics of organisms. We only have to think, for example, of the temporal scale of energy generation, metabolic reactions, transcriptional order, and cell proliferation and development. All these processes make evident the presence and ubiquity of ultradian oscillators in biology: with a period of about 40 minutes, the oxygen consumption and other metabolic processes in *Acanthamoeba castellanii*; similar ultradian clocks were observed in other protists (ciliates and flagellates) and yeast; a 40 minute cycle in general transcriptional activity in yeast; with a period of 69 minutes, respiration in *Dictyostelium*; 3 hour cycles of expression of the mammalian p53 protein; 2 hour periodicity in the expression of the Notch effector Hes1 in cultured cells; a 1.5-3 hour periodicity in the expression of NF-κB signaling molecule in mouse cells in culture, among many others (Lloyd & Murray, 2007; Paetkau et al., 2006).
The complex time structure of organisms requires the synchronized operation of multiple processes in many time domains. To focus exclusively on one time domain and thereby ignoring the full complexity of the system is to risk misconception of underlying mechanisms and to oversimplify the whole phenomenon. Several authors have suggested that at least some circadian pacemakers comprise coupled ultradian ones. Theodosios Pavlidis, in 1969 (Pavlidis, 1969, 1971), proposed the idea of generating slow rhythms from relatively fast biochemical processes by weak coupling of ultradian oscillators. Many other modes of coupling are possible, and the over all period of the whole may be longer or shorter than the free-running period of the longest or shortest component, respectively (Winfree, 1967, 2001).
The presence of 'beats' was noted in several experimental studies and models and it has been suggested as a mechanism for producing circadian oscillations. For example, Patekau

and collaborators (Paetkau et al., 2006) propose a model in which two independent transcriptional-translational oscillators with periods much shorter than 24 hours are coupled to drive a forced oscillator that has a circadian period, using mechanisms and parameters of conventional molecular biology. The *Drosophila* circadian clock can be modeled as a system of coupled ultradian ones based on data showing ultradian peaks in the power spectrum (Dowse & Ringo, 1987). Barrio and cols. (Barrio et al., 1997) developed a theoretical model of ensambles of mutually coupled ultradian oscillators to explain the generation of circadian rhythms in mammals. Díez-Noguera (Díez-Noguera, 1994) propose a functional model of the circadian system based on the degree of intercommunication in a complex system (the circadian pacemaker). The model was conceived to explain previous results concerning the maturation of motor activity in young rats. The maturation of the rhythm shows a predominance of ultradian components just after weaning, which disappear gradually when the circadian rhythm becomes apparent.

5. Experiments and mathematical models from the pacemaker crayfish

Crayfish is a nocturnal freshwater crustacean belonging to the Decapoda Order. With respect to the study of circadian rhythms crayfish has proved to be an excellent model due to its ability to survive in the non-natural conditions of the laboratory.
In this animal it has been detected a great variety of circadian rhythms in both behavior and physiological activity (Aréchiga et al., 1993). An example is the rest-activity (the motor) circadian rhythm and the circadian rhythm of sensitivity to light of retinular cells, (ERG circadian rhythm, (see Figure 2).

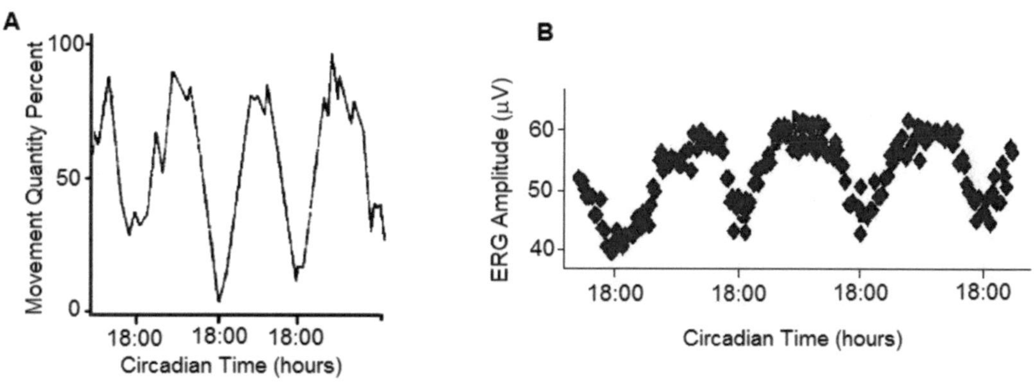

Fig. 2. Crayfish motor circadian rhythm (A) and ERG circadian rhythm (B).

5.1 Pacemaker organization for crustaceans

For crustaceans it has been proposed the existence of a multioscillatory pacemaker system (Aréchiga, 1993; Rodíguez-Sosa, 2008). To define a circadian system of multiple oscillators, identification of its individual components becomes the first task. It must be shown that each of these pacemakers is able to maintain a self-sustained circadian rhythmicity in isolation as well as being in synchrony within the whole circadian system.
Circadian rhythmicity has been demonstrated to be expressed in various isolated structures such as the isolated eyestalk (Sánchez & Fuentes-Pardo, 1977), the neurosecretory X-organ-

sinus gland system and in the retina-lamina ganlglionaris system (Aréchiga & Rodríguez-Sosa, 1998, 2002; Rodríguez-Sosa et al., 1994; Uribe et al., 1998, as cited in Rodríguez-Sosa, 2008). Another possible pacemaker for the crayfish circadian system is the supraesophageal ganglion. Its abblation supresses circadian rhythmicity, however, no experiments *in vitro* have been reported and some rhythms persists after the lesion (Hernández & Fuentes-Pardo, 2001). The way in which these pacemakers interact to generate a synchronous rhythmicity is still unknown (See Figure 3).

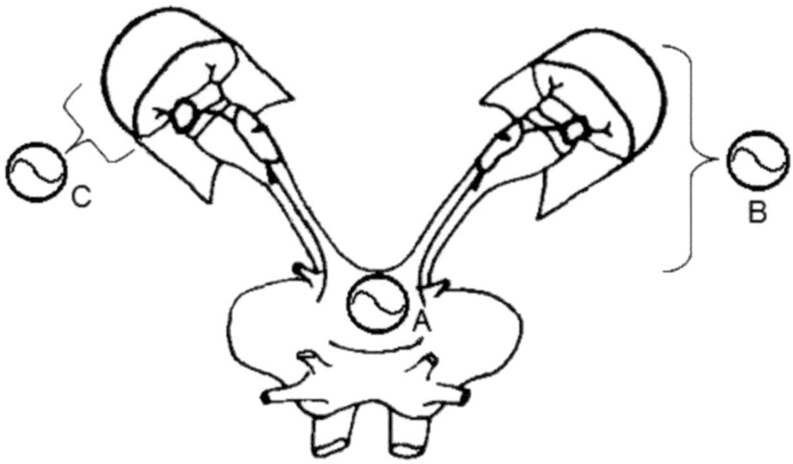

Fig. 3. Schematic representation of the crayfish cerebroid ganglion and eyestalks. A) Cerebroid ganglion, B) Eyestalk and C) Retina are the proposed pacemakers (Modified from Aréchiga et al., 1993).

Moreover, at present, there are no conclusive studies about the origin of the circadian oscillations in one of the pacemakers. An approach to this problem involves the study of the ontogeny of this circadian rhythm.

For the expression of a circadian pattern it is necessary that the anatomical substrate reaches maturity and establishes the necessary structural and physiological relationships between its parts. During development, different structures and functions begin to show some temporal organization that eventually will acquire circadian characteristics. This implies that underlying the sense of time of the organism there are a number of changes in its anatomical and functional organization in the pacemaker. Indeed, the organism exhibits successive changes in period, relative amplitude and activity level of their circadian rhythms during all the ontogeny process. It can be assumed that variation in these parameters involves changes in the structures that participate in the generation of the rhythm, namely, the pacemaker (Fanjul-Moles et al., 1987).

5.2 The presence of ultradian and circadian rhythms in the pacemaker emergent temporal patterns

Ultradian and circadian rhythms have been reported in various studies on crustaceans such as locomotor activity and the photoresponse amplitude in the crayfish retina or cardiac activity (Aguzzi et al.; Fanjul-Moles & Prieto-Sagredo, 2003; Miranda-Anaya et al., 2003b, as cited in Rodríguez-Sosa, 2008). The mechanisms underlying this interaction have been a matter of discussion in several reports. In what follows we are going to present our experimental results, interpretation and mathematical modeling.

Experimental data show that during crayfish ontogeny, before the complete maturation of its neuroendocrine system, there are only ultradian frequency oscillators in the pacemaker. Because of the influence of some neurosecretions, presumably the pigment dispersing hormone (PDH), high frequency oscillations progressively vanish until they completely disappear and the circadian oscillation appears (Figure 4).

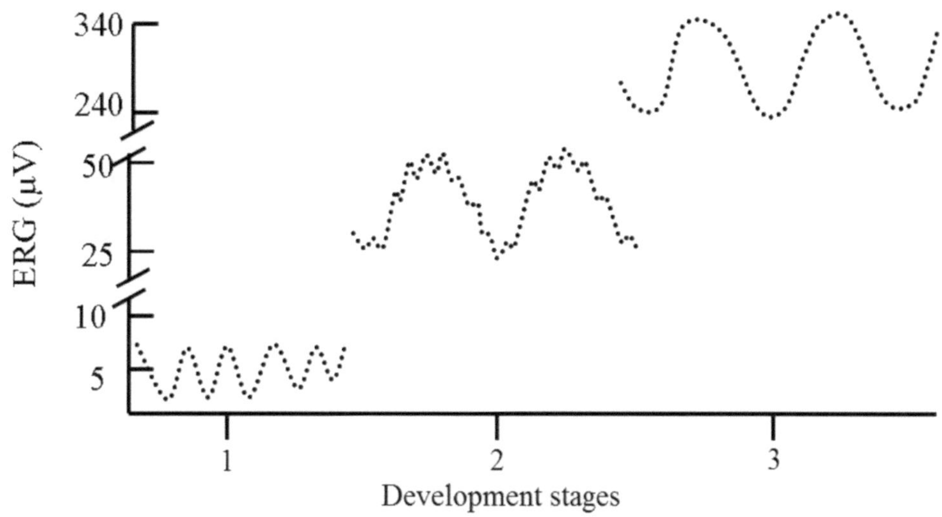

Fig. 4. Ontogeny of the ERG circadian rhythm. In very young crayfish (immediately after hatching), the ERG amplitude is very low (~4 μV) and shows clear ultradian fluctuations with a period ranging from 15 min to 4 h. Four weeks old crayfish express higher ERG amplitude (~50 μV) and, for the first time, the presence of a circadian oscillation. Older animals (around 5 months after hatching) show a progressive increment in ERG amplitude and period length, as well as a progressive disappearance of the high frequency cycles.

The four hour pattern (ultradian oscillations) found in the youngest crayfish is similar to the pattern found in the ERG amplitude recorded from the isolated eyestalk (a presumible pacemaker) of an adult crayfish (Sánchez & Fuentes-Pardo, 1976). In this experimental design, it could be observed that, superimposed on circadian variations in the ERG amplitude, there were high frequency cycles that seem to be correlated with the circadian time, since their amplitude depended on the phase of the circadian rhythm when they appeared.

Another experimental design in which ultradian oscillations appear superimposed to the ERG circadian rhythm was recorded from crayfish deprived of the sinus glands. A plausible interpretation to these results is that the organization of a circadian rhythm is produced as a consequence of the loss of a release from the sinus gland of a neurohormonal substance, presumptively PDH (Moreno-Sáenz et al., 1986).

In addition to the past scenarios, we have observed the presence of ultradian rhythms in experiments in which we used deuterium oxide (D_2O) in long term recordings of the ERG

(Fuentes-Pardo & Moreno-Sáenz, 1988). The authors analyzed the effect of deuterium oxide on the circadian oscillations obtained from both intact animal and isolated eyestalk. Results showed a direct relationship between the D_2O dose and the lengthen of period in both circadian and ultradian cycles. It was proposed that the lengthening of the circadian period is due to the effect of D_2O upon the high frequency oscillations. The lengthening produced by D_2O could result from the diffusion of this substance to all the cells, tissues and organs of the organism, particularly to the cells involved in the generation and expression of the ERG oscillatory activity. These cells would actually be the oscillators that reduce their oscillation frequency produced by the physicochemical changes of D_2O. The results allow us to propose that D_2O affects the oscillatory machinery by its well-established general property of slowing biochemical reaction kinetics due to the "heavy isotope effects".

Finally, the last scenario in which we have observed circadian and ultradian oscillations is when the ERG circadian rhythm recorded from a crayfish kept under constant darkness is perturbed by the presence of a light stimulus, this induces a phase change, an advance or a delay, that can be detected once the rhythm returns to a steady state. The sense and magnitude of change depend on the circadian time of stimulus application. It is worthwhile noticing that immediately after the light application, the ERG circadian rhythm shows a transitory stage characterized by the presence of irregular high frequency (ultradian) oscillations; the characteristics of these, particularly phase as well as the circadian moment when the stimulus was applied, seem to determine whether the rhythm will show advance or delay in the steady state (Fuentes-Pardo et al., 2008).

It is natural to conjecture that the ultradian rhythms observed in each and every one of the above experimental scenarios (ontogeny, sectioned eyestalk, sinus gland deprivation, D_2O and application of a light stimulus) appear as a consequence of the failure (or decreased velocity in the case of D_2O) of the release of PDH. The circadian rhythm in the pacemaker's crayfish is generated by weak coupling of ultradian oscillators between cells. Ultradian oscillation would become apparent under weak coupling or in absence of coupling. The pacemaker period would be a function of the coupling of the ultradian oscillators, increasing as the coupling decreasis.

In the next section we explore this possibility with a simple model.

6. Circadian behavior in the pacemaker emerging from the coupling of ultradian oscillators

As we saw in the previous section, in the ontogenesis of the crayfish circadian rhythm the experiments showed a global ultradian rhythm in very young individuals that evolves into a global circadian rhythm with an intermediate stage in which both rhythms are superposed. How could one construct a pacemaker model based on the coupling of many ultradian oscillators?

The coupling strength of the oscillators in the pacemaker should vary during the development of the rhythm: In the early stages, the coupling should be weak enough to preserve the ultradian character of the resulting output, but strong enough to synchronize all the oscillators (otherwise the result would be a practically constant signal, being the sum of many unsynchronized clocks). At the other end of the process, in the adult stage, the strength of the coupling should be able to produce a global circadian result. And it should also reproduce the intermediate step where both ultradian and circadian rhythms coexist!

In a first stage we have taken a different option, without denying that it would be interesting to search for a simple model whose individual oscillators and modes of coupling evolve naturally in the above manner. Our approach consists in assuming the existence of a well-defined ultradian rhythm in the pacemaker from the beginning of the ontogenesis and of a circadian rhythm that emerges gradually, but whose circadian character is well defined from its first appearance. We concentrate on modeling the relations between the two. This does not exclude the possibility that the circadian oscillator might be the result of the coupling of many ultradian oscillators (c.f. the following section).

The results of this approach can be found in (Lara-Aparicio et al., 1993; Fuentes-Pardo et al., 1995, 2005). The mathematical model has proved useful for the understanding of several characteristics of the circadian rhythm.

At this time we are asking if the pacemaker temporal pattern observed in the crayfish could be the result of the coupling of ultradian oscillators. In order to mimic the described behavior we have to take into account the maturation (hormonal) effect. So in the next, we are going to show how in a simple model, low frequency oscillatory behavior in a pacemaker can be obtained from the coupling of its components, each one being a high frequency oscillator.

In order to fix ideas we will consider that the systems consists of four nonlinear oscillators. In the absence of any coupling, we will simply assume that the oscillators are identical and whose dynamics is determined by the same function *f*.

In mathematical terms we have a system of four second order nonlinear differential equations in which x_i (i=1,...4) represents the "position" of the i-th oscillator:

$$\ddot{x}_1 = f_1(x_1, \dot{x}_1) + a_{12}x_2 + a_{13}x_3 + a_{14}x_4$$

$$\ddot{x}_2 = f_2(x_2, \dot{x}_2) + a_{21}x_1 + a_{23}x_3 + a_{24}x_4$$

$$\ddot{x}_3 = f_3(x_3, \dot{x}_3) + a_{31}x_1 + a_{32}x_2 + a_{34}x_4$$

$$\ddot{x}_4 = f_4(x_4, \dot{x}_4) + a_{41}x_1 + a_{42}x_2 + a_{43}x_3$$

In other words, even when in principle the f_i could be different, we take them as identical for the sake of simplicity. Moreover, the terms involving the coefficients a_{ij} (linear terms) represent the coupling among the different oscillators in the pacemaker. The coupling is directly related to the PDH presence (see Section 5.2). It is important to point out that in many physical systems, such as masses joined by springs or interacting pendulums the nature of the coupling is relatively well known. On the other hand, in the case of cells, the underlying interactions among cells is due to rather complex communication mechanisms, that in fact, constitute the subject of very active research.

In principle, we don't impose any specific functional form for *f* although later on we will consider it to be a van der Pol oscillator.

We now adopt the specific functional form for the terms in the equation responsible for the oscillatory dynamics:

$$f_i(x_i, \dot{x}_i) = \mu(1 - x_i^2)\dot{x}_i, \ i = 1, ...4.$$

In other words, each separate component is a van der Pol system.

In the following pictures (Figure 5), the behavior of a van der Pol oscillator is depicted. The illustration is taken from Weiisstein, Eric W. "van der Pol Equation." from MathWorld--A Wolfram Web Resource (http://mathworld.wolfram.com/vanderPolEquation.html) and we have left the notation as it appears there, i.e. x and y are taken as independent and dependent variables respectively instead of t and x, so that the van der Pol equation reads

$$y'' - \mu(1 - y^2)y' + y = 0.$$

Moreover, using the language of dynamical systems, each component has the structure of a relaxation oscillation which is very robust (a stable limit cycle). Essentially this means that if the system is perturbed it will recover its oscillations.

After writing the system as a collection of eight equations of first order, rather than four of second order we can plot the positions and velocities of the oscillators

In Figure 6 we show a simulation for this system in which both velocities and positions are represented. Notice that after a transient state, in which individual high frequency oscillations are observed, a regime in which low frequency oscillators appears.

It would be worthwhile, in future to prove if the different perturbations to the pacemaker that we observed experimentally can be modeled by our coupled high frequency oscillators.

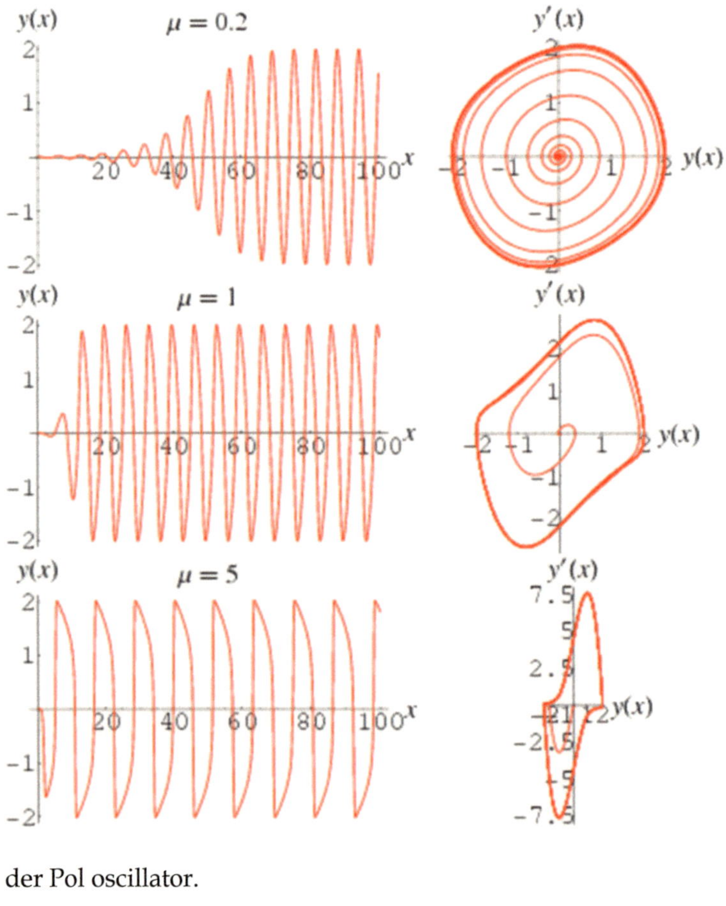

Fig. 5. Van der Pol oscillator.

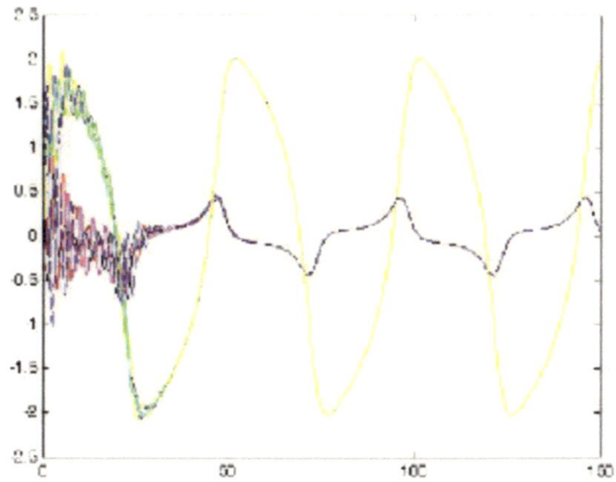

Fig. 6. Coupled oscillators.

7. Conclusion

The study of the emergent dynamics of circadian pacemaker illustrates the utility and even the necessity to develop mathematical models to understand the biological systems. Remarkable also is the interaction that can be observed among a biological theory, the experimental results, the mathematical model, and the mathematical theory.

In our work, mathematical models have been fundamental to understand the mechanism underlying to some phenomena and suggest us new experiments. When we propose and study the mathematical model to describe the ontogeny of crayfish circadian rhythm, immediately emerged many questions about the origin of circadian rhythms and the possible compatibility with the different proposals and explanations found in the literature.

At this moment our models have a qualitative character, but it is possible to refine them in order to obtain quantitative answers to some questions.

It is important to remember that, in spite of we want to make a simple model, the biological systems exhibits an extraordinary diversity and complexity. That is because is really hard to consider that the modeling process is finished.

8. Acknowledgments

This work was supported by IN228011 DGAPA grant.

9. References

Aréchiga H.; Fernández-Quiroz F.; Fernández de Miguel F. & Rodríguez-Sosa L. (1993). The circadian system of crustacean. *Chronobiology International*, Vol. 10, No. 1 (January 1993), pp. 1-19, ISSN 0742-0528

Barrio R. A.; Zhang L. & Maini P. K. (1997). Hierarchically coupled ultradian oscillators generating robust circadian rhythms. *Bulletin of Mathematial Biology*, Vol. 59, No. 3 (n.d.), pp. 517-532, ISSN 0092-8240

Díez-Noguera A. (1994). A functional model of the circadian system based on the degree of intercommunication in a complex system. American Journal of Physiology . Regulatory, Integrative and Comparative Physiology, Vol 267, No. 4 (October 1994), pp 1118-1135, ISSN 0363-6119

Dowse H. B. & Ringo M. (1987). Further evidence that the circadian clock in *Drosophila* is a population of coupled ultradian oscillators. *Journal of Biological Rhythms*, Vol. 2, No. 1 (March 1987), pp. 65-76, ISSN 0748-7304

Dunlap J. C. (1999). Molecular Bases for Circadian Clocks. *Cell*, Vol. 96, No. 2 (January 1999), pp 271-290, ISSN ISSN 0092-8674

Einstein, A. (1934). On the method of theoretical physics. *Phylosophy of Science*, Vol. 1, No. 2 (April 1934), pp. 163-169, ISSN 0031-8248

Fanjul-Moles M. L.; Moreno-Sáenz E.; Villalobos-Hiriart N. & Fuentes-Pardo B. (1987). ERG circadian rhythm in the course of ontogeny in crayfish. *Comparative Biochemistry and Physiology Part A*, Vol. 88, No. 2 (n.d.), pp. 213–219, ISSN 1095-6433

Fuentes-Pardo B.; Barriga-Montoya C; Lara-Aparicio M. & López de Medrano S (2008). Ultradian and Circadian Rhythms: Experiments and Models, In: *Ultradian Rhythms from Molecules to Mind*, D. Lloyd, E. Rossi , pp. 147-161, Springer, ISBN 978-1-4020-8351-8, New York

Fuentes-Pardo B.; Guzmán-Gómez A.; Lara-Aparicio M. & López de Medrano S. (2005). Modeling of biological rhythms, *Biological Rhythm Research*, Vol. 36, No. 1&2 (January 2005), pp. 3-8, ISSN 0929-1016

Fuentes-PardoB.,Lara-AparicioM.,LópezdeMedranoS.(1995).Perturbation of a circadian rhythm by single and periodic signals and its mathematical simulation. *Bulletin of mathematical biology*, Vol57, No. 2 (n.d.), pp. 175-89, ISSN 0092-8240

Fuentes-Pardo B. & Moreno-Sáenz E. (1988). Action of deuterium oxide upon the ERG circadian rhythm in crayfish *Procambarus bouvieri*. *Comparative Biochemistry and Physiology Part A*, Vol. 90, No. 3 (n.d), pp. 435–440, ISSN 1095-6433

Fuentes-Pardo B.; Barriga-Montoya C; Lara-Aparicio M. & López de Medrano S (2008). Ultradian and Circadian Rhythms: Experiments and Models, In: *Ultradian Rhythms from Molecules to Mind*, D. Lloyd, E. Rossi , pp. 147-161, Springer, ISBN 978-1-4020-8351-8, New York

Harmer S. L.; Panda S. & Kay S. (2001). Molecular bases of circadian rhythms. *Annual Review of Cell and Developmental Biology*, Vol. 17, No. () (November 2001), pp. 215-253, ISSN 1081-0706

Hernández O. H.& Fuentes-Pardo B. (2001) Cerebroid ganglion is the presumptive pacemaker of the circadian rhythm of the electrical response to light in the crayfish. Biological Rhythm Research, Vol. 32, No. 2 (n.d.), pp. 125-144, ISSN 1744-4179

Hodgkin, A. L.; Huxley A. F. & Katz B. (1952a). Measurement of current-voltage relations in the membrane of the giant axon of *Loligo*. *The Journal of Physiology*, Vol. 116, No. 4 (April 1952), pp 424-448, ISSN 0022-3751.

Hodgkin, A. L. & Huxley A. F. (1952b). Currents carried by sodium and potassium ions through the membrane of the giant axon of *Loligo*. *The Journal of Physiology*, Vol. 116, No. 4 (April 1952), pp 449-472, ISSN 0022-3751

Hodgkin, A. L. & Huxley A. F (1952c) The components of membrane conductance in the giant axon of *Loligo*. *The Journal of Physiology*, Vol. 116, No. 4 (April 1952), pp 473-496, ISSN 0022-3751

Hodgkin, A. L. & Huxley A.F. (1952d) The dual effect of membrane potential on sodium conductance in the giant axon of Loligo. *The Journal of Physiology*, Vol. 116, No. 4 (April 1952), pp 497-506, ISSN 0022-3751

Hodgkin, A. L. &. Huxley A. F. (1952e) A quantitative description of membrane current and its application to conduction and escitation in nerve. , *The Journal of Physiology*, Vol. 117, No. 4 (August 1952), pp 500-544.

Konopka R. J. & Benzer S. (1971). Clock mutants of *Drosophila melanogaster*. *Proceedings of the National Academy of Science of United States of America*, Vol. 68, No. 9 (September 1971), pp. 2112-2116, ISSN 0027-8424

Lara-Aparicio M.; López de Medrano S.; Fuentes-Pardo B. & Moreno-Sáenz E. (1993). A qualitative mathematical model of the ontogeny of a circadian rhythm in crayfish. *Bulletin of Mathematical Biology*, Vol. 55, No. 1 (n.d.), pp. 97-110, ISSN 0092-8240

Lloyd D. & Murray D. B. (2007). Redox rhythmicity: clocks at the core of temporal coherence. *BioEssays*, Vol. 29, No. 5 (May 2007), pp. 465-473, ISSN 1521-1878

Lloyd D.; Rossi E. L. & Roussel M. R. (2008). Introduction: The Temporal Organization of Living Systems from Molecule to Mind, In: *Ultradian Rhythms from Molecules to Mind*, D. Lloyd, E. Rossi , pp. 147-161, Springer, ISBN 978-1-4020-8351-8, New York

Moreno-Sáenz E.; Hernández-Falcón J. & Fuentes-Pardo B. (1986). Role of the sinus gland in crayfish circadian rhythmicity-II. ERG circadian rhythm. *Comparative Biochemistry and Physiology Part A*, Vol. 87, No. 1 (n.d.), pp. 119–125, ISSN 1095-6433

Murray J. D. (2003). *Mathematical Biology. I An Introduction* (3rd edition). Springer, ISBN 9780387952239, USA

Murray J. D. (2003). *Mathematical Biology. II Spatial Models and Biomedical Application* (3rd edition). Springer, ISBN 9780387952284, USA

Nitabach M. N.; Blau J. & Holmes T. C. (2002). Electrical silencing of *Drosophila* pacemaker neurons stops the free-running circadian clock. *Cell*, Vol. 109, No. 4 (May 2002), pp. 485-495, ISSN 0092-8674

Nitabach M. N.; Holmes T. C. & Blau J. (2005). Membranes, ions, and clocks: testing de Njus-Sulzman-Hastings model of the circadian oscillator. *Methods in enzymology*, Vol. 393, No () (n.d.), pp. 682-692, ISBN 978-0-12-182798-4

Nitabach M. N.; Wu Y.,Sheeba V.; Lemon W. C.; Strumbos J.; Zelensky P. K.; White B. H &, Holmes T. C. (2006). Electrical hyperexcitation of lateral ventral pacemaker neurons desynchronizes downstream circadian oscillators in the fly circadian circuit and induces multiple behavioral periods. *The Journal of Neuroscience*, Vol. 26, No. 2 (January 2006), pp. 479–489, ISSN 0270-6474

Nowak, M. (2006). *Evolutionary Dynamics. Exploring the equations of life* (1st edition). Belknap Press of Harvard University Press, ISBN 0674023382, Cambridge, Massachusetts

Paranjpe D. A. & Sharma V. K. (2005). Evolution of temporal order in living organisms. *Journal of Circadian Rhythms*, Vol. 3, No. 7 (May 2005), pp. 1-13, ISSN 1740-3391

Paetkau V.; Edwards R. & Illner R.(2006). A model for generating circadian rhythm by coupling ultradian oscillators. *Theoretical Biology and Medical Modelling*, Vol. 3, No. 12 (February 2006), pp. 1-10, ISSN 1742-4682

Pavlidis T. (1969). Populations of Interacting Oscillators and Circadian Rhythms. *Journal of Theoretical Biology*, Vol. 22, No. 3 (March 1969), pp. 418-436, ISSN 0022-5193

Pavlidis T. (1971). Populations of Biochemical Oscillators as Circadian Clocks. *Journal of Theoretical Biology*, Vol. 33, No. 2 (November 1971), pp. 319-338, ISSN 0022-5193

Rodríguez-Sosa L.; Calderón-Rosete G. & Flores G. (2008). Circadian and ultradian rhythms in the crayfish caudal photoreceptor. *Synapse*, Vol. 62, No. 9 (September 2008), pp 643-652, ISSN 1098-2396

Sánchez J. A. & Fuentes-Pardo B. (1977). Circadian rhythm in the amplitude of the electroretinogram in the isolated eyestalk of the crayfish. *Comparative Biochemistry and Physiology Part A*, Vol. 56, No. 4 (n.d.), pp. 601-605, ISSN 1095-6433

Winfree A. T. (1967). Biological Rhythms and the Behavior of Populations of Coupled Oscillators. *Journal of Theoretical Biology*, Vol. 16, No. 1 (July 1967), pp 15-42, ISSN 0022-5193

Winfree A. T. (2001). *The Geometry of Biological Time* (2nd edition). Springer-Verlag New York Inc, ISBN 9781441931962, New York

Zivkovic B. (June 2006). ClockTutorial #5: Circadian Organization, In: *Circadiana*, 05.04.11, Available from: http://circadiana.blogspot.com/2005/02/clocktutorial-5-circadian-organization.html

5

Non-Ultradian Cardiac Rhythms: Circadian Regulation of the Heart

Stephen Karaganis
Parker University
USA

1. Introduction

The heart undergoes relentless biophysical oscillations over the course of a life span in order to sustain life. The heart's continuous rhythm of beating consists of sustained, serial oscillations in ionic currents, membrane potential, and excitation-contraction coupling. The rhythm of its beats expresses a period range of 0.6-1 seconds in healthy adults. These high frequency ultradian (< 24 hr period) rhythms are the life blood of the body's most important myogenic oscillator and pump. However, these are not the only rhythms vital to the function of cadiac tissue, as the heart and other components of the cardiovascular system are under control of the body's circadian clock. This "clock" is not a singular entity, but rather consists of distributed oscillators which impose numerous biochemical and physiological rhythms with a periodicity of approximately 24 hours. Indeed, recent evidence has demonstrated that the very cells of the heart are circadian oscillators themselves.

Numerous studies of animal models, including humans, reveal that multiple processes of cardiac physiology are under control by the circadian system. Moreover, circadian control by the organismal "clock" encompasses multiple layers of regulation, extending, at its most reduced level, to the molecular clockworks residing within individual cardiomyocytes (Bray et al., 2008) and other cardiac cell types (Young, 2009). Coupling between cardiomyocytes at the tissue level results in a synchronized cardiac organ-clock. The cardiac clock functions in a semiautonomous manner in isolation from autonomic and humoral inputs. These "exogenous" inputs represent regulatory arms of the larger circadian system to which the cardiac clock is subject to control. The neurohumoral arms of the circadian system are driven by the neurocephalic circadian axis, the most important component of which (at least in mammals) resides in the suprachiasmatic nuclei of the hypothalamus. However, other cephalic components, including the eye and pineal, reinforce central and peripheral oscillations and maintain coupling between them, as well as with true exogenous factors such as light and dietary intake (Bell-Pedersen et al., 2005; Stratmann and Schibler, 2006). Together, these multiple systems interact to produce overt rhythms in cardiac physiology including rhythms of heart rate, contraction force, blood pressure, metabolism, gene expression, and more (Young, 2009).

Of particular clinical interest is the observation that multiple aspects of cardiac pathology fluctuate on a circadian basis. Numerous studies have documented daily oscillations in the occurrence of pathologic cardiac events (Elliott, 2001; Mahmoud at al., 2011). The collective impact of these time-of-day-dependent phenomena on human welfare and economics is likely enormous, though the etiology of this temporal dependence is not fully understood. Elucidation of the mechanisms underlying these time-dependent phenomena is no doubt complicated by the complex, hierarchical organization of the circadian system and its far-reaching presence across most tissues. In fact, it is not always clear what direct role circadian regulation plays in rhythmic features of cardiac physiology and pathology compared to indirect effects which may propagate between coupled organ systems. Moreover, not all such rhythms may necessarily be attributed to endogenous circadian control at all; rather, some rhythms may be driven independently by oscillating exposure to environmental factors themselves and not as zeitgebers (timekeepers or entrainment cues).

Understanding the role of the circadian system as a primary regulator of daily changes in cardiac physiology and pathophysiology is of both extreme scientific and clinical interest. Development of new therapeutic modalities, as well as improving standard ones, will require an unraveling of these intertwined regulatory processes, both direct and indirect, internal and external. This necessitates a deeper characterization of the role of circadian processes at multiple levels of cardiac function, from the cellular and molecular levels to the systems and organismal levels. The aim of this chapter, therefore, is to review the ever-increasing wealth of data on circadian control of the heart obtained from human and non-human animal models. I will explore many of the major findings to date at each hierarchical level of control to provide a broad view of how the circadian system regulates the physiology of the heart, contributes to its pathology, and adds to our current understanding of cardiovascular health.

2. The mammalian circadian clock

Circadian rhythms are defined as entrainable biological rhythms having an intrinsic periodicity under constant conditions (e.g. lighting conditions or temperature) of approximately 24 hours. Circadian clocks are ubiquitous amongst living organisms, and can be found across far-reaching taxa, including mammals, birds, lower vertebrates, invertebrates, non-animal multicellular organisms, and unicellular organisms (Bell-Pedersen et al., 2005). Among mammals, circadian clocks have been studied in numerous strains (both "normal" and pathological) of rodents, primarily in mice, rats, and hamsters, as well as other model systems, including humans (Martino and Sole, 2009).

These studies, along with studies of other vertebrate models (Bell-Pedersen et al., 2005), have demonstrated that numerous semi-autonomously operating clocks reside within a single mammalian organism. These clocks are distributed amongst most organs and tissues of the body, and can be reduced to the level of the individual cell (Stratmann and Schibler, 2006). These countless cellular clocks are biochemically coupled to produce coherent outputs at the tissue and organ levels, and govern a vast array of documented biochemical and physiological processes, including sleep-wake cycles, body temperature, metabolism, and cardiovascular functions to name a few.

2.1 Central physiological clocks

At the organismal level, central neural and peripheral clocks are organized in a hierarchical fashion, with intercellular communication being mediated by both neural and humoral mechanisms (Stratmann and Schibler, 2006). At the top of this hierarchy is the neurocephalic circadian axis, consisting of the hypothalamic suprachiasmatic nuclei (SCN) at its heart, along with the optic retinae and the epithalamic pineal gland (Bell-Pedersen et al., 2005).

The SCN, at the top of this neurohumoral triumvirate, is regarded as the "master pacemaker", as it synchronizes peripheral oscillators and dictates the appropriate phasing of "slave oscillators" subject to the regulatory arms of the central circadian axis. Consistent with the SCN's role as master pacemaker, its ablation abolishes multiple physiological and biochemical processes in multiple model species (Turek, 1985), and in rats loss of rhythms can be rescued by transplantation of intact SCN from donor rats (Ralph et al., 1990). Importantly, the period of host activity rhythms is imposed by the period of the donor animal in transplantation studies. Specifically, cardiovascular rhythms are under control of the SCN, as ablation of SCN abolishes rhythms in both blood pressure (Weaver, 1998) and heart rate (Warren et al., 1994) in rodents.

In vitro, individual cells of the SCN are capable of sustaining rhythms of multiple clock controlled outputs, including action potential firing rate, neuropeptide release, glucose uptake, and rhythms of gene expression (Bell-Pedersen et al., 2005; Quintero et al., 2003; Welsh et al., 1995). Intercellular coupling mechanisms within the SCN are unknown, though pathways coupling the SCN with other organs have been described. The SCN is part of a neuroendocrine feedback loop between the eyes and pineal gland, and these mutual interactions are necessary for entrainment or reinforcement of the hypothalamic clock.

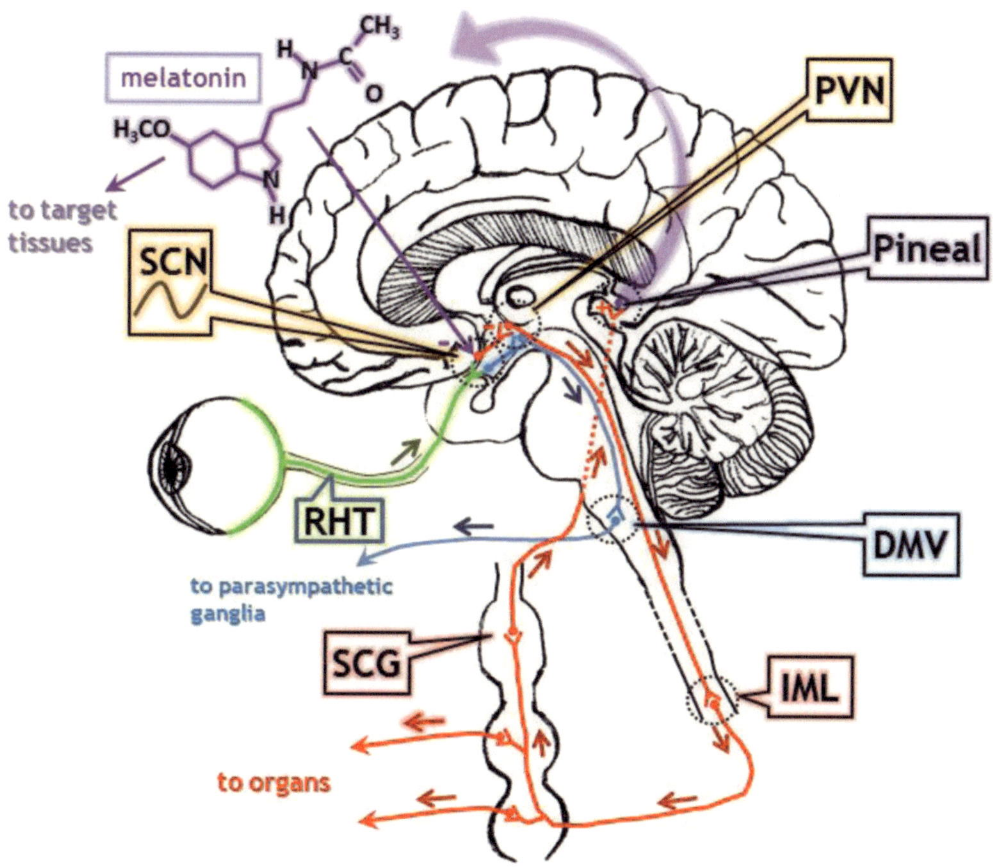

Fig. 1. Neuroendocrine pathways involving the SCN

As Figure 1 shows, light entrains the SCN via neural connections from the retinohypothalamic tract (RHT). In mammals, the SCN (and perhaps the retinae) is the only oscillator that is directly entrainable by light, although the pineal gland of many other vertebrate species is directly photoreceptive (Bell-Pedersen et al., 2005). The mammalian pineal, while not directly photosensitive, influences SCN activity by nightly secretion of the indoleamine hormone melatonin. The SCN is rich in melatonin receptors, and its activity is thus inhibited by melatonin during the dark period (Cassone et al., 1987). The neurohumoral feedback loop is closed by a polysynaptic pathway as follows. First order GABAergic neurons from the SCN synapse with neurons in the paraventricular nucleus (PVN) of the hypothalamus. Descending tracts from the PVN innervate targets in the intermediolateral cell column of the thoracic spinal cord, which in turn project to the superior cervical ganglia (SCG). Finally, sympathetic SCG neurons form noradrenergic synapses with the pineal gland, which possesses stimulatory β_2 adrenergic receptors (Moore, 1996).

The SCN regulates other peripheral organs (including the heart) by way of different autonomic efferents. In addition to sympathetic regulation by way of the IML, alternate SCN controlled efferent pathways arising from the PVN regulate parasympathetic ganglia by projecting to neurons in the dorsal motor nucleus of the vagus (DMV). It appears that separate populations of pre-autonomic cells in the SCN provide discreet control over symapathetic and parasympathetic pathways (Buijs et al., 2003).

2.2 Peripheral clocks

Previously it was believed that the master pacemaker within the SCN drove downstream oscillations in other tissues throughout the body, and that the molecular clockworks that underlie oscillator function were confined to this tissue. This view was largely based on studies which measured disruption of behavioural and physiological outputs of the organismal clock, and disruption of molecular rhythms in some tissues. It is now known that most tissues possess the same basic molecular machinery (i.e. "clock genes") as the hypothalamic pacemaker, and that many tissues (including the heart) can maintain functional oscillations in gene transcription and other processes in a semi-autonomous manner (Damiola et al., 2000; Oishi et al., 1998; Stratmann and Schibler, 2006).

Clock gene oscillations have been maintained in some peripheral tissues for periods of up to 20 days in culture, indicating a functional molecular clock is preserved *ex vivo* (Yoo et al., 2004). Other experiments have demonstrated that clock gene rhythms are not abolished in peripheral organs by SCN lesions, but that organs lose synchrony with one another, leading to altered phase relationships and disrupted coherent output *in vivo* (Guo et al. 2005, 2006; Yoo et al., 2004). Moreover, implementation of a restricted feeding paradigm (RF) competing with light cycles can uncouple rhythms in heart and liver from the SCN, without affecting the phase of the SCN itself (Damiola et al., 2000; Hara et al., 2001; Stokkan et al., 2001). As a result of these and other studies, the current prevailing view of the SCN as the body's circadian pacemaker is that its role is to synchronize, or entrain, functional peripheral oscillators throughout the body, rather than drive them directly.

2.3 Entrainment of peripheral clocks

As entrainable oscillators, peripheral tissues may be synchronized by neural or humoral signals, or by non-photic exogenous factors such as nutrient intake. Models using parabiosis between intact and SCN-lesioned mice demonstrate that some tissues, such as liver, can be entrained by humoral (or other non-neural) factors (Guo et al., 2005). Surpisingly, neither implantation of SCN tissue grafts nor non-neural cues from parabiotically linked mice are sufficient to rescue clock gene rhythms in other tissues, including cardiac tissue (Guo et al., 2005, 2006).

Food intake is a powerful zeitgeber for some peripheral tissues including the heart (Balsalobre et al., 2000; Le Minh et al., 2001; Stratmann and Schibler, 2006), and the heart can be regulated in discordance with the SCN under a restricted feeding schedule. The mechanism of food entrainment likely involves metabolic feedback into the transcriptional clock gene cycles, which in turn regulate multiple metabolic processes (Koshaka and Bass, 2007). Cellular redox state is known to modulate transcriptional clock gene regulation, and this may represent one or more pathways by which feeding induced metabolic changes can regulate the heart and other clocks (Rutter et al., 2001).

Plasma glucocorticoid levels are rhythmic in mammals (Stratmann and Schibler, 2006), and glucocorticoid signaling interacts with metabolic entrainment (Le Minh et al., 2001). Moreover, glucocorticoids are capable of phase shifting molecular rhythms in cardiac tissue and other peripheral tissues (Balsalobre, 2000). Plasma levels of epiniphrine and norepinephrine (NE) also show diurnal rhythms in humans (Sauerbier et al., 1977), and NE can entrain circadian clocks within cultured rat cardiomyocytes (Durgan et al., 2005). Thus, glucocorticoids, especially cortisol in humans, as well as catacholamines, represent other potential zeitgebers for peripheral oscillators. These may provide important mechanisms by which the SCN exerts control over the heart and other tissues (Stratmann and Schibler, 2006).

Nightly melatonin secretion by the pineal represents another humoral regulatory arm of the circadian system, though extra-pineal contributions to plasma melatonin levels are not fully characterized in mammals (Huether, 1993). Interestingly, recent evidence demonstrates mammalian cardiac tissue possesses active biosynthetic machinery necessary to produce melatonin (Sanchez-Hidalgo et al., 2009), suggesting that extra-pineal melatonin derived from cardiac tissue may act as a local autocrine or paracrine signal.

Numerous beneficial cardioprotective effects have been reported for melatonin (Reiter and Tan, 2009). Cardiovascular tissues express both MT1 and MT2 melatonin receptors throughout the body, and cardiomyocytes express membrane bound melatonin receptors both *in vivo* and *in vitro* (Pang et al., 1993; Peliciari-Garcia et al., 2011). The nuclear melatonin receptor RORa has been localized to heart as well (Naji et al., 2004), and cardiovascular modulation of heart rate in primates may involve activation of intracellular MT3 receptor quinone reductase 2 (QR2) (Inui and Hazeki, 2010). Because melatonin exerts non-receptor mediated effects on target tissues as well (as a powerful anti-oxidant and scavenger of free radicals), it is unclear which cardioprotective mechanisms may involve receptor-dependent or receptor-independent regulation.

2.4 Cellular and molecular clocks

The mammalian intracellular circadian clock is composed of a finely tuned molecular feeback loop (Figure 2). The major components of this feedback loop consist of "clock gene" products that either activate expression of other genes (positive elements) or inhibit gene expression (negative elements). The primary positive elements are encoded by the genes *clock* and *bmal1* (*brain and muscle ARNT-like protein 1*); these gene products contain a basic helix-loop-helix Per-ARNT-Sim (bHLH/PAS) domain, which allow them to heterodimerize in the cytoplasm, after which they translocate into the nucleus to activate gene transcription. CLOCK:BMAL1 heterodimers activate transcription of target genes (including other "clock genes" as well as "clock controlled genes", or "ccg's") by binding to consensus E-box sequences in their promoters (Muñoz and Balor, 2003).

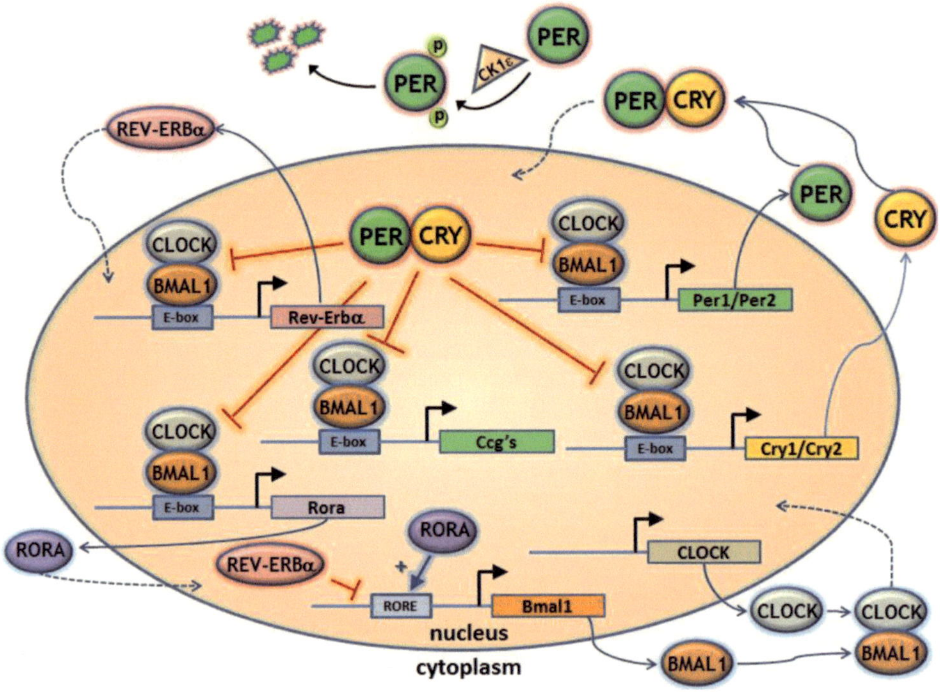

Fig. 2. Model of the intracellular molecular clock.

Two important targets of CLOCK:BMAL1 activation are the "negative" clock genes, *period* (*per*) and *cryptochrome* (*cry*). These phylogenetically conserved genes are preserved as core clock genes, although multiple mammalian orthologs of these genes have arisen as a result of gene duplications (Bell-Pedersen et al., 2005). Indeed, mammalian clock genes include three different *period* genes (*per1*, *per2*, and *per3*) and two *cryptochrome* genes (*cry1* and *cry2*). PER and CRY proteins heterodimerize in the cytoplasm and are then translocated into the nucleus, where they inhibit transcriptional activation by the CLOCK:BMAL1 complex. The negative elements close the loop, and robustness of the oscillations is enhanced by the positive limb. Accurate timekeeping is required to generate a ~24 hour period, and this requires precise timing of the feedback loop kinetics. This is mediated in part by the gene products of *casein kinase 1 epsilon* (*CK1ε*) and *casein kinase 1 delta* (*CK1δ*), which regulate stability and translocation of the PER:CRY complex via modulation of the PER phosphorylation state.

Redundancy is built into the circadian transcriptional loop by the presence of multiple functional isoforms of *period* and *cryptochrome* genes, as well as the gene for *neuronal PAS domain protein2* (*npas2*), whose protein product can substitute for CLOCK as a BMAL1 dimerization partner in some tissues (Reick et al., 2001). It is unclear what specific roles these partially redundant clock genes may have, however, and *per3* does not appear to be necessary for sustainment of the intracellular transcriptional oscillator (Ko and Takahashi, 2006). A fascinating study by Qi and Boatang showed that CLOCK protein localizes to the Z-disk of the cardiomyocyte sarcomere, and that translocation of CLOCK between the nucleus and cytoplasm is influenced by the activity of cross-bridge cycling (Qi and Boateng, 2006). Thus, cardiomyocyte activity may feed back into the core clock mechanism itself.

A secondary feedback loop is formed by activation of CLOCK:BMAL1 targets *rev-erbα* (an orphan nuclear receptor member) and *rora* (*retinoic acid-related orphan nuclear receptor*). REV-ERBα and RORA proteins competitively bind to retinoic acid-related orphan receptor response elements (ROREs) in the promotor of *bmal1*. These proteins have antagonistic functions, such that REV-ERBα represses *bmal1* transcription while RORA activates it. Furthermore, the kinetics of these protein activities differs, such that *bmal1* repression by REV-ERBα occurs more immediately, followed by a delayed activation by RORA (Ko and Takahashi, 2006). This secondary feedback loop is thought to stabilize the core transcriptional oscillator involving the *period* and *cryptochrome* genes (Preitner et al., 2002). Importantly, *rev-erbα* and *rora* genes have been shown to regulate pathways involved in cellular metabolism, which may have important consequences for cardiometabolic pathologies. These mechanisms are discussed in detail later. A third feedback loop (not illustrated) is based on transactivation of the *dec1* and *dec2* genes by the CLOCK:BMAL1 complex, followed by inhibition of CLOCK:BMAL1 by DEC1 and DEC2 proteins.

Most of this ensemble of clock genes has been shown to be rhythmically expressed in hearts of mammals and other animals (Cahill, 2002; Chong et al., 2003; Dardente, 2007), and clock gene mRNA rhythms have recently been measured in human hearts for *per1*, *per2*, and *bmal1*, but not *cry1*, which appears to be arrhythmic. (Leibetseder et al., 2009). Interestingly, the phases of clock gene mRNAs do not necessarily predict the phases of clock controlled outputs, and the phase angles between the core oscillator and outputs may be tissue specific (Karaganis et al., 2009).

Because the heart contains multiple cell types, including cardiomyocytes, epithelial cells, fibroblasts, and adipocytes, *in vivo* cardiac clock gene expression could reflect contributions of any one (or combinations) of these cell types. Indeed, functional clocks have been described in endothelia (Dermot et al., 2007; Takeda et al., 2007), adipose tissue (Zvonik et al., 2006), and fibroblasts (Welsh et al., 2004). However, rhythmic clock gene expression persists *in vitro* in isolated rat cardiomyocyte cultures (Durgan et al., 2005; Peliciari-Garcia, 2011), demonstrating the presence of a functional cardiomyocyte clock.

Intrerestingly, exogenously administered melatonin alters circadian expression of *rev-erbα* mRNA in rat cardiomyocyte cultures (Peliciari-Garcia et al., 2011). In addition to the membrane bound melatonin receptors, RORA has been described as a functional nuclear melatonin receptor, and may provide an important link between melatonin and regulation of peripheral oscillators, including the heart (Peliciari-Garcia et al., 2011). Other ROR members, including RORγ, may play in important role in peripheral oscillators as well (Ko and Takahashi, 2006).

2.5 The cardiac circadian transcriptome

Modern technology utilizing high density microarrays to report global gene transcription in murine models has tremendously expanded our understanding of the extent to which the circadian clock may regulate cellular function. Several laboratories have conducted microarray analyses to explore global cardiac gene expression in various normal and pathological murine models (Bray et al., 2008; Martino et al., 2007; Storch et al. 2002). The first such study to be conducted compared the circadian transcriptome between mouse heart and liver, and found that ~8% of cardiac genes (or 462 genes represented on the array) exhibited circadian oscillations (Storch et al. 2002). Other studies have yielded similar but more extensive estimates (up to 13% of heart genes rhythmic), or lower estimates (2-5% heart genes rhythmic) where greater stringencies were imposed on the analysis (Bray et al., 2008; Martino et al., 2007).

Gene ontology analysis from these studies reveals regulation across a wide array of molecular pathways, from genes involved in metabolism to cellular trafficking and cell death, to name a few. Surprisingly, although ~10% of genes were shown to be rhythmic in the liver (Storch et al., 2002), and these included similar functional gene categories as in the heart, there was very little overlap between individual genes showing circadian expression patterns in both tissues. In fact, only 39 genes showed similar circadian regulation in both heart and liver (Storch et al., 2002). This surprising result, along with microarray analyses of clock controlled transcriptomes in other tissues and organisms (Bailey et al., 2004, 2007; Duffield, 2003; Karaganis et al., 2008), have demonstrated that circadian regulation of gene transcription is both extensive and divergent. A key concept which has emerged from these studies is that circadian regulation of intracellular pathways is highly specific, and likely tuned to the particular demands and functions of a given tissue or organ. As we've seen, the heart is no exception.

Subsequent studies of murine cardiovascular tissue have confirmed and extended these observations, demonstrating that global regulation of clock controlled genes is divergent between closely related tissues or within different functional regions of the same organ (Bray et al., 2008; Martino et al., 2007). Separate analysis of rhythmic gene expression in atria and ventricles of mouse heart has demonstrated a surprising divergence in the apparent number of clock controlled genes expressed within these two tissues (Figure 3). In this study, which utilized mutants with cardiomyocyte specific clock disruption to identify intrinsically regulated ccg's (more on this later), 548 genes exhibited circadian transcriptional rhythms in the atria, compared to 176 genes in the ventricles (Bray et al., 2008).

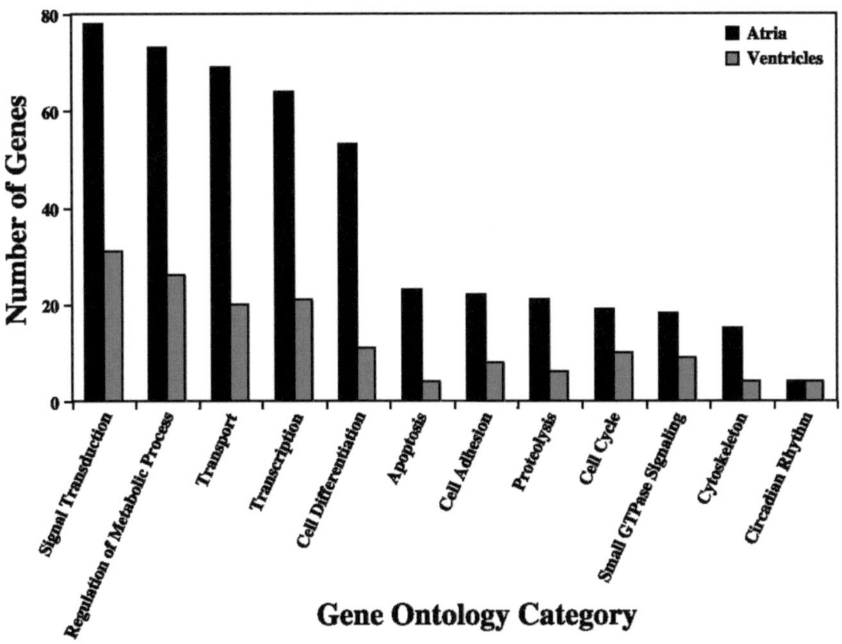

Fig. 3. Gene ontology of circadian regulated genes from atria and ventricles. From: Bray, et al., (2008). Disruption of the Circadian Clock Within the Cardiomyocyte Influences Myocardial Contractile Function, Metabolism, and Gene Expression. *American Journal of Physiology. Heart and Circulatory Physiology, Vol.* 294, pp.H1036–H1047, ISSN 1522-1539

Many of these genes could be expected to influence normal and pathological aspects of cardiophysiology, including genes affecting metabolism, contractile function, and cell growth or remodeling. It is worth mentioning a word of caution when interpreting the functional significance of these studies, however, since the behaviors of oscillating transcripts do not necessarily predict that final gene products will have similar protein expression profiles. Posttransciptional and posttranslational regulatory mechanisms, such as phosphorylation and ubiquitination may also be under clock control. The final relative phasing and amplitudes of protein expression may therefore arise from a complex interplay between regulatory pathways involving kinetics of gene transcription and translation, as well as mRNA and protein turnover via stability and degradation pathways. This point is highlighted by an important study conducted by the Hastings lab, which discovered extensive differences between circadian regulated transcription and protein levels in the mouse liver (Reddy et al., 2006). For instance, this study revealed that up to 20% of the hepatic proteome was rhythmic, while mRNA levels were rhythmic for less than half the number of these genes. Clearly, circadian regulation at the transcriptional level is an important mechanism of regulation by tissue clocks, but caution must be taken when extrapolating these findings to the protein level.

3. Circadian cardiovascular physiology and pathology

The circadian system regulates numerous cellular and molecular processes of cardiovascular function, including blood pressure, heart rate, contractility, vasomotor tone, blood clotting, and cardiovascular metabolism (Sole and Martino, 2009). It is presumed that normal function of these processes is necessary to maintain optimal health and longevity, and that disruption of circadian regulation of these processes can lead to both acute and chronic pathologies, some with potentially disastrous consequences. This section will describe some of the major features of cardiovascular function and pathology that may be regulated by the circadian clock.

Because other rhythmic environmental exposures and behaviours may drive physiological rhythms with similar periodicities maintained by the circadian clock, it is possible that some ~24 hour cardiovascular rhythms are not a result of circadian control (i.e., are not endogenously maintained rhythms). Moreover, because of the hierarchical organization of the organismal circadian system, measurable outputs may reflect different levels of control, ranging from local intrinsic oscillator function to systems level control by the neurohumoral arms of the SCN and other components of the circadian system.

Indeed, it is likely that many rhythmic processes of the cardiovascular system reflect combinatorial interactions between multiple oscillating systems, both intrinsic and extrinsic. For instance, platelet aggregability, a likely predisposing factor for acute ischemic cardiovascular incidents, is elevated as a result of morning standing and ambulation, but is not increased in the absence of morning activity (Andrews et al., 1996; Brezinski et al., 1988). In contrast, other predisposing factors for cardiac ischemia, such as oscillating fibrinolytic activity of endolthelial cells, may be regulated by circadian oscillators both intrinsic and extrinsic to the heart (Maemura et al, 2000).

3.1 Temporal variation in the timing of acute cardiovascular events

Several acute types of pathological cardiovascular events present in a circadian fashion. For example, the incidence of myocardial infarction in humans is much higher in the morning hours, peaking between 06:00-12:00, just as patients arise from bed, or soon before or after doing so (Cohen et al., 1997; Muller et al., 1985). In contrast, the incidence of infarcts reaches a nightly trough during the hours between 03:00-06:00. Overall, infarcts are approximately three fold more likely to occur during the morning than during night.

Other related cardiovascular events that peak in the early or late morning hours include deadly ventricular arrhythmias (Tofler et al., 1995), defibrillation threshold (Venditti et al., 1996) atrial and ventricular refractoriness (Kong et al., 1995; Simantirakis et al., 2001), ischemic stroke (Argentine et al., 1990), rupture of aortic aneurysm or aortic dissection (Manfredini et al., 2004; Mehta et al., 2002; Sumiyoshi et al., 2002) and sudden cardiac death (Mahmoud at al., 2011; Muller et al., 1987). Some cardiovascular events, such as atrial arrhythmias (Deguchi et al., 2009; Sandberg et al., 2010) or thromboembolic stroke (Marshal, 1977) may peak at other times of day. Comorbid conditions, such as obstructive sleep apnea (OSA), may influence the timing of cardiovascular events, and contribute to pathological circadian disruption (Kuniyoshi et al., 2008).

3.2 Circadian regulation of heart rate and blood pressure

Heart rate (HR) and blood pressure (BP) both exhibit diurnal rhythms in humans, peaking the during the day when humans are active, or during the active nocturnal phase in rodent models (Mansoor et al., 1994; Millar-Craig et al., 1978; Reilly et al., 2007; Weber et al., 2002). HR and BP are lowest during nighttime, but begin to rise in the early morning hours in anticipation of waking. These rhythms coincide with rhythms in autonomic tone, with the sympathetic system dominating during the day, and the parasympathetic system dominating at night. The adaptive value of these daily rhythms is obvious, in that elevated HR and BP allow the body to carry out the physical demands associated with daily activities, while a nightly reduction in the levels of these processes allows the sleeping body to save energy and shift its focus to other important demands, such as cellular upkeep, tissue remodelling, or other restorative processes (Sole and Martino, 2009). Importantly, the timing of these cardiovascular rhythms is slightly phase advanced relative to the sleep/wake cycles (i.e. cardiovascular rhythms anticipate transitions between activity phases), allowing for a smooth transition between these alternating states.

The importance of maintaining these diurnal cardiovascular rhythms is evident when comparing variants of hypertensive patients, known as "dippers" and "non-dippers". In some hypertensive patients ("dippers"), normal amplitude circadian rhythms are maintained, albeit over an elevated baseline. Other hypertensive patients, so called "non-dippers", express a continuously high blood pressure through the active and sleep phases. This latter group, having disrupted blood pressure rhythms, are at greater risk for developing other cardiovascular diseases and suffering organ damage (Mancia and Parati, 2000; Verdicchia et al., 1990, 1993). Classification of hypertensive patients as non-dippers is based on having less than a 10% decrease in blood pressure at night, since most normotensive patients exhibit a >10% change. Some studies, however, have shown that blood pressure rhythm amplitudes are distributed normally throughout a given population, indicating that a 10% threshold is an arbitrary cutoff value (Mancia and Parati, 2000).

Other important, related cardiovascular changes exhibit daily rhythms as well, including vascular resistance and tone, although studies have produced conflicting results about how vascular resistance changes throughout the day (Elherik et al., 2002; Kawano et al., 2002; Otto et al., 2004; Shaw et al., 2001), and differential, tissue specific vasomotor control may occur throughout the body.

4. Evidence linking cardiovascular rhythms and pathology with intrinsic oscillators

It is unclear to what extent daily variations in heart rate and blood pressure are due to intrinsic cardiac oscillators or exogenous factors. Because peripheral vascular clocks have been described (Dermot et al., 2007), and given the presence of circulating zeitgebers (Guo et al., 2004), it is possible that many rhythms of normal and pathological cardiovascular function can be attributed to these dispersed signals or to behavioural patterns. Until recently, diurnal rhythms in acute cardiovascular events have been attributed solely to the stress of awakening and the accompanying morning surge in blood pressure. In light of the discoveries of intrinsic cardiovascular clocks, however, these phenomena are currently being re-examined, and it is now clear that at least some of these diurnal pathologies result from a contribution of local, intrinsic circadian regulation.

4.1 Lessons from clock mutants

Several studies have shown disrupted cardiovascular rhythms in animal models possessing mutations in core clock gene components. For example, heart rate (HR) and arterial blood pressure (BP) rhythms (assayed by radiotelemetry) are abolished in *bmal1* knockout mutants (*bmal1*$^{-/-}$) even a under light:dark (LD) cycle, and *bmal1*$^{-/-}$ mice are hypotensive (Curtis et al., 2006). On the other hand, dominant negative *clock*$^{\Delta19}$ mutants express a less severe phenotype, showing partial disruption of HR and BP rhythms (Curtis et al., 2006). Disruption of the negative limb of the core molecular clock also disrupts cardiovascular rhythms, as baseline rhythms in HR and BP (measured by vascular pressure transducers) were lost in both *cry1*$^{-/-}$ and *cry2*$^{-/-}$ mice under free-running conditions in constant darkness (Masuki et al., 2005).

Because these mutants have deficient clocks in all tissues, including the SCN, it is impossible to determine through these studies whether loss of intrinsic cardiac oscillators contribute to these phenotypes. To resolve this issue, ME Young and colleagues have generated mutant mice containing a cardiomyocyte-specific *clock*$^{\Delta19}$ mutation, called CCM mice. By comparing various measures of cardiac function and global gene expression between wild type and CCM mice *in vivo* and *ex vivo*, this group has identified multiple putative pathways through which the intrinsic cardiomyocyte clock might regulate cardiovascular function and dysfunction (Bray et al., 2008; Durgan et al., 2006).

For example, *in vivo* heart function is altered in CCM mice, which show diminished HR rhythms, sinus brachycardia, reduced cardiac output, and other functional differences (Bray et al., 2008). Experiments utilizing an *ex-vivo* cardiac perfusion system demonstrate the normal heart undergoes circadian rhythms in cellular metabolism and contractile function in response to cardiac workload (Durgan et al., 2007). CCM mice show abolished rhythms in triglyceride synthesis, reduced cardiac efficiency, and chronically elevated fatty acid oxidation (Bray et al., 2008). Additionally, while normal hearts exhibit an increased responsiveness to fatty-acids during the active period, which persists *in vitro*, this rhythm is abolished in CCM hearts (Durgan et al., 2006). In agreement with this role of the cardiomyocyte clock as a regulator of cellular metabolism, genes regulating both lipid and glycogen metabolism where found to be regulated by the cardiomyocyte clock (Bray et al., 2008), and cardiac responsiveness to a high fat diet is altered in CCM mice (Tsai et al., 2009).

A working model proposed by Young and colleagues is that the cardiomyocyte circadian clock gates lipid metabolic pathways to balance β-oxidation rates with fatty acid supply in a manner that is appropriate to the time of day. During the active period, when metabolic energy requirements are high, transcriptional responsiveness to fatty-acids is increased, allowing induction of triglyceride synthesis and fatty acid oxidation. This allows the heart to accommodate diurnal changes in circulating fatty-acids levels as a result of feeding or fasting status. This elevated transcriptional response at a time of day when fatty acid levels are high is necessary, since excess fatty acids can otherwise be shunted into harmful "lipotoxic" pathways. Thus, exposing the heart to an excess of lipids at an inappropriate time of day (when the transcriptional machinery is not primed for healthy lipid metabolism) can cause contractile dysfunction, as in diabetes mellitus (Young et al., 2002).

Interestingly, *rev-erbα* is known to be an important regulator of lipid metabolism, in addition to its role as a core clock gene (Duez and Staels, 2008). It functions to control intracellular triglyceride metabolism and β-oxidation pathways as well as plasma lipid and lipoprotein metabolism. Additionally, *rev-erbα* is implicated as a mediator of vascular inflammation, and has been speculated to play a role in the development of metabolic disorders, including obesity and diabetes. *Rev-erbα* could therefore contribute to the development of cardiovascular pathologies through multiple levels of control

4.2 Disruption of circadian cycles has cardiovascular consequences

Shift work has long been hypothesized to be a risk factor for cardiovascular disease and other chronic conditions in humans. Shift workers develop a non-dipper blood pressure profile and may be at increased risk for hypertension (Mosendane, 2008). Additionally, increased risk for metabolic disturbances have been reported for shift workers, including dyslipidaemia, metabolic syndrome, and diabetes, although a recent thorough review shows epidemiological evidence for metabolic and cardiovascular disease is inconsistent (Wang et al., 2011). However, the suggestive evidence warrants further study of these associations. The etiology of cardiovascular disease in shift workers, if present, is unknown. While there are many confounding factors associated with shift work (such as poor diet and higher smoking prevalence), circadian dyssynchrony has logically been proposed as a causative factor.

Several experimental animal studies support the hypothesis that circadian system perturbations cause or exacerbate cardiovascular disease and reduce longevity. In one such study, cardiomyopathic Syrian hamsters (a model for congestive heart failure) were subjected to weekly reversals of LD cycles, resulting in major disruptions of circadian body rhythms (Plamen et al., 1998). Rhythm-disturbed animals experienced a median 11% decrease in life span compared with controls.

Hamsters heterozygous for the *tau* mutation (a point mutation in the *CK-1ε* gene) have shortened periods and are unable to entrain properly to a normal 24 hour LD cycle. Fascinating studies have revealed that +/*tau* mutants have reduced longevity under a standard photoperiod, and longevity can be rescued in aged hamsters where normal SCN tissue has been grafted into the mutant host (Hurd and Ralph, 1998; Ralph and Menaker, 1988). Interestingly, *tau*/*tau* homozygotes are spared these deleterious effects as they cannot entrain at all under these conditions and can simply free-run. This observation demonstrates that internal desynchronisation of the circadian clock, and not the *tau* mutation *per se*, has pathological consequences.

A compelling recent study has demonstrated that mortality in rhythm perturbed +/*tau* hamsters coincides with major cardiomyopathy and renal disease (Martino et al., 2008).

Moreover, +/*tau* animals raised in a shorter photoperiod matching their endogenous period phenotype were protected from these deleterious effects, and were clinically no different than wild type animals. In addition, this research group showed that lesion of the SCN in young mutants protected mice from the onset of pathological cardiac hypertrophy under a disruptive light cycle. Collectively, these results provide powerful evidence that internal dissonance from the SCN pacemaker is harmful, and indeed worse than complete loss of the pacemaker itself.

Another study by Martino et al. compared global rhythmic gene transcription in heart and aorta in normal (sham operated) mice with those in an induced cardiovascular disease state (Martino et al., 2007). The rhythmic heart transcriptome was biphasic, as described elsewhere (Bray et al., 2008), and was highly similar to the aortic transcriptome, with an overall conserved phase angle, but somewhat phase delayed (Figure 4).

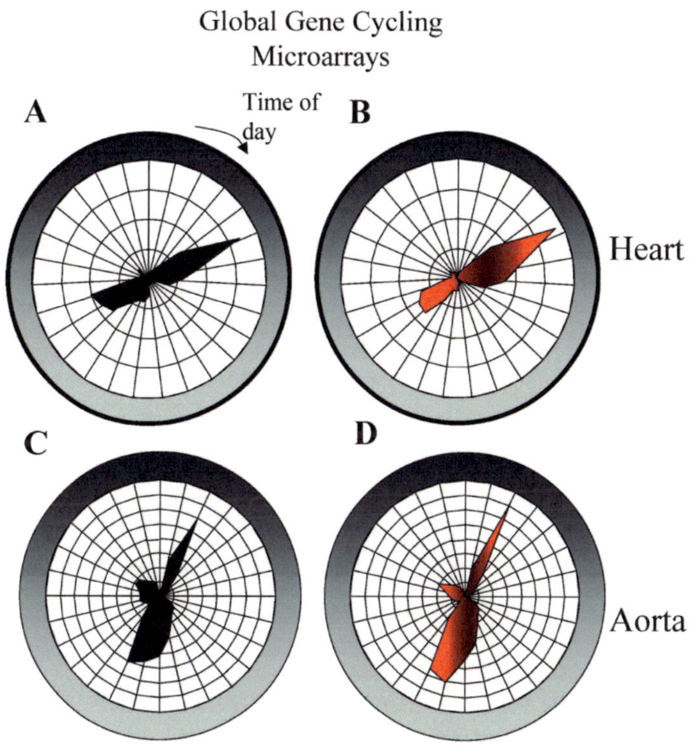

Fig. 4. Phase plots of circadian transcriptomes in heart and aorta. Reprinted from: Martino, et al., (2007). Disturbed Diurnal Rhythm Alters Gene Expression and Exacerbates Cardiovascular Disease With Rescue by Resynchronization. *Hypertension*, Vol.49, pp.1104-1113, ISSN 1524-4563

Remarkably, pressure overload induced hypertrophy (via transaortic constriction, or TAC) had no apparent effect on global circadian gene transcription in either the heart or aorta. However, TAC mice subjected to disruptive photoperiods exhibited abnormal adaptive responses to the disease state, such as vascular thinning and muscular atrophy as opposed to compensatory hypertrophy in the non-disrupted cohorts. Rhythm disturbed TAC mice also exhibited altered cardiac rhythms of genes important for regulating hypertrophy, blood pressure, and fibrosis, as well as altered clock gene rhythms in both the heart and SCN. Furthermore, a rescue protocol implementing a restorative photoperiod reversed pathological loss of compensatory responses including cardiomyocyte hypertrophy and perivascular fibrosis (Martino et al., 2007). Therefore, it must be concluded that the circadian clock regulates compensatory cardiac tissue remodeling secondary to the primary cardiovascular disease state.

5. Therapeutic implications and future directions

5.1 Preventative chronotherapeutic applications

Our expanding current understanding of the circadian system's role in regulating cardiovascular function should, in principle, open new avenues for chronotherapeutic applications. Perhaps the simplest application is chronobiological awareness. All patients, and especially those with predisposing health risk factors, may benefit by practicing good "sleep hygiene". This refers to maintaining a regular sleep/wake schedule by going to bed and rising at regular times, and ensuring a full night's sleep. Patients should be screened for sleep apnea, which of course should be treated if found.

Unnecessary phase shifts, for instance due to traveling or late nights out, should be minimized. Re-entrainment after disruptive phase shifts, as in jet lag, can be facilitated using supplemental melatonin. This may be especially beneficial in frequent travelers. New melatonergic agonists, such as, *ramelteon* and *tasimelteon*, have different pharmacological properties and may provide alternative therapeutic effects. (Singh et al., 2010). The availability of alternative treatments offers the promise of individualized chronotherapies.

If at all possible, shift work should be avoided in patients with cardiovascular disease or with strong predisposing factors. If changing hours is not permissible, negative effects might be mitigated by chronobiological awareness and focus on making healthy pro-active lifestyle choices, such as maintaining proper diet and exercise regimes and undergoing regular physical exams. While these are good general preventative recommendations for any patient, a greater appreciation for the health benefits of circadian chronosynchrony may increase compliance, and can be aided by both an increase in doctor awareness and patient education.

5.2 Chronotherapeutic interventions

Multiple recent studies have shown a strong time-dependent efficacy for administration of anti-hypertensive medications, including beta blockers, calcium channel blockers, angiotensin-converting enzyme (ACE) inhibitors, and angiotensin II receptor blockers (ARB's) (Takeda and Maemura, 2010). Chronotherapy was shown to be especially useful in patients with resistant hypertension, and more beneficial than changing drug combinations (Hermida et al., 2008). Anti-hypertensive chronotherapy, in conjunction with the benefits of ambulatory blood pressure monitoring in candidate patients (Mancia and Parati, 2000), could provide effective new means of tailoring treatment to subjects with different blood pressure profiles.

Chronic nightly melatonin administration has also been reported to reduce hypertension in human male patients (Scheer et al., 2004). In addition to its acute soporific, phase-shifting, and anti-hypertensive effects, melatonin has powerful cardioprotective benefits. This may be due in part to melatonin's properties as a potent anti-oxidant, but studies using a perfused rat heart system have demonstrated a possible receptor dependent protection against ischemia/reperfusion injury (Genade et al., 2008). Clinical trials are underway to test the effectiveness of melatonin in treating human patients with ischemic heart disease (Dominguez-Rodriguez, 2007; 2010).

Mechanisms underlying circadian variation in cardiac arrhythmias are not understood, and chronotherapeutic studies for treating cardiac arrhythmias are lacking. However, circadian expression of voltage gated K^+ channel mRNA and protein levels (for *Kkv1.5* and *Kv4.2*) has been detected in rat heart (Yamashita et al., 2003), and more recently for L-type voltage gated Ca^{2+} channels (*VGCCa1C* and *VGCCa1D*) in embryonic chick heart (Ko et al., 2010). As we gain new understanding of how the cardiomyocyte circadian clock gates electrophysiological membrane properties, the way will be paved for the development of new chronotherapies targeting cardiac arrhythmias.

Perhaps the ultimate frontier of circadian chronotherapy lies in gene transfer techniques. Although current gene transfer methods are inefficient and risky, the field of gene therapy is in its infancy, and should be expected to mature as technical difficulties are resolved. Several labs have already employed these methods to treat hypertension in rat models, and other models of gene chronotherapy for the treatment of cardiovascular disease are under development (Lin et al., 1995, 1998; Murakami et al., 1999; Wang et al., 2004; Yla-Herttuala, 2000).

5.3 Future avenues of research

Much has been learned about the intimate partnership between circadian oscillators and cardiovascular health, and much is still to be learned. Fruitful avenues of research have employed circadian mutants, animal disease models, and a variety of *ex vivo* and *in vivo* preparations. Classical circadian research methods, such as surgical grafting, ablation, and cycle disruption, have been used to great new effect, in concordance with modern molecular tools such as mutant construction, and microarray analysis. This multi-pronged approach has revolutionized our understanding of peripheral oscillators, and energized a new paradigm for studying systems biology.

These same approaches and model systems will no doubt continue to produce valuable new knowledge, while advanced technologies promise to forge new inroads in the quest to unravel cardiovascular clocks. Adaptations of molecular manipulation techniques will allow valuable tissue specific knockdown and overexpression experiments to be conducted in parallel with genetic knockouts. Tissue and cell specific genetic engineering, side by side with improved biological assays, should allow us to continue to dissect the circadian code, gene by gene, protein by protein. The circadian proteome must be characterized and reconciled with the mosaic of divergent circadian transcriptomes. As new therapies are investigated, and epidemiological data are collected, we will continue to bridge the gap between laboratory animal and human patient.

6. Conclusion

As we've seen in this review, circadian rhythms are woven into the dynamic fabric of temporal cardiac homeostasis. Governance of this complexly balanced tapestry is shared between a synchronous cooperation between distributed, intrinsic oscillators and the master pacemaker within the SCN. Discordance between system components can cause cardiovascular dysfunction, and exacerbate pre-existing disease. While we continue to unmask the role of circadian rhythms in cardiovascular function, the impetus will increase for application of circadian principles into clinical practice. As our fourth dimensional view of human medicine matures, we will more clearly see how circadian regulation of the heart is an indispensable feature of healthy cardiovascular function.

7. Acknowledgment

Financial support for production of this document was provided in part by Parker University. I thank Monica Karaganis for help with art production and formatting of this document, and I thank Carolyn Omo for assistance in locating manuscripts. Lastly, I thank Dr. Farshid Marzban for his support and for providing scholarly input.

8. References

Andrews, N.; Gralnick, H.; Merryman, P.; Vail, M.; Quyyumi, A. (1996). Mechanisms Underlying the Morning Increase in Platelet Aggregation: A Flow Cytometry Study. *Journal of the American College of Cardiology*, Vol.28, pp.1789-1795

Argentino. C.; Toni, D.; Rasura, M.; Violi, F.; Sacchetti, M.; Allegretta, A.; Balsano, F.; Fieschi, C. (1990). Circadian Variation in the Frequency of Ischemic Stroke. *Stroke*, Vol.21, pp.387-389

Bailey, M.; Beremand, P.; Hammer, R.; Reidel, E.; Thomas, T.; & Cassone, V. (2004). Transcriptional Profiling of Circadian Patterns of mRNA Expression in the Chick Retina. *Journal of Biological Chemistry*, Vol.279, No.50, pp.52247-52254

Balsalobre, A.; Brown, S.; Marcacci, L.; Tronche, F.; Kellendonk, C.; Reichardt, H.; Schutz, G.; Schibler, U. (2000). Resetting of Circadian Time in Peripheral Tissues by Glucocorticoid Signaling. *Science*, Vol.289, pp.2344-2347

Bell-Pedersen, D.; Cassone, V.; Earnest, D.; Golden, S.; Hardin, P.; Thomas, T.; Zoran, M. (2005). Circadian Rhythms from Multiple Oscillators: Lessons from Diverse Organisms. *Nature Reviews: Genetics*, Vol.6, No.7, pp.544-556

Bass, J. & Martino, T. (2007). A Sense of Time: How Molecular Clocks Organize Metabolism. *Trends in Endocrinology and Metabolism*, Vol.18, No.1, pp.4-11

Bray, M.; Shaw, C.; Moore, M.; Garcia, R.; Zanquetta, M.; Durgan, D.; Jeong, W.; Tsai, J.; Bugger, H.; Zhang, D.; Rohrwasser, A.R.; Rennison, J.; Dyck, J.; Litwin, S.; Hardin, P.; Chow, C.; Chandler, M.; Abel, D. & Young, M. (2008). Disruption of the Circadian Clock Within the Cardiomyocyte Influences Myocardial Contractile Function, Metabolism, and Gene Expression. *American Journal of Physiology. Heart and Circulatory Physiology, Vol.* 294, pp.H1036–H1047, ISSN 1522-1539

Brezinski, D.; Tofler, G.; Muller, J.; Pohjola-Sintonen, S.; Willich, S.; Schafer, A.; Czeisler, C.; Williams, G. (1988). Morning Increase in Platelet Aggregability: Association With Assumption of the Upright Posture. *Circulation*, Vol.78, pp.35-40

Buijs, R.; la Fleur, S.; Wortel, J.; Van Heyningen, C.; Zuiddam, L.; Mettenleiter, T.; Kalsbeek, A.; Nagai, K.; Niijima, A. (2003). The Suprachiasmatic Nucleus Balances Sympathetic and Parasympathetic Output to Peripheral Organs Through Separate Preautonomic Neurons. *The Journal of Comparative Neurology*, Vol.464, No.1, pp.36- 48

Cahill, G. (2002). Clock Mechanisms in Zebrafish. *Cell Tissue Research*, Vol.309, No.1, pp.27- 34.

Cassone, V.; Roberts, M.; Moore, R. (1987). Melatonin Inhibits Metabolic Activity in the Rat Suprachiasmatic Nuclei. *Neuroscience Letters*, Vol.81, pp.29-34

Chong, N.; Chaurasia, S.; Haque, R.; Klein, D. & Iuvone, P. (2003). Temporal-Spatial Characterization of Chicken Clock Genes: Circadian Expression in Retina, Pineal Gland, and Peripheral Tissues. *Journal of Neurochemistry*, Vol.85, No.4, pp.851-860

Cohen, M.; Rohtla, K.; Lavery, C.; Muller, J.; Mittleman, M. (1997). Metaanalysis of the Morning Excess of Acute Myocardial Infarction and Sudden Cardiac Death. *American Journal of Cardiology*, Vol.79, pp.1512-1516

Curtis, A.; Cheng, Y.; Kapoor, S.; Reilly, D.; Price, T.; Fitzgerald, G. (2007). Circadian Variation of Blood Pressure and the Vascular Response to Asynchronous Stress. *Proceedings of the National Academy of Sciences of the United States of America*, Vol.104, No.9, pp.3450-3455

Dardente, H. & Cermakian, N. (2007). Molecular Circadian Rhythms in Central and Peripheral Clocks in Mammals. *Chronobiology International*, Vol.24, No.2, pp.195- 213

Deguchi, Y.; Amino, M.; Adachi, K.; Matsuzaki, A.; Iwata, O.; Yoshioka, K.; Watanabe, E.; Tanabe, T. (2009). Circadian distribution of paroxysmal atrial fibrillation in patients with and without structural heart disease in untreated state. *Annals of Noninvasive Electrocardiology*, Vol.14, No.3, pp.280-289

Dominguez-Rodriguez, A.; Abreu-Gonzalez, P. (2010). Myocardial Ischemia-Reperfusion Injury: Possible Role of Melatonin. *World Journal of Cardiology, Vol.*2, No.8, pp.233- 236

Dominguez-Rodriguez, A.; Abreu-Gonzalez, P.; Garcia-Gonzalez, M.; Kaski, J.; Reiter, R.; Jimenez-Sosa, A. (2007). A Unicenter, Randomized, Double-Blind, Parallel-Group, Placebo-Controlled Study of Melatonin as an Adjunct in Patients with Acute Myocardial Infarction Undergoing Primary Angioplasty: The Melatonin Adjunct in the Acute Myocardial Infarction Treated with Angioplasty (MARIA) Trial: Study Design and Rationale. Contemporary Clincal Trials, Vol.28, No.4, pp.532-539

Duez, H. & Staels, B. (2009). Rev-erb-a: An Integrator of Circadian Rhythms and Metabolism. *Journal of Applied Physiology*, Vol.107, No.6, 1972-1980

Durgan, D.; Hotze, M.; Tomlin, T.; Egbejimi, O.; Graveleau, C.; Abel, E.; Shaw, C.; Bray, M.; Hardin, P.; Young, M. (2005). The Intrinsic Circadian Clock within the Cardiomyocyte, *American Journal of Physiology: Heart and Circulatory Physiology*, Vol.89, pp.H1530–H1541

Durgan, D.; Moore, M.; Ha, N.; Egbejimi, O.; Fields, A.; Mbawuike, U.; Egbejimi, A.; Shaw, C.; Bray, M.; Nannegari, V.; Hickson-Bick, D.; Heird, W.; Dyck, J.; Chandler, M.; Young, M. (2007). Circadian Rhythms in Myocardial Metabolism and Contractile Function: Influence of Workload and Oleate. *American Journal of Physiology: Heart and Circulatory Physiology*, Vol.293, No.4, pp.H2385-H2393

Duffield, G. (2003). DNA Microarray Analyses of Circadian Timing: The Genomic Basis of Biological Time. *Journal of Neuroendocrinology*, Vol.15, pp.991-1002

Elherik, K.; Khan, F.; McLaren, M.; Kennedy, G.; Belch, J. (2002). Circadian Variation in Vascular Tone and Endothelial Cell Function in Normal Males. *Clinical Science (London, England)*, Vol.102 pp.547-552

Elliot, W. (2001). Cyclic and Circadian Variations in Cardiovascular Events. *American Journal of Hypertension*, Vol.14, pp.291S-295S

Genade, S.; Genis, A.; Ytehus, K.; Huisamen, B.; Lochner, A. (2008). Melatonin Receptor-Mediated Protection Against Myocardial Ischaemia/Reperfusion Injury: Role of its Anti-Adrenergic Actions. *Journal of Pineal Research*, Vol.45. No.4, pp.449-458

Hermida, R.; Ayala, D.; Fernandez, J.; Calvo, C. (2008). Chronotherapy Improves Blood Pressure Control and Reverts the Nondipper Pattern in Patients with Resistant Hypertension. *Hypertension*, Vol.51, pp.69-76

Huether, G. (1993). The contribution of extrapineal sites of melatonin synthesis to circulating melatonin levels in higher vertebrates. *Experientia*, Vol.49, No.8, pp.665-670

Hurd M., & Ralph, M. (1998). The Significance of Circadian Organization for Longevity in the Golden Hamster. *Journal of Biological Rhythms*, Vol. 13, pp.430-436

Inui, Y.; Hazeki, O. (2010). Acute Effects of Melatonin and its Time of Administration on Core Body Temperature and Heart Rate in Cynomolgus Monkeys. *The Journal of Toxicological Sciences*, Vol.35, No.3, pp.383-91

Karaganis, S.; Kumar, V.; Beremand, P.; Bailey, M.; Thomas, T. & Cassone, V. (2008). Circadian Genomics of the Chick Pineal Gland In Vitro. *BMC Genomics*, Vol.9, No.206

Karaganis, S.; Bartell, P.; Shende, V.; Moore, A.; Cassone, V. (2009). Modulation of Metabolic and Clock Gene mRNA Rhythms by Pineal and Retinal Circadian Oscillators. *General and Comparative Endocrinology*, Vol.161, No.2, pp.179-192

Kawano, H.; Motoyama, T.; Yasue, H.; Hirai. N.; Waly, H.; Kugiyama, K.; Ogawa, H. (2002). Endothelial Function Fluctuates with Diurnal Variation in the Frequency of Ischemic Episodes in Patients with Variant Angina. *Journal of the American College Cardiology*, Vol.40, pp.266-270

Klein, D.; Moore, R.; & Reppert, S. (Ed(s).). (1991). *Suprachiasmatic Nucleus: the Mind's Clock*, Oxford University Press, ISBN 0-19-506250-7, 200 Madison Avenue, New York, New York 10016

Ko, C.; Takahashi, J. (2006). Molecular Components of the Mammalian Circadian Clock. *Human Molecular Genetics*, Vol.15, pp.R271-277

Kong, T.; Goldberger, J.; Parker, M.; Wang, T.; Kadish, A. (1995). Circadian Variation in Human Ventricular Refractoriness. *Circulation*, Vol.92, pp.1507-1516

Kuniyoshi, F.; Garcia-Touchard, A.; Gami, A.; Romero-Corral, A.; van der Walt, C.; Pusalavidyasagar, S.; Kara, T.; Caples, S.; Pressman, G.; Vasquez, E.; Lopez- Jimenez, F.; Somers, V. (2008). Day-Night Variation of Acute Myocardial Infarction in Obstructive Sleep Apnea. *Journal of the American College of Cardiology*, Vol.52, pp.343-346

Le Minh, N.; Damiola, F.; Tronche, F.; Schutz, G.; Schibler, U. (2001). Glucocorticoid Hormones Inhibit Food-Induced Phase-Shifting of Peripheral Circadian Oscillators. *The EMBO Journal*, Vol.20, pp.7128-7136

Leibetseder, V.; Humpeler, S.; Svoboda, M.; Schmid, D.; Thalhammer, T.; Zuckermann, A.; Marktl, W.; Ekmekcioglu, C. (2009). Clock Genes Display Rhythmic Expression in Human Hearts. *Chronobiology International*, Vol.26, No.4, pp.621-636

Lin, K.; Chao, J.; Chao, L. (1995). Human Atrial Natriuretic Peptide Gene Delivery Reduces Blood Pressure in Hypertensive Rats. *Hypertension*, Vol.26, pp.847-853

Lin, K.; Chao, J.; Chao, L. (1998). Atrial Natriuretic Peptide Gene Delivery Attenuates Hypertension Cardiac Hypertrophy and Renal Injury in Salt Sensitive Rats. *Human Gene Therapy*, Vol.9, pp.1429-1438

Maemura, K.; de la Monte, S.; Chin, M.; Layne, M.; Hsieh, C.; Yet, S.; Perrella, M.; Lee, M. (2000). CLIF, A Novel Cycle-Like Factor, Regulates the Circadian Oscillation of Plasminogen Activator Inhibitor-1 Gene Expression. *The Journal of Biological Chemistry*, Vol.275, pp.36847-36851

Mahmoud, K.; de Smet, B.; Zijlstra, F.; Rihal, C.; Holmes, D. (2011). Sudden Cardiac Death: Epidemiology, Circadian Variation, and Triggers. *Current Problems Cardiology,* Vol.36, No.2, pp.56-80

Mancia, G.; Parati, G. (2000). Ambulatory Blood Pressure Monitoring and Organ Damage *Hypertension,* Vol.36, pp.894-900

Manfredini, R.; Boari, B.; Gallerani, M.; Salmi, R.; Bossone, E.; Distante, A.; Eagle, K.; Mehta, R. (2004). Chronobiology of Rupture and Dissection of Aortic Aneurysms. *Journal of Vascular Surgery,* Vol.40, pp.382-388

Mansoor, G.; McCabe, E.; White, W. (1994). Long-Term Reproducibility of Ambulatory Blood Pressure. *Journal of Hypertension,* Vol.12, pp.703-708

Marshall, J. (1977). Diurnal Variation in Occurrence of Strokes. *Stroke,* Vol.8, pp.230-231

Martino, T.; Tata, N.; Belsham, D.; Chalmers, J.; Straume, M.; Lee, P.; Pribiag, H.; Khaper, N.; Liu, P.; Dawood, F.; Backx, P.; Ralph, M. & Sole, M. (2007). Disturbed Diurnal Rhythm Alters Gene Expression and Exacerbates Cardiovascular Disease With Rescue by Resynchronization. *Hypertension,* Vol.49, pp.1104-1113, ISSN 1524-4563

Martino, T.; Oudit, G.; Herzenberg, A.; Tata, N.; Koletar, M.; Kabir, G.; Belsham, D.; Backx, P.; Ralph, M. & Sole, M. (2008). Circadian Rhythm Disorganization Produces Profound Cardiovascular and Renal Disease in Hamsters. *American Journal of Physiology. Regulatory, Integrative, and Comparative Physiology,* Vol.294, pp.R1675- R1683

Martino, T. & Sole, M. (2009). Molecular Time: An Often Overlooked Dimension to Cardiovascular Disease. *Circulation Research,* Vol.105, pp.1047-1061, ISSN 1524-4571

Masuki, S.; Todo, T.; Nakano, Y.; Okamura, H.; Nose, H. (2005). Reduced Alpha- Adrenoceptor Responsiveness and Enhanced Baroreflex Sensitivity in Cry- Deficient Mice Lacking a Biological Clock. *The Journal of Physiology,* Vol.566, pp.213- 24

Mehta, R.; Manfredini, R.; Hassan, F.; Sechtem, U.; Bossone, E.; Oh, J.; Cooper, J.; Smith, D.; Portaluppi, F.; Penn, M.; Hutchison, S.; Nienaber, C.; Isselbacher, E.; Eagle, K. (2002). Chronobiological Patterns of Acute Aortic Dissection. *Circulation,* Vol.106, pp.1110-1115

Millar-Craig, M.; Bishop, C.; Raftery, E. (1975). Circadian Variation of Blood-Pressure. *Lancet,* Vol.1, pp.795-797

Moore, R. (1996). Neural Control of the Pineal Gland. *Behavioral Brain Research,* Vol.73, pp.125-130

Mosendane, T.; Mosendane, T.; Raal, F. (2008). Shift Work and its Effects on the Cardiovascular System. *Cardiovascular Journal of Africa,* Vol.19, No.4, pp.210-215

Muller, J.; Stone, P.; Turi, Z.; Rutherford, J.; Czeisler, C.; Parker, C.; Poole, W.; Passamani, E.; Roberts, R.; Robertson, T. (1985). Circadian Variation in the Frequency of Onset of Acute Myocardial Infarction. *The New England Journal of Medicine,* Vol.313, pp.1315-1322

Muller, J.; Ludmer, P.; Willich, S.; Tofler, G.; Aylmer, G.; Klangos, I.; Stone, P. (1987). Circadian Variation in the Frequency of Sudden Cardiac Death. *Circulation,* Vol.75, pp.131-138

Muñoz, E. & Baler, R. (2003). The Circadian E-box: When Perfect is Not Good Enough. *Chronobiology International,* Vol.20, No.3, pp.371-388

Naji, L.; Carillo-Vico, A.; Guerrero, J.; Calvo, J. (2004). Expression of Membrane and Nuclear Melatonin Receptors in Mouse Peripheral Organs. Life Sciences, Vol.74, No.18, pp.2227-2236

Otto, M.; Svatikova, A.; Barretto, R.; Santos, S.; Hoffmann, M.; Khandheria, B.; Somers, V. (2004). Early Morning Attenuation of Endothelial Function in Healthy Humans. *Circulation*, Vol.109, pp.2507-2510

Pang, S.; Dubocovich, M. & Brown, G. (1993). Melatonin Receptors in Peripheral Tissues: A New Area of Melatonin Research. *Biological Signals*, Vol.2, No.4, pp.177-180

Peliciari-Garcia, R.; Zanquetta, M.; Andrade-Silva, J.; Gomes, D.; Barreto-Chaves, M.; Cipolla-Neto J. (2011). Expression of Circadian Clock and Melatonin Receptors Within Cultured Rat Cardiomyocytes. *Chronobiology International*, Vol.28, No.1, pp.21-30

Penev, P.; Kolker, D.; Zee, P. & Turek, F. (1998). Chronic Circadian Desynchronization Decreases the Survival of Animals with Cardiomyopathic Heart Disease. *American Journal of Physiology*, Vol.275, pp.H2334-H2337

Preitner, N.; Damiola, F.; Lopez-Molina, L.; Zakany, J.; Duboule, D.; Albrecht, U. & Schibler, U. (2002). The Orphan Nuclear Receptor REV-ERBalpha Controls Circadian Transcription Within the Positive Limb of the Mammalian Circadian Oscillator. *Cell*, Vol.110, pp.251-260

Qi, L.; Boateng, S. (2006). The circadian protein Clock Localizes to the Sarcomeric Z-Disk and is a Sensor of Myofilament Cross-Bridge Activity in Cardiac Myocytes. *Biochemical and Biophysical Research Communications*, Vol.351, pp.1054-1059

Quintero, J.; Kuhlman, S.; McMahon, D. (2003).The Biological Clock Nucleus: A Multiphasic Oscillator Network Regulated by Light. *Journal of Neuroscience*, Vol.23, pp.8070-8076

Ralph, M. & Menaker, M. (1988). A Mutation of the Circadian System in Golden Hamsters. *Science*, Vol.241, pp. 1225-1227

Ralph, M.; Foster, R.; Davis, F.; Menaker, M. (1990).Transplanted Suprachiasmatic Nucleus Determines Circadian Period. Science, Vol.247, pp.975-978

Reick, M.; Garcia, J.; Dudley, C. & McKnight, S. (2001). NPAS2: An Analog of Clock Operative in the Mammalian Forebrain. *Science*, Vol.293, pp.437-438

Reilly, D.; Westgate, E.; FitzGerald, G. (2007). Peripheral Circadian Clocks in the Vasculature. *Arteriosclerosis, Thrombosis, and Vascular Biology*, Vol.27, pp.1694-1705

Reiter, R. & Tan, D. (2009). Melatonin and Cardiac Pathophysiology. *Heart Metabolism*, 44:31–34

Rutter, J.; Reick, M.; Wu, L.; McKnight, S. (2001). Regulation of Clock and NPAS2 DNA Binding by the Redox State of NAD Cofactors. *Science*, Vol.293, pp.510-514

Sanchez-Hidalgo, M.; de la Lastra, C.; Carruscosa-Salmoral, M.; Naranjo, M.; Gomez- Corvera, A.; Caballero, B.; Guerrero, J. (2009). Age-Related Changes in Melatonin Synthesis in Rat Extrapineal Tissues. *Experimental Gerontology*. Vol.44, pp.328-334

Sandberg, F.; Bollmann, A.; Husser, D.; Stridh, M.; Sörnmo, L. (2010). Circadian Variation in Dominant Atrial Fibrillation Frequency in Persistant Atrial Fibrillation. *Physiological Measurments*, Vol.31, No.4, pp.531-542

Sauerbier, I.; von Mayersbach, H. (1977). Circadian Variation of Catecholamines in Human Blood. *Hormone and Metabolic Research*, Vol.9, 529-30

Scheer, F.; Van Montfrans, G.; van Someren, E.; Mairuhu, G. & Buijs, M. (2004). Daily Nighttime Melatonin Reduces Blood Pressure in Male Patients With Essential Hypertension. *Hypertension*, Vol.43, pp.192-197

Shaw, J.; Chin-Dusting, J.; Kingwell, B.; Dart, A. (2001). Diurnal Variation in Endothelium-Dependent Vasodilatation is Not Apparent in Coronary Artery Disease. *Circulation*, Vol.103, pp.806-812

Simantirakis, E.; Chrysostomakis, S.; Marketou, M.; Kochiadakis, G.; Vardakis, K.; Mavrakis, H.; Vardas, P. (2001). Atrial and Ventricular Refractoriness in Paced Patients: Circadian Variation and Its Relationship to Autonomic Nervous System Activity. *European Heart Journal*, Vol.22, pp.2192-2200

Srinivasan, V.; Singh, J.; Pandi-Perumal, S.; Brown, G.; Spence, D. & Cardinali, D. (2010). Jet Lag, Circadian Rhythm Sleep Disturbances, and Depression: The Role of Melatonin and its Analogs. *Advances in Therapy*, Vol.27, pp.796-813.

Storch, K.; Lipan, O.; Leykin, I.; Viswanathan, N.; Davis, F.; Wong, W.; Weitz, C. (2002). Extensive and Divergent Circadian Gene Expression in Liver and Heart. *Nature*, Vol.417, pp.78-83

Stratmann, M.; Schibler, U. (2006). Properties, Entrainment, and Physiological Functions of Mammalian Peripheral Oscillators. *Journal of Biological Rhythms*, Vol.21, pp.494-506

Sumiyoshi, M.; Kojima, S.; Arima, M.; Suwa, S.; Nakazato, Y.; Sakurai, H.; Kanoh, T.; Nakata, Y.; Daida, H. (2002). Circadian, Weekly, and Seasonal Variation at the Onset of Acute Aortic Dissection. *The American Journal of Cardiology*, Vol.89, pp.619- 623

Takeda, N.; Maemura, K.; Horie, S.; Oishi, K.; Imai, Y.; Harada, T.; Saito, T.; Shiga, T.; Amiya, E.; Manabe, I.; Ishida, N. & Nagai, R. (2007). Thrombomodulin is a Clock- Controlled Gene in Vascular Endothelial Cells. *Journal of Biological Chemistry*, Vol.282, pp.32561-32567

Tofler, G.; Gebara, O.; Mittleman, M.; Taylor, P.; Siegel, W.; Venditti, F.; Rasmussen, C.; Muller, J. (1995). Morning Peak in Ventricular Tachyarrhythmias Detected by Time of Implantable Cardioverter/Defibrillator Therapy. The CPI Investigators. *Circulation*, Vol.92, pp.1203-1208

Tsai, J.; Kienesberger, P.; Pulinilkunnil, T.; Sailors, M.; Durgan, D.; Villegas-Montoya, C.; Jahoor, A.; Gonzalez, R.; Garvey, M.; Boland, B.; Blasier, Z.; McElfresh, T.; Nannegari, V.; Chow, C.; Heird, W.; Chandler, M.; Dyck, J.; Bray, M.; Young, M. (2010). Direct Regulation of Myocardial Triglyceride Metabolism by the Cardiomyocyte Circadian Clock. *The Journal of Biological Chemistry*, Vol.285, No.5, pp.2918-2929

Turek, F. (1985). Circadian Neural Rhythms in Mammals. *Annual Review of Physiology*,Vol.47, pp.49-64

Venditti, F.; John, R.; Hull, M.; Tofler, G.; Shahian, D.; Martin, D. (1996). Circadian Variation in Defibrillation Energy Requirements. *Circulation*, Vol.94, pp.1607-1612

Verdecchia, P.; Schillaci, G.; Guerrieri, M.; Gatteschi, C.; Benemio, G.; Boldrini, F.; Porcellati, C. (1990). Circadian Blood Pressure Changes and Left Ventricular Hypertrophy in Essential Hypertension. *Circulation*, Vol.81, pp.528-536

Verdecchia, P.; Schillaci, G.; Zampi, I.; Gatteschi, C.; Battistelli, M.; Bartoccini, C.; Porcellati, C. (1993). Blunted Nocturnal Fall in Blood Pressure in Hypertensive Women with Future Cardiovascular Morbid Events. *Circulation*, Vol.88, pp.986-992

Wang, Z.; Chen, L.; Wan, C.; Qu, Y.; Cornelissen, G.; Halberg, F. (2004). In Vitro Circadian ANP Secretion by Gene Transferring Cells Encapsulated in Polycaprolactone Tubes: Gene Chronotherapy. *Peptides*, Vol.25, No.8, pp.1259-1267

Wang, X.; Armstrong, M.; Cairns, B.; Key, T.; Travis, R. (2011). Shift Work and Chronic Disease: the Epidemiological Evidence. *Occupational Medicine*, Vol.61, pp.78-89

Warren, W.; Champney, T.; Cassone, V. (1994).The Suprachiasmatic Nucleus Controls the Circadian Rhythm of Heart Rate via the Sympathetic Nervous System. *Physiology and Behavior*, Vol.55, No.6, pp.1091-1099

Weaver, D. (1998). The Suprachiasmatic Nucleus: A 25-year Retrospective. *Journal of Biological Rhythms*, Vol.13, pp.100-112

Weber, M. The 24-Hour Blood Pressure Pattern: Does it Have Implications for Morbidity and Mortality? *The American Journal Cardiology*, Vol.89, pp.27A-33A

Welsh, D.; Logothetis, D.; Meister, M.; Reppert, S. (1995). Individual Neurons Dissociated from Rat Suprachiasmatic Nucleus Express Independently Phased Circadian Firing Rhythms. *Neuron*, Vol.14, pp.697-706

Welsh, D.; Yoo, S.; Liu, A.; Takahashi, J.; Kay, S. (2004). Bioluminescence Imaging of Individual Fibroblasts Reveals Persistent, Independently Phased Circadian Rhythms of Clock Gene Expression. *Current Biology*, Vol.14, pp.2289-2295

Yla-Herttuala, S.; Martin, J. (2000). Cardiovascular Gene Therapy. *Lancet*, Vol.355, pp.213- 222

Young, M.; McNulty, P. & Taegtmeyer, H. (2002). Adaptation and Maladaptation of the Heart in Diabetes: Part II: Potential Mechanisms. *Circulation*, Vol.105, pp.1861-1870

Young, M. (2009). Anticipating Anticipation: Pursuing Identification of Cardiomyocyte Circadian Function. *Journal of Applied Physiology*, Vol.107, pp.1339-1347

Zvonic, S.; Ptitsyn, A.; Conrad, S.; Scott, L.; Floyd, Z.; Kilroy, G.; Wu, X.; Goh, B.; Mynatt, R.; Gimble, J. (2006). Characterization of Peripheral Circadian Clocks in Adipose Tissues. *Diabetes*, Vol.55, pp.962-970

Part 3

Indications, Complications and Other Clinical Concerns with Implantable Electronic Devices

6

Cardiac Resynchronization in Mildly Symptomatic Heart Failure Patients

Paolo Pieragnoli, Giuseppe Ricciardi,
Gemma Filice, Antonio Michelucci and Luigi Padeletti
University of Florence,
Italy

1. Introduction

Despite advances in detection and therapy heart failure remains a major and growing social problem.
The Framingham Heart Study (Lloyd-Jones et al., 2002) demonstrated that one out of five 40 year-old adults will develop heart failure symptoms at some point in their lifetime.
In the United States (Lloyd-Jones et al., 2010), there are 5 million heart failure patients in a total population of 294 million and in Europe; there are 10 million heart failure patients in a total population of 666 million (Mosterd A et al.,1999). Health-care expenditure for heart failure typically accounts for 1% to 2% of total health costs, of which hospitalizations constitute 60% to 70% (Berry C et al., 2001; Rydén-Bergsten & Andersson, 1999).

2. Clinical profiles and prognosis in heart failure

Heart failure is a syndrome rather than a primary diagnosis and has many potential etiologies, various clinical features, and numerous clinical subsets; some patients never develop cardiac dysfunction, and others with cardiac dysfunction may or not develop clinical heart failure.
Heart failure is a progressive disorder that is frequently preceded by asymptomatic left ventricular (LV) systolic dysfunction. In the early stages of LV systolic dysfunction individuals are typically asymptomatic, partly because of compensatory mechanisms involving the autonomic nervous system, neurohormones, and changes in the cardiac structure and function.
Whether the dysfunction is primarily systolic, diastolic or combined, it leads to neurohormonal and circulatory abnormalities, usually resulting in characteristic symptoms such as fluid retention, shortness of breath, and fatigue, especially on exertion. The severity of clinical symptoms may vary substantially during the course of the disease and may not correlate with changes in underlying cardiac function. Although the mechanisms responsible of heart failure progression to a symptomatic state are not clear, many modifiable factors have been identified that predispose or aggravate the remodelling process and the development of cardiac dysfunction. Treatment of systemic hypertension, with or without LV hypertrophy, reduces the development of heart failure.
In patients with atherosclerotic cardiovascular disease the prevention of myocardial infarction is of crucial importance, since its occurrence confers an 8-to 10-fold increase in the risk of subsequent heart failure (Lindenfeld et al., 2010).

Others modifiable risk factors include anemia, diabetes, hyperlipidemia, obesity, valvular abnormalities, alcohol, certain illicit drugs, some cardiotoxic medications, and diet.

Cardiac resynchronization therapy by means of cardiac biventricular stimulation has proved to be an essential therapy for heart failure, especially in highly symptomatic patients with LV systolic dysfunction.

In fact, current guidelines recommend cardiac resynchronization therapy in patients with left ventricular ejection fraction (LVEF) <35%, QRS prolongation (> = 120ms), and New York Heart Association (NYHA) class III or IV heart failure.

These recommendations are consequent to multiple prospective, randomized trials demonstrating the benefits of cardiac resynchronization therapy in advanced heart failure: symptoms can be reduced and exercise capacity improved, overall mortality decreased and LV function increased. In particular cardiac resynchronization therapy was able to slow heart failure progression.

Therefore, it appeared reasonable to test cardiac resynchronization therapy in patients who have structural heart disease but have not yet developed severe heart failure symptoms, especially considering the relatively high percentage of mortality and hospitalizations in mild symptomatic heart failure patients (Zannad et al., 2011). The possibility of using cardiac resynchronization therapy in this population justifies an attempt to define and identify mild symptomatic patients.

The current American College of Cardiology/American Heart Association (ACC/AHA) practice guidelines for heart failure (Hunt et al., 2009) divide cardiovascular disorders into four stages, the first two of which (A and B) do not include symptomatic patients.

Stage A denotes a high risk for heart failure but without evidence of structural heart disease and includes individuals with hypertension, diabetes or known atherosclerotic disease. Stage B includes individuals with cardiac abnormalities "structural heart disease but without symptoms". Stage C includes individuals with symptomatic heart failure with underlying structural heart disease. Stage D includes individual with advanced structural heart disease and refractory symptoms of heart failure requiring specialized interventions.

In a study of a community cohort, Ammar et al. (Ammar et al., 2007) provided information regarding the prevalence and the mortality associated with each heart failure stage, giving prognostic validation to heart failure staging.

Participants were classified according to their medical history, symptoms questionnaire, physical examination, and echocardiogram. In the cohort, 32% were normal, 22% were stage A, 34% were stage B, 12% were stage C, and 0.2% were stage D. Mean B-type natriuretic peptide concentrations (pg/ml) increased by stages: stage 0= 26, stage A=32, stage B= 53, stage C= 137 and stage D=353.

Survival at 5 years was 99% in normal subjects, 97% in stage A, 96% in stage B, 75% in stage C, and 20% in stage D.

Before ACC/AHA decided to adopt heart failure stages, classification focused solely on the patients' clinical symptoms, using the NYHA functional classification (class I-IV). In NYHA classification all patients had structural heart disease and class I included asymptomatic patients, while class II included mildly symptomatic patients.

Baldassseroni et al. (Baldasseroni et al., 2002) analyzed data from the Italian Network on Cardiac HF Registry including 5517 unselected patients with cardiac heart failure due to various causes and found that NHHA class I-II was present in 71% of all patients and in 67,2% of left bundle branch block (LBBB) patients.

Moreover the authors indicated that the presence of LBBB is an unfavorable prognostic marker in patients with cardiac heart failure and the negative effect does not depend on age, cardiac heart failure severity, or drug prescriptions.

When combining ACC/AHA and NYHA classifications, NYHA class I can be included in Stage B and NYHA class II-III in Stage C (see table 1). It should be considered however that these stages included both patients with systolic and diastolic LV dysfunction. Instead, studies which evaluated the role of cardiac resynchronization therapy in asymptomatic or mildly symptomatic heart failure enrolled only patients with systolic LV dysfunction. Some previous studies can be analyzed in order to define percentage prevalence and characteristics of patients with systolic LV dysfunction in NYHA functional class I and II.

A recent metanalysis (T.J. Wang et al., 2003) reported a prevalence of asymptomatic LV systolic dysfunction varying from 0.9% to 12.9%.

The prevalence of asymptomatic LV systolic dysfunction was twofold to eightfold higher in men than in women and higher in the elderly. Moreover the prevalence was highest among individuals with known coronary heart disease, ranging from 4.8% to 8.5%.

In SOLVD study (Studies of LV Dysfunction prevention), the development of heart failure was analyzed in patients with asymptomatic LV systolic dysfunction defined by an LVEF < 35%. Among the total population 30% in the placebo group compared with 21% in the enalapril group developed heart failure over a period of 8.3 years. In the Framingham study, a mortality rate of 40% in asymptomatic patients with a marginally reduced LVEF (<50%) was found over a period of 5 years.

Iuliano et al. (Iuliano et al., 2002) performed a retrospective analysis to examine the association between QRS prolongation (>120 ms) and mortality in patients with a LVEF <40% and reported that NYHA I and II classes were present respectively in 1,2 % and 54 % of all patients and in 1,4% and 48 % of patients with QRS > 120 ms. Moreover they concluded that QRS prolongation is an independent predictor of both increased total mortality and sudden death in patients with heart failure.

Edelmann et al. (Edelmann et al., 2011) evaluated data of 4259 patients with preserved or reduced LVEF. NYHA I and II classes were present respectively in about 7-8% and 50% of population with reduced LVEF. Moreover the authors underlined how comorbidities can condition symptoms appearance.

De Marco et al. (De Marco et al., 2004) analyzed data of 11804 patients with left ventricular dysfunction (LVEF < 40%). Percentages of NYHA I and II classes proved to be respectively 19, 5 % and 50, 8 %.

On the basis of these data it can be noted that the number of mildly symptomatic heart failure patients with systolic dysfunction is comparable to the number of highly symptomatic patients who at present have the widest indication for cardiac resynchronization therapy. This is very important considering the influence of heart failure therapy on health-care costs in terms of devices and hospitalization.

3. Therapy of heart failure

Obviously the first approach in asymptomatic or mildly symptomatic patients is medical therapy. In fact angiotensin converting enzyme inhibitors, angiotensin receptor blockers, and B- blockers have been proven to provide cardiovascular benefit to patients at any stage of heart failure.

ACC/AHA Stage		NYHA Functional Class	
Stage	Description	Class	Description
A	Patients at high risk of developing HF because of the presence of conditions that are strongly associated with the development of HF. Such patients have no identified structural or functional abnormalities of the pericardium, myocardium, or cardiac valves and have never shown signs or symptoms of HF.	No comparable functional class	
B	Patients who have developed structural heart disease that is strongly associated with the development of HF but who have never shown signs or symptoms of HF.	I (Mild)	No limitation of physical activity. Ordinary physical activity does not cause undue fatigue, palpitation, or dyspnea.
C	Patients who have current or prior symptoms of HF associated with underlying structural heart disease.	II (Mild)	Slight limitation of physical activity. Comfortable at rest, but ordinary physical activity results in fatigue, palpitation, or dyspnea.
		III (Moderate)	Marked limitation of physical activity. Comfortable at rest, but less than ordinary activity causes fatigue, palpitation, or dyspnea.
D	Patients with advanced structural heart disease and marked symptoms of HF at rest despite maximal medical therapy and who require specialized interventions.	IV (Severe)	Unable to carry out any physical activity without discomfort. Symptoms of cardiac insufficiency at rest. If any physical activity is undertaken, discomfort is increased.

ACC/AHA - American College of Cardiology/American Heart Association; HF - heart failure; NYHA - New York Heart Association

Table 1. ACC/AHA vs NYHA Classification of Heart Failure

Even if medical treatment of heart failure improves prognosis and reduces symptoms by impeding molecular disease mechanisms, reversing self-propelling neurohormonal reactions and reducing afterload burden, drugs cannot abolish electrical dyssynchrony or resynchronize mechanical delay.
Therefore any intervention despite optimal heart failure medication capable of slowing or even reversing disease progression, thereby reducing hospitalizations may help to reduce healthcare costs in these patients. Cardiac resynchronization therapy can be considered an intervention of this type. Some studies have indicated the utility of cardiac resynchronization therapy in these patients determining an enlargement of cardiac resynchronization therapy indications. A synthesis of these studies is reported in table 2 and 3 and a more detailed description of them in the following paragraphs.

4. Cardiac resynchronization therapy

4.1 Contak CD

Contak CD was the first study which investigates in NYHA I/II the effect of cardiac resynchronization therapy with defibrillator (CRT-D) compared with defibrillator (ICD) only to stratify NYHA I/II and NYHA III/IV heart failure patients with or without cardiac resynchronization therapy. Enrollment criteria were an LVEF ≤35% and a QRS width ≥ 120ms. The total population consisted of 490 patients, 32% of whom were in NYHA class II at the time of study enrollment, LBBB was present in 55%, and the mean QRS width was 160ms. During follow-up in patients in NYHA class II at baseline no significant symptomatic improvement was achieved in the cardiac resynchronization therapy group compared with the control group. Nonetheless in NYHA class II patients, cardiac resynchronization therapy was linked to significant improvement in LV dimension but not in LVEF over either 3 or 6 months.
This study was limited by the presence of the patients' clinical instability (passing from a NYHA functional class to another), by the presence of suboptimal medical therapy at enrollment, and by a major change in trial design midway through the investigation resulting in a combination of the 3- and 6-month control period from two different phases of study in the data analysis, and by difficulties inherent in subgroup analysis.

4.2 Miracle ICD-II

Miracle ICD-II examines the effect of CRT-D compared with ICD only exclusively in NYHA II patients with an indication for ICD therapy. LVEF was ≤35 and QRS ≤ 130 ms. Primary end points in this trial were cardiac function tests, NYHA classification and quality of life. There was only a 6 months follow up. Results of function tests were not significantly different in CRT-D patients compared with those receiving ICD alone. However, cardiac resynchronization therapy produced significant improvement in LV systolic and diastolic volumes and left ventricular ejection fraction indicating that cardiac resynchronization therapy promotes reverse remodelling even in patients with less symptomatic heart failure. The fact that these effects did not improve exercise capacity is not completely unexpected because patients with mildly symptomatic heart failure usually have better-preserved exercise tolerance than those with advanced heart failure. Nevertheless, the beneficial impact of cardiac resynchronization therapy on parameters that characterize adverse cardiac remodelling is interesting and important and should be put into perspective.

TRIAL	CONTAK CD (Higgins 2003)	MIRACLE ICD II (Abraham, 2004)	REVERSE (Linde, 2008)
Number of patients	581	186	610
Follow-up (months)	6	6	12
Ejection Fraction (%)	≤ 35	≤ 35	≤ 40
QRS (ms)	≥ 120	≥ 130	≥ 120
Cardiac rhythm (for inclusion)	sinus	sinus	sinus
NYHA class (%) I	-	-	18
II	32	100	82
III	60	-	-
IV	8	-	-
Mean QRS (ms)	160	166	153
LBBB (%)	54	88,2	NR
Primary End-point	HF clinical composite response	Change in peak VO2	HF clinical composite response
Secondary End-point	VO2, NYHA class, quality of life, 6 min WT, LV volumes, LVEF	VE/VCO2, NYHA class, quality of life, 6 min WT, LV volumes, LVEF	LVESVi, LVEF
Results	CRT improves functional status	No change primary end-point, improvements in secondary end-points	No change primary end-point, improvements in secondary end-points

AF – atrial fibrillation; AFl – atrial flutter; CRT – cardiac resynchronization therapy; HF – heart failure; LV – left ventricle; LVEF – left ventricular ejection fraction; LVESVi – left ventricular endsystolic volume indexed; VO2 - peak oxygen consumption; NR – not reported.

Table 2. Characteristics of clinical trials evaluating effects of cardiac resynchronization therapy in asymptomatic or mild symptomatic heart failure patients with left ventricular dysfunction

TRIAL	REVERSE European (Daubert, 2009)	MADIT-CRT (Moss, 2009)	RAFT (Tang, 2010)
Number of patients	262	1820	1798
Follow-up (months)	24	28	40
Ejection Fraction (%)	≤ 40	≤ 30	≤ 30
QRS (ms)	≥ 120	≥ 130	≥ 120 / ≥ 200 paced
Cardiac rhythm (for inclusion)	sinus	sinus	sinus, paced / persistent AF, Afl
NYHA class (%) I	17	15	-
II	83	85	80
III	-	-	20
IV	-	-	-
Mean QRS (ms)	153	158	158
LBBB (%)	NR	70	72
Primary End-point	HF clinical composite response events	Death from any cause, non fatal heart failure events	Death from any cause, HF hospitalization
Secondary End-point	LVESVi, LVEF	Recurring HF events, echocardiographic changes at 1 year	Death from any cause, death from any cardiovascular cause, HF hospitalization
Results	CRT better in terms of primary and secondary end-points	CRT better in terms of primary and secondary end-points	CRT improves HF and mortality

AF - atrial fibrillation; AFl - atrial flutter; CRT - cardiac resynchronization therapy; HF - heart failure; LV - left ventricle; LVEF - left ventricular ejection fraction; LVESVi - left ventricular endsystolic volume indexed; VO2 - peak oxygen consumption; NR - not reported.

Table 3. Characteristics of clinical trials evaluating effects of cardiac resynchronization therapy in asymptomatic or mild symptomatic heart failure patients with left ventricular dysfunction

These findings motivated three studies: the Resynchronization Reverse Remodeling in Systolic LV dysfunction (REVERSE), the Multicenter Automatic Defibrillator Implantation With cardiac resynchronization therapy (MADIT-CRT), and the Resynchronization /defibrillation for Ambulatory heart failure Trial (RAFT) trials which all aimed at assessing whether cardiac resynchronization therapy improves the clinical condition and prevents disease progression in such heart failure patients.

4.3 REVERSE

REVERSE was a multicenter, randomized, double-blind controlled study enrolling 610 patients during the scheduled follow-up period of 12 months; 419 with cardiac resynchronization therapy (or CRT-D) switched on and 191 with cardiac resynchronization therapy switched off. Patients were required to be in sinus rhythm, in NYHA class I (17%) or class II (83%) for at least 3 months before enrollment; LVEF had to be ≤ 40%, LV end-diastolic dimension ≥ 55mm, and QRS duration ≥120ms. European patients (n=261) enrolled in 35 centers had to be followed up for 24 months within their randomized group.

All patients had been receiving optimal medical therapy for heart failure, including stable doses of an angiotensin-converting enzyme inhibitor or angiotensin II receptor blocker and a beta-blocker for at least 3 months. Patients were excluded if they had been classified as NYHA functional class III or IV or had been hospitalized for heart failure in the 3 months before enrollment.

The primary end point of this study was defined as a heart failure composite response, with response groups classified as "worsened" (death, hospitalization for heart failure, crossover because of worsening heart failure, worsening NYHA class, or worsened heart failure determined by patient global assessment score), "improved" or unchanged.

Secondary end points were LV volumes, LVEF, and heart failure hospitalization. Other endpoints took into consideration 6-minute walk test, quality-of-life scores, and episodes of ventricular tachycardia or ventricular fibrillation. A CRT-D device was implanted in 82% of the CRT-ON and 85% of the CRT-OFF group. About 20% were women, 56% had ischemic cardiomyopathy, mean QRS duration was 153ms, and mean LVEF was 26%.

The REVERSE trial showed for the first time that cardiac resynchronization therapy improves ventricular structure and function (a significant decrease in LV end-diastolic and end-systolic volume indexes, as well as an increase in LVEF) in patients with asymptomatic and mildly symptomatic heart failure. In contrast, there was no significant difference between the percentage of patients who worsened in the composite primary end point compared with the percentage of patients who remained unchanged or improved. In addition, REVERSE demonstrates a significant reduction in heart failure morbidity defined as the need for hospitalization in patients with worsening heart failure in as much as in patients with active cardiac resynchronization therapy there was a statistically significant 53% relative risk reduction in time to first heart failure hospitalization. Finally, REVERSE found no significant improvement in quality of life or exercise capacity with cardiac resynchronization therapy which is not surprising in a group of patients with little functional impairment at baseline.

Out of the 262 European patients, who remained in their double-blind assignment for 24 months, 180 were assigned to CRT-ON and 82 to CRT-OFF. In contrast to the main study 19% patients worsened with CRT-ON compared with 34% with CRT-OFF (p=0.01).

However, no difference in 6-minute walk distance, quality of life, or NYHA classification was observed between the two groups. LV end-systolic volume index decrease by a mean of 27.5 ± 31.8 mL/m^2 in the CRT-ON group compared with 2.7 ± 25.8 mL/m^2 in the CRT -OFF group ($p<0.0001$). Reverse remodelling by cardiac resynchronization therapy was thus progressive, with the greatest effect during the first 6 months and further improvement developing over the following 12 months. This progressive reverse remodelling was accompanied by a significant delay in time to first heart failure hospitalization or death (HR 0.38; p= 0.003) with cardiac resynchronization therapy, suggesting that cardiac resynchronization therapy prevents the progression of disease in patients with asymptomatic or mildly symptomatic LV dysfunction when it is utilized for a period of 1 to 2 years.

We have to consider that the baseline characteristics in the European cohort of REVERSE had some key differences with respect to the North American subgroup. The European group had a lower proportion of ischemic cardiomyopathy, a lower incidence of prior myocardial infarction, a lower body mass index and longer average QRS duration.

4.4 MADIT–CRT

MADIT–CRT was designed to determine whether CRT-D in high-risk, relatively asymptomatic patients with ischemic and nonischemic cardiomyopathy would significantly reduce the combined end point of all-cause mortality or heart failure events, whichever of the two occurred first, as compared with ICD therapy alone. The secondary objectives were measures of reverse remodelling after 12 months and all-cause mortality was one of the tertiary end points.

In order to satisfy inclusion criteria, patients with ischemic causes had to be classified as in NYHA class I or II, and those with nonischemic causes had to be classified as in NYHA class II. All patients had to have LVEF <30% and sinus rhythm with QRS > 130 ms. MADIT-CRT had a group sequential design as in other MADIT trials. Randomization to arms was done on a 3:2 basis, and patients were stratified by ischemic or nonischemic cardiomyopathy in each study center.

Secondary endpoint was recurrent heart failure events; tertiary end point was focused particularly on LV volume and LVEF changes assessed by echocardiography 1 year after enrollment.

The study population consisted of 1820 patients (1089 in the CRT-D arm and 731 in the ICD-only arm); 25% were female, 45% had nonischemic cardiomyopathy, the mean LVEF was 24%, the mean QRS duration was 158 ms, and 70% of the patients had an LBBB configuration. The average follow-up for all patients was 2.4 year.

During follow-up the primary end point occurred in 187 out of 1089 patients in the CRT-D group (17.2%) and 185 out of 731 patients in the ICD-only group (25.3%). There was not a significant difference in benefit between patients with ischemic cardiomyopathy and those with nonischemic cardiomyopathy. The superiority of cardiac resynchronization therapy was driven by a 41% reduction in the risk of heart failure events, a finding that was evident primarily in a prespecified subgroup of patients with a QRS duration of 150 ms or more. An analysis of the Kaplan-Meier estimate of heart failure survival probability shows that there was already an early diverging of curves in favour of CRT-D after 2 months.

The annual mortality rate (3%) was equally low in both arms of randomization.

Moreover a significant reverse LV remodelling was found at 1 year with a mean increase in LVEF of 11%, and a drop in both mean LV end-diastolic volume (52 ml), and in LV end-systolic volume (57 ml). These analyses prove that CRT-D can induce a significant reversal of the structural remodelling process, even in patients without or with only mild symptoms of heart failure (NYHA I/II). A slight but still significant reduction in mitral regurgitation was noticed in the CRT-D arm.

Exercise capacity, measured by a 6-minute walk test, did not improve with CRT-D; both quality-of- life scores showed a trend toward improved scores, but the difference before and after cardiac resynchronization therapy was not significant. The biomarker brain natriuretic peptide was significantly reduced in CRT-D patients (-35 pg/dl) but not in the ICD-only arm.

Therefore MADIT-CRT clearly demonstrated that heart failure progression can be prevented within 2.5 years of follow-up in patients with structural heart disease without or with only mild symptoms of heart failure at the time of CRT-D.

Prevention of heart failure progression is combined with reverse ventricular remodelling. Since patients in NYHA I/II or stage B heart failure have almost no limitations on their exercise capacity and have a relatively low overall mortality rate, it is difficult to demonstrate a significant increase in exercise capacity or decrease in overall mortality within a relatively short time.

4.5 RAFT

In conclusion **RAFT** study enrolled 1798 patients in NYHA class II or III heart failure, with a LVEF of 30% or less, and an intrinsic QRS duration of 120 ms or more, or a paced QRS duration of 200 ms or more, in order to receive either an ICD alone or a CRT-D. The primary outcome was death from any cause or hospitalization for heart failure.

The primary outcome, death or hospitalization for heart failure occurred in 364 out of 904 patients (40.3%) in the ICD group, as compared with 297 out of 894 patients (33.2 %) in the CRT-D group ($p<0.001$). The time to the occurrence of the primary out-come was significantly prolonged in the CRT-D group ($p<0.001$).

During the course of the trial the mortality rate in the two groups was 23.5 %(422 out of the 1798 patients).

In the CRT-D group, the 5-year actuarial rate of death was 28.6%, as compared with 34.6% in the ICD group. The time until death was significantly prolonged (relative risk reduction, 25%) in the CRT-D group ($p=0.003$).

The number of patients who were hospitalized for heart failure was lower in the CRT-D group, with 174 patients hospitalized (19.5%), as compared with 236 (26.1%) in the ICD group ($p<0.001$).

However, the number of device-related hospitalizations was higher in the CRT-D group, with 179 hospitalizations (20%) as compared with 110 (12.25) in the ICD group ($p<0.001$).

Among patients with NYHA class II heart failure and among those with class III heart failure, the two study interventions were associated with similar reductions in the risk of death or hospitalization for heart failure, death from any cause, and hospitalization for heart failure.

5. Concluding remarks

Taking these studies into consideration, cardiac resynchronization therapy in mild systolic heart failure results in reverse remodelling and clinical improvements comparable to those we see in advanced heart failure stages. In particular cardiac resynchronization therapy proved to be advantageous especially in patients with a prolonged QRS (> 150 ms) which probably indicates the existence of ventricular dyssynchrony. This should be considered even in the light of a recent study (Bleeker et al., 2006) which demonstrated that the severity of baseline LV dyssynchrony, assessed with color-coded tissue Doppler imaging, was comparable between patients in NYHA class II and those in NYHA classes III to IV. In their study NYHA II class patients showed a significant improvement in LVEF and reduction in LV end-systolic volume after cardiac resynchronization therapy, similar to the one in patients in NYHA classes III to IV. Cardiac resynchronization therapy should therefore be considered in patients with a reduced LVEF, wide QRS (and/or dyssynchrony), and minimal or asymptomatic heart failure in addition to optimal medical therapy. All these data confirm the pertinence of the recent update on cardiac resynchronization therapy guidelines which included indications for mildly symptomatic heart failure patients. Further reinforcement of this consideration derives from the fact that cardiac resynchronization therapy has been considered a cost-effective intervention for patients with mildly symptomatic heart failure and for asymptomatic patients with left ventricular dysfunction and previous heart failure symptoms.

Another aspect that should be analyzed is the rationale for the combined use of cardiac resynchronization therapy and ICD in these heart failure patients. This is particularly important in as much as sudden death is the leading cause of mortality in mild systolic heart failure (MERIT HF, 1999). Therefore, the potentially greatest benefit of ICDs is likely to be conferred on patients with mild-to- moderate heart failure.

The Sudden Cardiac Death in Hearth Failure (SCD-HeFT) trial showed a lowering of all-cause mortality by ICD therapy in patients with mild-to-moderate heart failure and LVEF <35%. The risk reduction was limited to functional class II patients. No treatment benefit was observed among the 30% of patients who were in NYHA functional class III.

EVADEF study demonstrated that ICD implantation effectively reduces sudden cardiac death so that mildly symptomatic patients tend to die of progressive heart failure.

Finally, Gold et al. (Gold et al., 2011.) studied a patient population receiving CRT-D devices (83 % out of the entire REVERSE cohort) and concluded that cardiac resynchronization therapy did not affect the overall frequency of ventricular tachyarrhythmias even if this arrythmia increased in CRT-ON patients without reverse remodelling, whereas it decreased in those with reverse remodelling. In their opinion these data could rise the issue of whether or not ICD backup is chronically needed in those patients with normalization of LV structure and function with cardiac resynchronization therapy. However the incidence of ventricular arrhythmias was similar in NYHA I and II patients, and in those with ischemic or nonischemic cardiomyopathy as well. Accordingly, neither the etiology nor the severity of heart failure was able to predict which patients were more likely to experience appropriate ICD therapy thereby benefiting from ICD backup with cardiac resynchronization therapy. Thus the authors concluded that further confirmation of their results are needed before a strategy of excluding ICD backup in certain mild symptomatic cardiac resynchronization therapy patients can be recommended.

Thus on the basis of these remarks it is difficult to affirm at present, that the use of cardiac resynchronization therapy in mildly symptomatic heart failure patients should not be combined with ICD.

6. References

Abraham, W.T. et al., 2004. Effects of cardiac resynchronization on disease progression in patients with left ventricular systolic dysfunction, an indication for an implantable cardioverter-defibrillator, and mildly symptomatic chronic heart failure. *Circulation*, 110(18), pp.2864-2868.

Al-Majed, N.S. et al., 2011. Meta-analysis: Cardiac Resynchronization Therapy for Patients With Less Symptomatic Heart Failure. *Annals of Internal Medicine*, 154(6), pp.401-412.

Ammar, K.A. et al., 2007. Prevalence and prognostic significance of heart failure stages: application of the American College of Cardiology/American Heart Association heart failure staging criteria in the community. *Circulation*, 115(12), pp.1563-1570.

Anand, I.S. et al., 2009. Cardiac resynchronization therapy reduces the risk of hospitalizations in patients with advanced heart failure: results from the Comparison of Medical Therapy, Pacing and Defibrillation in Heart Failure (COMPANION) trial. *Circulation*, 119(7), pp.969-977.

Anon, 1992. Effect of enalapril on mortality and the development of heart failure in asymptomatic patients with reduced left ventricular ejection fractions. The SOLVD Investigattors. *The New England Journal of Medicine*, 327(10), pp.685-691.

Anselmino, M. et al., 2009. Optimization of cardiac resynchronization therapy: echocardiographic vs semiautomatic device algorithms. *Congestive Heart Failure (Greenwich, Conn.)*, 15(1), pp.14-18.

Baldasseroni, S. et al., 2002. Left bundle-branch block is associated with increased 1-year sudden and total mortality rate in 5517 outpatients with congestive heart failure: a report from the Italian network on congestive heart failure. *American Heart Journal*, 143(3), pp.398-405.

Bardy, G.H. et al., 2005. Amiodarone or an implantable cardioverter-defibrillator for congestive heart failure. *The New England Journal of Medicine*, 352(3), pp.225-237.

Berry, C., Murdoch, D.R. & McMurray, J.J., 2001. Economics of chronic heart failure. *European Journal of Heart Failure: Journal of the Working Group on Heart Failure of the European Society of Cardiology*, 3(3), pp.283-291.

Bleeker, G.B. et al., 2006. Cardiac resynchronization therapy in patients with systolic left ventricular dysfunction and symptoms of mild heart failure secondary to ischemic or nonischemic cardiomyopathy. *The American Journal of Cardiology*, 98(2), pp.230-235.

Cleland, J.G. et al., 2001. The CARE-HF study (CArdiac REsynchronisation in Heart Failure study): rationale, design and end-points. *European Journal of Heart Failure: Journal of the Working Group on Heart Failure of the European Society of Cardiology*, 3(4), pp.481-489.

Cleland, J.G.F. et al., 2008. Patients with heart failure who require an implantable defibrillator should have cardiac resynchronisation routinely. *Heart (British Cardiac Society)*, 94(8), pp.963-966.

Coceani, M., 2010. Guideline challenge: has CRT earned a Class I recommendation? *Circulation. Heart Failure*, 3(3), pp.460-461.

Cohn, J.N. & Tognoni, G., 2001. A randomized trial of the angiotensin-receptor blocker valsartan in chronic heart failure. *The New England Journal of Medicine*, 345(23), pp.1667-1675.

Daubert, C. et al., 2009. Prevention of disease progression by cardiac resynchronization therapy in patients with asymptomatic or mildly symptomatic left ventricular dysfunction: insights from the European cohort of the REVERSE (Resynchronization Reverses Remodeling in Systolic Left Ventricular Dysfunction) trial. *Journal of the American College of Cardiology*, 54(20), pp.1837-1846.

Daubert, J Claude, Leclercq, C. & Mabo, P., 2009. Cardiac resynchronization therapy in combination with implantable cardioverter-defibrillator. *Europace: European Pacing, Arrhythmias, and Cardiac Electrophysiology: Journal of the Working Groups on Cardiac Pacing, Arrhythmias, and Cardiac Cellular Electrophysiology of the European Society of Cardiology*, 11 Suppl 5, pp.v87-92.

De Marco, T et al., 2004. Confusion at large: incorrect assignment of patients to the AHA/ACC stages of heart failure in the ADVANCENT Registry. *Journal of Cardiac Failure*, 10 suppl 4, S96. Abstract 288.

Dickstein, K. et al., 2008. ESC guidelines for the diagnosis and treatment of acute and chronic heart failure 2008: the Task Force for the diagnosis and treatment of acute and chronic heart failure 2008 of the European Society of Cardiology. Developed in collaboration with the Heart Failure Association of the ESC (HFA) and endorsed by the European Society of Intensive Care Medicine (ESICM). *European Journal of Heart Failure: Journal of the Working Group on Heart Failure of the European Society of Cardiology*, 10(10), pp.933-989.

Dickstein, K. et al., 2010. 2010 Focused Update of ESC Guidelines on device therapy in heart failure: an update of the 2008 ESC Guidelines for the diagnosis and treatment of acute and chronic heart failure and the 2007 ESC guidelines for cardiac and resynchronization therapy. Developed with the special contribution of the Heart Failure Association and the European Heart Rhythm Association. *European Heart Journal*, 31(21), pp.2677-2687.

Edelmann, F. et al., 2011. Contribution of comorbidities to functional impairment is higher in heart failure with preserved than with reduced ejection fraction. *Clinical Research in Cardiology: Official Journal of the German Cardiac Society*. Available at: http://www.ncbi.nlm.nih.gov/pubmed/21416189.

Ekman, I., Kjörk, E. & Andersson, B., 2007. Self-assessed symptoms in chronic heart failure--important information for clinical management. *European Journal of Heart Failure: Journal of the Working Group on Heart Failure of the European Society of Cardiology*, 9(4), pp.424-428.

Exner, D.V., 2009. Is it time to expand the use of cardiac resynchronization therapy to patients with mildly symptomatic heart failure? *Journal of the American College of Cardiology*, 54(20), pp.1847-1849.

Foley, P.W.X. et al., 2009. Long-term effects of upgrading from right ventricular pacing to cardiac resynchronization therapy in patients with heart failure. *Europace: European Pacing, Arrhythmias, and Cardiac Electrophysiology: Journal of the Working Groups on Cardiac Pacing, Arrhythmias, and Cardiac Cellular Electrophysiology of the European Society of Cardiology*, 11(4), pp.495-501.

Gold, M.R. et al., 2011. The impact of cardiac resynchronization therapy on the incidence of ventricular arrhythmias in mild heart failure. *Heart Rhythm: The Official Journal of the Heart Rhythm Society*, 8(5), pp.679-684.

Goldberg, L.R. & Jessup, M., 2006. Stage B heart failure: management of asymptomatic left ventricular systolic dysfunction. *Circulation*, 113(24), pp.2851-2860.

Goldenberg, I. et al., 2010. Long-term benefit of primary prevention with an implantable cardioverter-defibrillator: an extended 8-year follow-up study of the Multicenter Automatic Defibrillator Implantation Trial II. *Circulation*, 122(13), pp.1265-1271.

Hasan, A., 2011. Does cardiac resynchronization therapy prevent heart failure? *Current Heart Failure Reports*, 8(1), pp.4-6.

Higgins, S.L. et al., 2003. Cardiac resynchronization therapy for the treatment of heart failure in patients with intraventricular conduction delay and malignant ventricular tachyarrhythmias. *Journal of the American College of Cardiology*, 42(8), pp.1454-1459.

Hunt, S.A. et al., 2009. 2009 focused update incorporated into the ACC/AHA 2005 Guidelines for the Diagnosis and Management of Heart Failure in Adults: a report of the American College of Cardiology Foundation/American Heart Association Task Force on Practice Guidelines: developed in collaboration with the International Society for Heart and Lung Transplantation. *Circulation*, 119(14), pp.e391-479.

Iuliano, S. et al., 2002. QRS duration and mortality in patients with congestive heart failure. *American Heart Journal*, 143(6), pp.1085-1091.

Jessup, M., 2009. MADIT-CRT--breathtaking or time to catch our breath? *The New England Journal of Medicine*, 361(14), pp.1394-1396.

Klapholz, M., 2009. Beta-blocker use for the stages of heart failure. *Mayo Clinic Proceedings. Mayo Clinic*, 84(8), pp.718-729.

Klein, H.U., 2010. Cardiac resynchronization therapy in asymptomatic or mildly symptomatic heart failure patients. *Current Treatment Options in Cardiovascular Medicine*, 12(5), pp.431-442.

Landolina, M. et al., 2007. Comparison of the effects of cardiac resynchronization therapy in patients with class II versus class III and IV heart failure (from the InSync/InSync ICD Italian Registry). *The American Journal of Cardiology*, 100(6), pp.1007-1012.

Leclercq, C., Mabo, P. & Trochu, J.N., 2008. Cardiac resynchronization for asymptomatic or mildly symptomatic heart failure: a bridge too far? *Journal of the American College of Cardiology*, 52(23), pp.1844-1846.

Linde, C. et al., 2008. Randomized trial of cardiac resynchronization in mildly symptomatic heart failure patients and in asymptomatic patients with left ventricular dysfunction and previous heart failure symptoms. *Journal of the American College of Cardiology*, 52(23), pp.1834-1843.

Linde, C. & Daubert, C., 2010. Cardiac resynchronization therapy in patients with New York Heart Association class I and II heart failure: an approach to 2010. *Circulation*, 122(10), pp.1037-1043.

Linde, C. et al., 2010. Cost-effectiveness of cardiac resynchronization therapy in patients with asymptomatic to mild heart failure: insights from the European cohort of the REVERSE (Resynchronization Reverses remodeling in Systolic Left Ventricular Dysfunction). *European Heart Journal*. Available at: http://www.ncbi.nlm.nih.gov/pubmed/21112898.

Lindenfeld, J., Albert, N.M., Boehmer, J.P., Collins, S.P., Ezekowitz, J.A., Givertz, M.M., Katz, S.D., Klapholz, M., Moser, D.K., Rogers, J.G., Starling, R.C., Stevenson, W.G., Tang, W.H.W., Teerlink, J.R. & Walsh, M.N., 2010a. HFSA 2010 Comprehensive Heart Failure Practice Guideline. *Journal of Cardiac Failure*, 16(6), pp.e1-194.

Lindenfeld, J., Albert, N.M., Boehmer, J.P., Collins, S.P., Ezekowitz, J.A., Givertz, M.M., Katz, S.D., Klapholz, M., Moser, D.K., Rogers, J.G., Starling, R.C., Stevenson, W.G., Tang, W.H.W., Teerlink, J.R. & Walsh, M.N., 2010b. HFSA 2010 Comprehensive Heart Failure Practice Guideline. *Journal of Cardiac Failure*, 16(6), pp.e1-194.

Lloyd-Jones, D.M. et al., 2002. Lifetime risk for developing congestive heart failure: the Framingham Heart Study. *Circulation*, 106(24), pp.3068-3072.

Lloyd-Jones, D. et al., 2010. Heart disease and stroke statistics--2010 update: a report from the American Heart Association. *Circulation*, 121(7), p.e46-e215.

Marijon, E. et al., 2010. Predictors for short-term progressive heart failure death in New York Heart Association II patients implanted with a cardioverter defibrillator--the EVADEF study. *American Heart Journal*, 159(4), pp.659-664.e1.

Metoprolol CR/XL Randomised Intervention Trial in Congestive Heart Failure (MERIT-HF), 1999. Effect of metoprolol CR/XL in chronic heart failure: Metoprolol CR/XL Randomised Intervention Trial in Congestive Heart Failure (MERIT-HF). *Lancet*, 353(9169), pp.2001-2007.

Miyazaki, C. et al., 2008. Comparison of echocardiographic dyssynchrony assessment by tissue velocity and strain imaging in subjects with or without systolic dysfunction and with or without left bundle-branch block. *Circulation*, 117(20), pp.2617-2625.

Moss, A.J., 2008. Life versus death. *Circulation*, 117(15), pp.1912-1913.

Moss, A.J. et al., 2009. Cardiac-resynchronization therapy for the prevention of heart-failure events. *The New England Journal of Medicine*, 361(14), pp.1329-1338.

Mosterd, A. et al., 1999. Prevalence of heart failure and left ventricular dysfunction in the general population; The Rotterdam Study. *European Heart Journal*, 20(6), pp.447-455.

Myrvang, H., 2011. Device therapy: Adding CRT to ICD improves outcomes in patients with NYHA class II and III heart failure. *Nature Reviews. Cardiology*, 8(1), p.4.

Ng, K. et al., 2007. The benefits of biventricular pacing in heart failure patients with narrow QRS, NYHA class II and right ventricular pacing. *Pacing and Clinical Electrophysiology: PACE*, 30(2), pp.193-198.

Reynolds, C.R. & Gold, M.R., 2010. Cardiac resynchronization therapy in mild heart failure: a review of the REVERSE and MADIT-CRT trials. *Current Cardiology Reports*, 12(5), pp.367-373.

Rickard, J. & Wilkoff, B.L., 2011. Pivotal trials of cardiac resynchronization therapy: evolution to therapy in mild heart failure. *Journal of Interventional Cardiac Electrophysiology: An International Journal of Arrhythmias and Pacing*. Available at: http://www.ncbi.nlm.nih.gov/pubmed/21373899.

Rydén-Bergsten, T. & Andersson, F., 1999. The health care costs of heart failure in Sweden. *Journal of Internal Medicine*, 246(3), pp.275-284.

Singh, J.P. et al., 2011. Left Ventricular Lead Position and Clinical Outcome in the Multicenter Automatic Defibrillator Implantation Trial-Cardiac Resynchronization Therapy (MADIT-CRT) Trial. *Circulation*, 123(11), pp.1159-1166.

St John Sutton, M. et al., 2009. Cardiac resynchronization induces major structural and functional reverse remodeling in patients with New York Heart Association class I/II heart failure. *Circulation*, 120(19), pp.1858-1865.

Steffel, J. & Hürlimann, D., 2009. Current practice of cardiac resynchronization therapy (CRT) in the real world: insights from the European CRT survey. *European Heart Journal*, 30(20), pp.2433-2435.

Strauss, D.G. et al., 2011. An ECG index of myocardial scar enhances prediction of defibrillator shocks: an analysis of the Sudden Cardiac Death in Heart Failure Trial. *Heart Rhythm: The Official Journal of the Heart Rhythm Society*, 8(1), pp.38-45.

Tang, A.S.L. et al., 2010. Cardiac-resynchronization therapy for mild-to-moderate heart failure. *The New England Journal of Medicine*, 363(25), pp.2385-2395.

Turschner, O. et al., 2010. Criteria for patient selection in cardiac resynchronization therapy. *Future Cardiology*, 6(6), pp.871-880.

Van Bommel, R.J. et al., 2010. Critical appraisal of the use of cardiac resynchronization therapy beyond current guidelines. *Journal of the American College of Cardiology*, 56(10), pp.754-762.

Wang, N.C. et al., 2008. Clinical implications of QRS duration in patients hospitalized with worsening heart failure and reduced left ventricular ejection fraction. *JAMA: The Journal of the American Medical Association*, 299(22), pp.2656-2666.

Wang, T.J. et al., 2003. The epidemiology of "asymptomatic" left ventricular systolic dysfunction: implications for screening. *Annals of Internal Medicine*, 138(11), pp.907-916.

Warner Stevenson, L., 2003. The points for pacing. *Journal of the American College of Cardiology*, 42(8), pp.1460-1462.

Zannad, F. et al., 2011. Eplerenone in patients with systolic heart failure and mild symptoms. *The New England Journal of Medicine*, 364(1), pp.11-21.

Zaręba, W., 2010. Comparison of clinical trials evaluating cardiac resynchronization therapy in mild to moderate heart failure. *Cardiology Journal*, 17(6), pp.543-548.

7

Infections of Permanent Transvenous Pacemakers - Etiology, Medical Treatment and Optimal Surgical Techniques

Maria A. Gutierrez-Martin, Juan Gálvez-Acebal, Omar A. Araji, Nuria Miranda-Balbuena and Jose M. Barquero
Virgen Macarena University Hospital, Seville, Spain

1. Introduction

Intracardiac electrostimulation devices have achieved remarkable progresses in the treatment of patients with heart disorders, with an increasing number of implants in recent years. One of the most relevant complications are device-related infections that are increasing significantly; what is more, the rate of increase in device-related infections per year has been disproportionally higher than the rate of newly implanted devices. Such infections are caused mainly by *staphylococci* and are associated with the formation of biofilms on the device. Diagnosis requires both a well-defined etiology, with the obtainment of appropriate samples, and a well-established location (catheter lead and/or endocardium) in order to carry out the most appropriate therapeutic strategy, which usually requires both a complete device withdrawal and a correct antibiotic treatment. But there is still no consensus about the most appropriate antibiotic pattern, particularly in relation to its duration, and the best time to reintroduce a new device.

2. Epidemiology and incidence

Pacemaker infections are infrequent but there has been an increase over last years, with an older population associated to an increment in morbidity and mortality rates and in financial cost. In a retrospective analysis of the National Hospital Discharge Survey database (Voigt et al., 2010) from 1996 through 2006, a 57% increment in cardiac device-related infections was registered. A population-based study in Olmsted County Minnesota calculated an incidence of permanent pacemaker and implantable cardioverter defibrillator infection of 1.9 per 1000 device-years (95% confidence interval (CI) 1.1-3.1). The incidence of pocket infection was 1.37 per 1000 device-years (95% CI 0.62 - 3.05) and pocket infection with bacteremia or device-related endocarditis occurred in 1.14 per 1000 devices-year (95% CI 0.47 - 2.74) (Uslam et al, 2007). Another prospective multicenter study in France observed an incidence of pacemaker related infective endocarditis of 0.39 cases per 1000 devices-year (Duval et al, 2004).
Nowadays, the estimated average cost of medical and surgical treatment of this kind of infections is $25,000 (Daouriche, 2004). Treatment of pacemaker-related infections typically requires a two-stage surgical approach, with complete removal of the implanted system

followed by insertion of a new one; so major costs are derived from hospitalization, diagnostic procedures, intravenous antibiotics and commonly two surgical procedures with a new device.

3. Pathogenesis

Staphylococci are the mean etiological agents (60-80%) and include *Staphylococcus aureus* and coagulase-negative *staphylococci* with meticillin-resistant strains in some institutions. Gram negative bacilli represent 5-10% of cases and another 10% are negatives cultures (Table 1). Rarely fungi or mycobacteria are etiological agents.

Early infections are acquired by contamination of cutaneous microbiota when pacemaker is implanted or generator is revised (Da Costa et al., 1998). When microorganisms adhere to device's surface, biofilms are formed (Daouriche, 2001). The biofilm is an extraordinarily complex structure formed by a community of microorganisms, involved in a molecular matrix. Their training begins with the adhesion of the microorganisms to the surface of the biomaterial through nonspecific physicochemical forces and bacterial structures called adhesins, which are different depending on the microbial agent involved. The bacterial inoculum needed to cause infection is several thousand times lower in the presence of prosthetic material. Once the organism is attached to the surface it produces a matrix, which in the case of *Staphylococcus epidermidis* is composed of a gelatinous substance called slime, which consists mostly of polysaccharides (polysaccharide intercellular adhesion). Subsequently, depending on the interaction between the microorganisms and the host defense systems, there will be or not a progression in the formation of a mature biofilm. Periodically shedding fragments of the biofilm with the more superficially located organisms liberated in the cardiovascular system will result in symptoms (Vila et al., 2008).

The microorganisms located within biofilms are protected from host defense mechanisms and are resistant to the action of antimicrobials. This resistance is determined by different mechanisms such as reduced diffusion of drugs, altered growth rate of microorganisms, resistance mechanisms expressed in planktonic bacteria, genetic elements transfer and biomaterial own action. In these circumstances it is common that the antimicrobial minimum inhibitory concentration for the organisms inside the biofilm is thousands times higher than for the microorganisms located on the surface (Rodríguez-Martínez & Pascual, 2008).

If pocket infections persist they may progress by catheter leads to a systemic infection with bloodstream and/or endocardium affectation. In other cases, this systemic involvement is caused by a different focus bacteremia that colonizes the leads, as can occur in health-care related procedures like vascular catheter related bacteremia (Uslan et al., 2009; Chamis et al., 2001).

There are many risk factors for pacemaker devices infection. One retrospective study observed that long-term corticoid use (OR: 13.9; 95%CI 1.44-20.29) and the presence of more than two pacing leads (OR: 5.41; 95%CI: 1.44-20.29) were independent risk factors for pacemakers infections; in contrast, antimicrobial prophylaxis prior to implantation was a protective one (OR: 0.087; 95%CI: 0.016-0.48) (Sohail et al., 2006). Another prospective multicenter study observed that the occurrence of infection was positively correlated with fever within 24 hours before the implantation procedure (OR: 5.83; 95%CI, 2.00-16.98), use of temporary pacing before the implantation procedure (OR: 2.46; 95%CI: 1.09-5.13) and early reinterventions (OR: 15.04; 95%CI: 6.7-33.73); however, implantation of a new system (OR: 0.46; 95%CI 0.24-0.87) and antibiotic prophylaxis (OR: 0.4; 95%CI: 0.18-0.86) were negatively correlated with risk of infection (Klug et al., 2006).

Microorganism	Sohail et al N=189	Alarcón et al N=243	Catanchin et al N=39	Chua et al N=123
Staphylococcus aureus	29%	20%	60%	24%
Coagulase-negative *staphylococci*	42%	42%	32%	68%
Other Gram positive cocci	4%	3%	4%	NR
Gram negative bacilli	9%	9%	4%	17%
Fungal	2%	1%	-	NR
Polymicrobial	7%	9%	-	13%
Culture negative	7%	13%	36%	NR

Table 1. Etiology of intracardiac electronic devices infections in clinical series.

4. Clinical manifestations

There are local and systemic infections. Local infections affect only generator's pocket and are expressed by local inflammatory symptoms like pain, tenderness, erythema and purulent drainage. In another cases exteriorization of the device material could be the only manifestation. Some patients with localized pocket infection have bacteremia without lead affectation. One study observed that local manifestations at the site of pacemaker implantation are associated with infection of the intravascular part of the leads in 79% of patients, and no clinical observations or laboratory investigations permitted identification of these patients with negative lead cultures (Klug et al., 2004).
Systemic infections affect the intravascular catheter lead and/or endocardium; they are manifested by fever, pulmonary embolism, severe sepsis and metastatic infections (Table 2). In many cases, local and systemic symptoms coexist, but there can also exist a systemic infection without any local symptomatology; which is more frequent in late infections. Sometimes, the diagnosis of recurrent pneumonia is made due to recurrent embolisms from catheter's tip or tricuspid vegetations. Since this is a bacteriemic infection, metastatic infections are frequent such as septic arthritis, osteomyelitis or endophthalmitis. In a recent international cohort of 2781 episodes of infective endocarditis, 10% of them were device-related endocarditis (Murdoch et al., 2009). When endocarditis is present, it is right-sided with tricuspid valve or

Clinical variable	Range %
Fever	80-100
Murmur on examination	20-43
Local findings	45
Pulmonary embolism	29-33
Anemia	66
Leukocytosis	59
High erythrocyte sedimentation rate	59
Positive blood cultures	77-95
Positive swab cultures from generator-pocket	61
Lead vegetation	85-92
Valve vegetation	90-100

Table 2. Clinical features in intracardiac device-related endocarditis in different series (N=180) (Sohail et al., 2008; Massoure et al., 2006; Duval et al., 2004; Del Río et al., 2003)

mural endocardium affected. Only in exceptional cases mitral and/or aortic valves are affected. In left-sided endocarditis systemic embolism, stroke, congestive heart-failure and metastatic infections are more frequent and have a more severe prognosis.
Leukocytosis with neutrophilia, elevation of the C-reactive protein or another acute phase reactant are the main altered laboratory parameters.

5. Diagnosis

The diagnostic must be microbiological and anatomical. The main procedures are blood cultures and culture of exudates of the pocket. Any purulent drainage should be properly processed for staining and suitable cultures. Bacteremia is present in many patients with systemic infections and sometimes in local infections too, so blood cultures are crucial for diagnostic, perhaps previous to any antimicrobial treatment. Bacteremia can be detected even in patients without fever. The sonication of extracted device can be a useful method that allows the recovering of microorganisms that cannot be isolated by conventional methods. Despite this, the results obtained with these methods must be interpreted with caution in the appropriate clinical context, because they can have an uncertain clinical significance or can be the result of a contamination (Mason et al., 2011; Rohacek et al., 2010).
Transesophageal echocardiography is a good diagnostic procedure to detect leads involvement because it has a higher sensibility to detect vegetations than transthoracic echocardiography. These vegetations are usually located on the distal extreme of the lead, and/or the endocardium, generally at the level of the tricuspid valve, but in some patients they may also exist in the endocardial wall and the mitral or aortic valves (Victor et al., 1999). The vegetations may be single or multiple and often easily distinguishable from the strands that are filamentous structures attached to the electrodes without clinical relevance (Kerut et al., 2007). In other occasions the affectation of the lead adopts an aspect of thickening or sleeve (Klug et al., 2007). In patients with cardiac prosthetic valves, the involvement of the same should be ruled out by transesophageal echocardiography, especially when the causative agent is *S aureus* (Habib et al., 2010).

6. Medical treatment

Antimicrobial agents are one of the main elements of treatment, along with early and complete withdrawal of the device. Antibiotic regimen depends on the location of the infection and its severity. In local infections may be sufficient to use oral antibiotics for several days, while severe and/or systemic infections, as those with bacteremia or endocarditis, require intravenous antibiotics for several weeks.
In critically ill patients empirical use of these drugs is justified, especially in systemic infections, in patients with significant comorbidities and when a high risk of complication development exists. In these cases antibiotics associations directed against the main organisms should be used. Since *Staphylococcus aureus* and coagulase-negative *Staphylococci* are the main microorganisms involved and, depending on each institution, the number of meticillin-resistant strains may be high, it is recommended the use of glycopeptides such as vancomycin or teicoplanin associated with a drug active against gram-negative bacilli, which depends on the epidemiology of each institution and include cefazidime, cefepime, piperacillin + tazobactam or carbapenems (Mermel et al., 2009).

Vancomycin should be used according to current recommendations, which means that there should be given an initial loading dose adjusted to patient's weight in seriously ill patients (25-30 mg/Kg) and continue with the following doses adjusted to renal function and serum trough levels (15-20 µg/ml) (Ryback et al., 2009).

The association of aminoglycosides is not well established, since we only have evidence of a decrease in bacteremia duration in some cases, but it is also associated with more adverse effects, especially nephrotoxicity (Cosgrove et al., 2009).

Once culture results are obtained, treatment should be adjusted depending on the isolated organisms and their antimicrobial susceptibility. Thus, in the case of methicillin-sensitive *Staphylococcus aureus* (MSSA) the drug of choice should be cloxacillin or nafcillin in appropriate doses. In methicillin-resistant *Staphylococcus aureus* (MRSA), drug selection depends on the minimum inhibitory concentration (MIC) against vancomycin: strains with MIC $\leq$ 1 µg/ml should continue with vancomycin at appropriate doses, whereas strains with MIC $\geq$ 1 µg/ml require an alternative to vancomycin (Soriano et al., 2008). In these cases, the most employed drugs are daptomycin and linezolid. Daptomycin is a lipopeptide antibiotic rapidly bactericidal on most of gram-positive cocci, including drug-resistant strains; a recent clinical trial demonstrated it is not inferior to antistaphylococal penicillin or vancomycin in patients with bacteremia and right-sided endocarditis by MSSA and MRSA, using a dose of 6 mg/Kg/day (Fowler et al., 2006). However, some therapeutic failures on this drug at low doses advise for the use of greater doses between 8 and 10 mg/Kg/day. Linezolid an oxazolidinone antibiotics exhibit bacteriostatic activity against many Gram-positive cocci and provide the advantage of having a high bioavailability which permits an oral administration and do not require dose adjustment for renal insufficiency; although prolonged treatment may have more side effects such as myelosuppression or neuropathy. For patients allergic to beta-lactam antibiotics glycopeptides are the drugs of choice. There are other alternatives as dalbavancin, telavancin, ceftobiprole or trimethoprim-sufametoxazole but the experience is limited.

Infections caused by coagulase-negative staphylococci should follow a similar attitude. In methicillin-sensitive strains, oxacillin or nafcillin are the drugs of choice; whereas in strains resistant to methicillin, use of vancomycin is preferred, although it is still not clear which role do new drugs play in these cases. New drugs such as daptomycin or linezolid are of great interest due to the activity of some of these drugs in bacterial biofilms, and maybe the need for device removal could be avoided in the future, at least in selected cases (Parra et al., 2010).

The use of rifampicin is controversial since it has not been proven to increase its clinical efficacy and, in turn, it is associated with an increased number of adverse reactions and interactions with other drugs such as oral anticoagulants, used regularly in this population. On the other hand, there is a theoretical advantage in its use when a more intense action on microorganisms located inside the biofilm is required. However, device removal is necessary in most cases to eradicate the infection and after its extraction, rifampicin benefits do not appear to outweigh risks, so its use is discouraged (Perlroth et al., 2008).

Directed treatment for gram negative microorganisms depends on the characteristics of each center. In general quinolones, cotrimoxazole, amoxicilin + clavulanate or cephalosporins, could be useful. However there is a gradual increase in infections caused by multidrug resistant pathogens as gram-negative bacilli-producing β-lactamases by different mechanisms, so it may be necessary to employ more complex treatments (Table 3). Once again, the complete removal of the device facilitates eradication (Rodríguez-Baño et al., 2010).

There is no consensus on the optimal duration of medical treatment. It is possible that in infections involving only the generator pocket, several days treatment duration may be sufficient. In systemic infections the antimicrobial regimen depends on the type of organism, site of infection (pacemaker lead versus endocardium) and the effective withdrawal of the infected device. In the published series, the average treatment duration was of 4-6 weeks, although in the series of Dumont et al., they describe 8 patients treated during 8.2 ± 5.4 days without recurrence (Dumont et al., 2003). Commonly, 2 weeks of parenteral therapy after device removal may be enough if there are no septic complications, whereas when there is device-related endocarditis or a complicated *Staphylococcus aureus* bacteremia, it is necessary to prolong this treatment for 4 weeks. In patients who can not remove the system completely due to their comorbidity and/or technical difficulties, they may require prolonged treatment with antibiotics for several months or even a lifetime (chronic suppressive therapy); in these cases the objective would be to keep localized the infection in the system, avoiding a possible dissemination. This should be exceptional and restricted to selected patients, but is expected to increase in coming years (Baddour, 2001; Baddour et al., 2010).

Microorganism	**Antibiotic**
Staphylococcus aureus and Coagulase negative Staphylococci Meticillin sensible	Cloxacillin or nafcillin
Staphylococcus aureus meticillin resistant MIC vancomycin > 1 µg/ml MIC vancomycin < 1 µg/ml	 Daptomycin. Linezolid Vancomycin
Coagulase negative *Staphylococii* meticilin resistant	Vancomycin
Enterococcus faecalis	Penicillin, Ampicillin
Enterobacter sp, *Serratia* sp, *Citrobacter freundii*, *Morganella* sp	Cefepime, carbapenems Fluorquinolones
Pseudomonas aeruginosa	Cefepime, Ceftazidime, aztreonam Piperacillin+tazobactam, carbapenems (except ertapenem) Fluorquinolones

Table 3. Directed antimicrobial therapy for systemic infections. Abbreviations: MSSA, meticillin-sensible Staphylococcus aureus; MRSA, meticillin-resistant Staphylococcus aureus; MIC, minimal inhibitory concentration.

7. Surgical techniques

Although randomized trials comparing lead extraction to conservative management are lacking, observational studies have clearly demonstrated the role of extraction in case of infections of pacemakers; because mortality rates of device-related endocarditis treated only with antibiotics are very high, as much as 66% in some series.

Like in any other surgical procedure, the best way of treating an infectious complication is avoiding it with a good prevention, consisting in a strict aseptic manipulation of a patient without signs of infection anywhere and employing periprocedural prophylactic antibiotics. A standard regimen includes administration of 2 g of cefazolin intravenously one hour before the procedure, or vancomycin, 90 to 120 minutes before surgery, if the patient is

penicillin allergic or in centers where oxacillin resistance among staphylococci is high (Bertaglia et al., 2006).
Superficial wound infections that do not involve the device do not require extraction and can be managed with oral antibiotherapy; but, in general, foreign body infection requires removal of the entire system to ensure a complete eradication and to prevent the recurrence of infection. When there is a localized pocket infection, there is still controversy with which is the best way to approach. The NASPE 2000 guidelines accept a conservative treatment consistent in device removal cutting the exposed parts of the leads; an attitude that is proving to be unsuccessful and increases the risk of recurrence or spreading of the infection and patient's mortality (Chua et al., 2000). What is more, the recent AHA scientific statement and update (Baddour et al., 2010) does not include this approach.
The first techniques employed for extraction of a transvenous lead were external traction with counter weights or open cardiac surgery with inflow occlusion or cardiopulmonary bypass. In 1988 Byrd and his colleagues (Smith et al., 1994) incorporated a percutaneous technique for lead extraction attempted via the implant vein using locking stylets and dilator sheaths or via the femoral vein using snares, retrieval baskets, and sheaths. After this introduction, cardiac pacemaker lead extraction techniques have improved and there are currently many options to select.

7.1 Direct traction

Direct traction techniques consist in lead traction with standard or locking stylets without countertraction. Care must be taken not to compromise the integrity of the lead, because this difficult the removal and increases the risk of complications or incomplete extraction. To avoid this risk, forceful traction is contraindicated and any lead that cannot be freed from tissue without distortion or stretching should be extracted with countertraction techniques.

7.1.1 Simple traction

Simple traction is the first employed and most basic lead extraction technique. The lead exits via the implant vein using standard non-locking stylets and fixation screw retraction clips. A modification consists on prolonged graded traction with increasing weights that are connected to the proximal end of the lead. Although it can be performed in any case, best results are obtained when used with recently implanted leads (less than one or two years).
When removing older leads, excessive traction may result in coil rupture, leaving fragments in the cardiovascular system with subsequent thrombotic or infectious complications. Unopposed traction can also lead to invagination of the myocardium, myocardial rupture, arrhythmia, hypotension or acute severe tricuspid regurgitation secondary to valve leaflet avulsion (Farooqi et al., 2010).
Rosenheck et al. (2002) employed lead rotation during simple traction technique in 89 patients with 113 lead extractions. Removal was fully completed in 97 (85.8%) leads with a 6.9% of partial and an 8% of unsuccessful removal rate. The only predictor of successful removal was lead age and there was only a small asymptomatic pericardial effusion in one patient.

7.1.2 Locking stylet

This technique uses a special traction device to assist in the removal of cardiac leads. This specialized stylet wire can be inserted through a cardiac lead's conductor lumen once the proximal connector has been removed. The stylet can then be locked into position, firmly grasping the distal end of the lead or anywhere along the conductor coil. This technique prevents the risk of elongation of the lead body and coil during exertion, ensuring that the entire lead is removed. Compared to simple traction, the use of a locking stylet results in extraction of greater number of intact leads (Kennergren et al., 2000) and a reduced risk of rupture.

The use of a locking stylet is limited when the conductor is broken or central lumen distorted, and has similar complications than simple traction such as myocardial invagination or rupture.

Alt et al. (1996) described the experience gathered between 1990 and 1994 by seven European centers regarding a locking stylet for removal of 150 leads. Complete removal was possible in 122 cases (81%) and in 18 cases (12%) a partial removal was obtained. Failure to remove the lead with the extraction stylet was experienced in 10 cases (7%). There were no major complications or deaths.

7.2 Lead extraction sheaths

7.2.1 Telescoping sheaths

The function of telescoping sheaths is to mechanically disrupt the fibrosis and provide a passage to remove a lead. The use of a sheath is a two-staged process: counterpressure and countertraction (Byrd & Wilkoff, 2000). In the first stage, the sheath is pushed along the lead while a similar traction is applied to the locking stylet to avoid a tear through the vascular wall. The second stage is initiated when the sheath has been advanced to the lead tip-myocardial interface and countertraction is employed. In this stage, traction is placed on the lead while countertraction is utilized in the sheath to minimize the risk of myocardial invagination or rupture. Care must be taken to maintain the sheath angle in parallel with the lead to minimize the risk of vascular lesion. Although counter traction prevents invagination of the myocardium, perforation of the myocardium is still possible. Major risks associated with this technique involve vascular lesion and myocardial perforation.

Results using conventional sheaths are reported in the U.S. Lead Extraction Database (Smith et al., 1994; and Byrd et al., 1999), with a complete removal rate of 86.8% and partial removal rate of 7.5%. Major complications occurred in 2.5% (haemopericardium, tamponade, haemothorax and one death).

7.2.2 Electrosurgical sheaths

The electrosurgical sheath (fig. 1) uses radiofrequency energy, similarly to a surgical cautery tool. It consists on two electrodes settled on the beveled tip of a sheath and the radiofrequency energy is conducted between the bipolar electrodes. It is used to locally dissect the binding tissue that surrounds and anchors transvenous leads. The tapered distal end of the sheath can also be used to mechanically disrupt these adhesions, like a conventional one; and dislocation of the tip is achieved with countertraction.

In the Excl trial (Farooqi et al., 2010) 287 leads in 166 patients were extracted with bipolar electrosurgical sheaths; 96% of leads were completely removed, 4% partially removed and only one lead could not be removed (laser sheath as an adjunct was used in 2% of cases). Major complications included three cardiac tamponade, one haemothorax and an arteriovenous fistula.

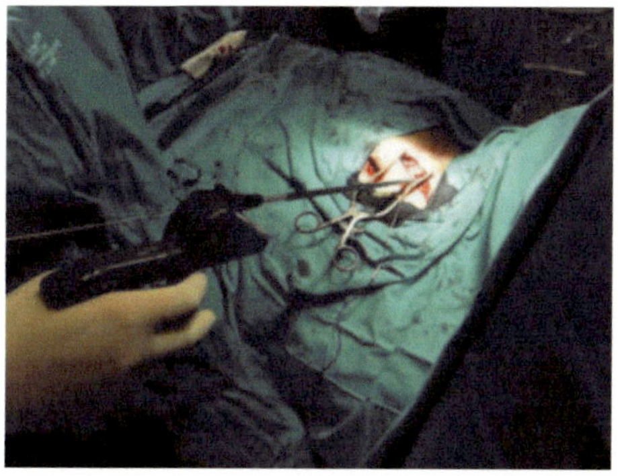

Fig. 1. Intraoperative image of a lead extraction with an electrosurgical sheath.

Compared to laser ablation, electrosurgical sheaths are designed to be more supple so that may be easier to maneuver. The radiofrequency energy is confined to less than one fourth of the circumference of the sheath allowing a directed and careful dissection of the tissue and reducing the chance of vascular damage; but in the other hand this directional control reduces the cutting efficacy through the fibrosis (Verma & Wilkoff, 2004).

7.2.3 Laser ablation

The Excimer laser sheath consists on a circumferential thin layer of optical fibers that run along the sheath and finish at the distal tip producing a ring of laser light in pulses to a tissue depth of 100 µm, dissolving the nearest fibrous tissue adherent to leads. Thus, fibrous tissue encapsulating the lead body is removed in a controlled manner and occluded vasculature can be re-canalised (Farooqi et al., 2010).

The outer layer of the sheath is made of plastic and acts as a support for maneuvering the laser but for mechanical countertraction too. Compared to electrosurgical sheaths, the circumferencial cutting is more powerful for extraction of multiple leads or with older implantation date, and in veins occluded by clot and fibrosis too. On the other hand, this circumferential cutting increases the risk of venous laceration, especially at the superior vena cava.

Appropriate sizing of the laser sheath and a proper traction/countertraction technique are crucial to prevent complications. A coaxial orientation of the sheath and lead, with the leading edge of the sheath oriented away from the wall of the vessel decreases the risk of vascular injury; and we must be careful not to advance the outer sheath more deeply than the laser sheath to avoid pinching the vascular wall (Henrikson & Brinker, 2008).

Major complications associated with laser-assisted lead extraction include: major venous injury, arrhythmia, myocardial tear, pneumothorax, hemothorax, arteriovenous fistula, tricuspid valve injury and pulmonary embolus (Lawton et al., 2006).

The total initial experience of laser lead extraction in the U.S. (Byrd et al., 2002) was reported on 2561 pacing and defibrillator leads from 1684 patients at 89 sites, with a procedural success rate of 90%, a major complication rate (tamponade, hemothorax, pulmonary embolism, lead migration, and death) of 1.9% and an in-hospital death rate of 0.8%. The latest report about laser lead extraction is the LExICon study (Wazni et al., 2010), an observational retrospective study of 2405 consecutive laser-assisted lead extractions in 13 sites in the U.S. and Canada. In this study, the most common indication for extraction was infection and a 96.5% of leads were completely removed, with a procedural failure rate that statistically increased when leads were implanted for more than 10 years. The clinical success rate was of 97.7% (resolution of clinical goals associated with the indication for lead removal), and failure to achieve it was associated with body mass index <25 kg/m^2 and low extraction volume centers. Major adverse events (any complication related to the procedure that required procedural intervention or transfusion to prevent death, threat to life, or any complication related to the procedure that resulted in death or serious harm to bodily function or structure) occurred in 1.4% of procedures, with a death rate of 0.28%; and were associated with body mass index <25 kg/m^2. Indicators of all-cause in-hospital mortality were pocket infections, device-related endocarditis, diabetes and creatinine ≥ 2.0; with an overall in-hospital mortality of 1.86%, a higher rate than the one presented by Byrd et al in 2002 and that reflects the complex comorbid condition of this patient population, especially device-related endocarditis. In this study, the all-cause in-hospital mortality rate for the device-related endocarditis population was 4.3%, 1.7% for pocket infection and 0.3% for all noninfected patients, proving the seriousness of deep advanced and pocket infections.

Moon et al. (2002), found three independent predictors of the need for laser-assist during lead extractions: prolonged implant duration, nonseptic leads and necessary or discretionary versus mandatory indications.

7.3 Femoral and transjugular extraction techniques

The preferred via for lead extraction is the same transvenous access by which they were implanted, usually subclavian, cephalic or axillary veins. However, when removing broken or cut leads with free ends and when the primary approach via the implant vein fails, a femoral or transjugular access is the procedure of choice.

The internal jugular transvenous access was described by Mazetti et al. (2008), and, although their experience was based only on 18 patients and 22 leads, they achieved a high success rate with very few complications.

Lead extraction using the femoral vein is called "the inferior approach" and probably it is the most versatile approach for lead removal. There are two fundamental snaring techniques (Belott, 2007): a direct approach in which, once the lead is grabbed with a snare, an attempt is made to remove the lead by traction; and a two-step process, by first pulling either the proximal or distal end of the lead into the inferior vena cava and secondly, snaring the free end and pulling it for its removal. There are many tools for femoral lead extraction; the more advanced one is the Byrd Femoral Work Station (Cook Vascular Inc., Leechburg, PA).

Recently (Fischer et al., 2009), it has been described a simple and safe technique of transfemoral lead snaring to assist lead extraction and maintain vascular access in the setting of venous occlusion, when the distal lead tip pulls free of the myocardium before an extraction sheath is passed beyond the point of venous obstruction.

Finally, both the transjugular and transfemoral approaches have the same potential complications of cardiac or vascular perforations.

7.4 Surgical lead removal and other techniques

An open heart surgical approach for lead removal should be limited to two scenarios:

1. Patients with significant retained hardware after percutaneous removal failure.

2. Lead vegetations greater than 2 cm in diameter, because of concern of pulmonary embolism with percutaneous procedures. This is not a definitive indication because there is some experience in transvenous lead extraction with large vegetations without precipitating a pulmonary embolism or, even having evidence of it, neither survival nor length of hospital stay has been affected by this complication (Meier-Ewert et al., 2003).

In some cases, a combined technique is the best treatment option. Removal of the distal end of the lead by sternotomy and cardiopulmonary bypass due to the presence of large vegetations; and a simultaneous percutaneous procedure for extraction of the proximal end, due to severe fibrosis around the lead at the venous system, that precluded its traction from the atrium.

Although the currently recommended treatment for pacemaker infection is complete removal, both surgery and percutaneous techniques are complex and of very high risk in some patients with many comorbidities, in these cases, less invasive techniques have been applied at some centers:

- Closed irrigation system (Hurst et al., 1986), they treated 19 patients for infected or eroded permanent pacemaker pockets with local debridement and insertion of a closed irrigation system using a solution of tyloxapol and tobramycin. Successful eradication of the infection, without complete replacement of the pacemaker system, was achieved in all cases.
- Placement of an antibiotic-releasing envelope to treat an infected pacemaker pocket: only one case report has been described in the literature (Lopez, 2010), with good results.
- Vacuum-assisted system for pacemaker infection: Satsu & Onoe (2010) describe the application of vacuum-assisted therapy for treating four patients with infected permanent pacemaker with good results.

7.5 Selection of percutaneous lead extraction technique in permanent transvenous pacemaker infections

Extraction of recently implanted cardiac rhythm devices (less than one year) is commonly a safe and easy procedure which consists in pulse generator removal and direct lead traction. However, chronically implanted leads become encapsulated by fibrotic attachments along any length of the lead where there is contact with the vein, valve or endocardial structures. In these cases, percutaneous lead extraction has become the preferred method to remove leads with a rate of success in centers with a high-volume case load of 95-97% and high rates of resolution of infection. On the other side, these procedures are associated with complications rates between 0 and 11% and involve significant risks such as cardiac tamponade, hemothorax, pulmonary embolism, lead migration, pneumonia and death.

Every of these previous described techniques remain useful and its employment depends on the indication and the experience of each center, but there are some recent reviews that may be of interest in selecting one or another technique. They are summarized in next table (Table 4). Anyway, it is important to emphasize that operator experience is vital in determining success as familiarity of a wide array of techniques will increase the likelihood of uncomplicated extraction.

Mathur et al. (2003), made a retrospective analysis of various conventional techniques for lead extraction, obtaining good results and a low complication rate. They conclude that the only independent predictor associated with successful lead extraction with these techniques was a shorter dwell time. Success rates for leads in situ for greater than six years considerably decreased in their study.

Reference	Techniques	Results	Complications
Mathur et al Retrospective analysis hospital database 1986-1999	158 leads extracted in 80 patients: - Simple traction 16.4% - Locking stylet 6.1% - Telescoping sheath 67.3% - Transfemoral approach 6.1% - Thoracotomy 4.8%	Success at 1st procedure 87.7% - Cephalic approach 90% - Transfemoral approach 56% - Thoracotomy 75% Complete lead removal 86.7% Lead remnants 7.3% Complete lead remaining 6.1%	Deaths - 0 Tamponade - 1 Stroke - 1 Pulmonary embolism - 1 Significant bleeding 12%
Centella et al Retrospective analysis of their experience 1989-2006	314 leads extracted in 187 patients: -Symple traction 44 leads -Telescoping sheath 34 patients -Electrosurgical sheath 80 patients	Complete extraction 96.8% 48 patients required a second technique for lead remnant removal	Deaths - 1 Tamponade - 1 Sepsis – 1 Pulmonary embolism – 1 Severe tricuspid insufficiency – 1
Rusanov et al Retrospective analysis of a single operator experience 1993-2008	Percutaneous techniques 88.8% - Simple traction - Locking stylet - Telescoping sheath Open surgical approach 11.2% - No CPB 4.2% - CPB 6.3%	Complete extraction 86.2% Partial success (<4cm retained) 9.2% Failure to extract (>4cm retained) 4.6%	Pneumothorax – 2 (surgical approach) Persistent infection – 1 (percutaneous) Tamponade – 1 (surgical approach) No procedure-related deaths
Neuzil et al Prospective randomized study 2.5 years	161 leads implanted for at least 6 months in 120 patients: - 84 leads extracted with radiofrequency sheaths - 77 leads extracted with telescoping sheaths	Radiofrequency extraction: - Complete success 93% - Partial success 7% Standard extraction: - Complete success 73% - Partial success 14%	Pulmonary embolism – 2 Sepsis – 3 Blood transfusion requirement – 3 No procedure-related deaths
Wilkoff et al Randomized trial (PLEXES) 1995-1996	301 patients with 465 leads: - laser extraction: 244 leads - non-laser: 221 leads	Complete extraction: - laser 94% - non-laser 64% Partial extraction: - laser 2.5% - non-laser 1.8% Failure: - laser 3.3% - non-laser 34% Clinical success: - laser 94.8% - non-laser 95.9%	Tamponade – 2 (laser) Hemothorax – 1 (laser) Valve damage – 1 (laser) Procedure-related death – 1 (laser)
Verma & Wilkoff Retrospective study 1998-2001	450 consecutive lead extractions: - 354 laser-assisted - 96 radiofrequency-assisted	Procedure time lower in radiofrequency group Fluoroscopy time reduced in radiofrequency group	No complications in radiofrequency group Two deaths in laser group Success rates comparables in both groups

Table 4. Contemporary reviews of different transvenous lead extraction techniques.

In the same manner, Centella et al. (2007) revised their experience with percutaneous lead extraction between 1989-2006, using conventional techniques and electrosurgical sheaths. A statistically significant relation is observed between younger patients and major complication development, as well as with endocarditis being the indication for lead removal.

Rusanov et al. (2010), describe a single operator experience with percutaneous and open surgical techniques for lead removal in 143 endocardial leads. Complete radiographic success was achieved for 131 leads with a low rate of major complications. They also describe an interesting multistage procedure for patients with purulent wounds: first they exteriorize the generator and irrigate and débride the pocket while initiate or continue antibiotherapy. In a second stage, when wound cultures are negative, they perform lead extraction with a caudal approach. They refer an accelerated wound healing with this technique.

Neuzil et al. (2010) performed a prospective randomized study comparing conventional telescoping sheaths lead extraction results with electrosurgical sheaths one. They obtained statistically significant differences in success rates between both techniques, in favour of the electrosurgical system. They also observed a significant reduction in the time of traction with this technique.

Another prospective randomized study is the PLEXES study (Wilkoff et al., 1999), which compares lead extraction results using conventional or laser techniques. Extraction efficacy was significantly higher in patients randomized to laser-assisted removal, with shorter mean procedure duration. Complication rates were not significantly different between both groups, with an incidence in the laser group below 2%.

Verma & Wilkoff (2004) performed a retrospective review of 450 lead extractions in their institution and concluded that electrosurgical sheath appeared to have success rates comparable to laser sheath; although there was a selection bias because laser had been selected for more challenging lead extraction cases. Based on their experience, they recommend the use of radiofrequency sheaths, especially in patients at higher risk of complications; and they employ laser techniques as first option for cases requiring extraction of multiple leads, defibrillator leads, older implantation date ones and in occluded veins.

Regarding to the removal of infected leads, there are some data suggesting that leads associated with systemic sepsis may be easier to extract with little effort (Moon et al., 2002) and that infected leads that are difficult to remove and require electrosurgical or laser sheaths, are unlikely to be infected at their endocardial tip with some reported data suggesting that tip-only retentions at incomplete extractions do not develop recurrence of infection and do well without another intervention requirement (Kratz & Toole, 2010).

Finally, there is a short experience in relation to coronary sinus lead extraction. In many cases, this leads are extracted with simple traction but there are some reports of laser sheath employment for coronary sinus lead removal.

8. Conclusion

According to the increasing use of cardiac implantable electrophysiological devices, associated infectious complications are increasing, so that the most common essential indication for lead extraction remains infected systems. This can be a life-threatening complication associated with significant morbidity and mortality and its management

represents a difficult challenge for cardiology, cardiac surgery and infectious diseases specialists.
Although we dispose of a wide range of antibiotics to face pacemaker infections, the treatment of choice in device-related infections requires its complete removal. Considering that are healthcare-related infections, an increasing number of episodes caused by multiresistant microorganism strains is expected, so a better knowledge of the role of new antimicrobials is mandatory. We also need to investigate which is the appropriate duration of antibiotic therapy as well as the optimal time for a new device implantation.
Nowadays, there are many surgical tools to remove infected leads with high success rates. This sort of techniques must be performed at tertiary referral centers with a high volume demand on these procedures and with a cardiac surgeon as the primary operator or aware of the procedure at least. With a well-structured team and the availability of different surgical lead extraction techniques, the rate of major complications is very low.

9. References

Almirante, B. & Miró, JM. (2008). Infecciones asociadas a las válvulas protésicas cardiacas, las prótesis vasculares y los dispositivos de electroestimulación cardiacos. *Enf Infect Microbiol Clin*, (Nov 2008), Vol.26, No.10, pp.647-664, ISSN 0213-005X

Alt, E.; Neuzner, J.; Binner, L.; Göhl, K.; Res, JC.; Knabe, UH.; Zehender, M. & Reinhardt, J. (1996). Three-year experience with a stylet for lead extraction: a multicenter study. *Pacing Clin Electrophysiol*, Vol.19, No.1, (Jan 1996), pp. 18-25, ISSN 0147-8389

Baddour, LM. (2001). Long-term suppressive antimicrobial therapy for intravascular device-related infections. *Am J Med Sci*; Vol.322, No.4, (Oct 2001), pp.209-212, ISSN 1538-2990

Baddour, LM.; Epstein, AE.; Erickson, CC.; Knight, BP.; Levison, ME.; Lockhart, PB.; Masoudi, FA.; Okum, EJ.; Wilson, WR.; Beerman, LB.; Bolger, AF.; Mark Estes, NA.; Gewitz, M.; Newburger, JW.; Schron, EB. & Taubert, KA. (2010). Update on cardiovascular implantable electronic device infections and their management: a scientific statement from the American Heart Association. *Circulation*, Vol.121, pp. 458-477, ISSN 1524-4539

Belott, PH. (2007). Lead extraction using the femoral vein. *Heart Rhythm*, Vol.4, No.8, (August 2007), pp. 1102-1107, ISSN 1556-3871

Bertaglia, E.; Zerbo, F.; Zardo, S.; Barzan, D.; Zoppo, F. & Pascotto, P. (2006). Antibiotic prophylaxis with a single dose of cefazolin during pacemaker implantation: incidence of long-term infective complications. *Pacing Clin Electrophysiol*, Vol.29, No.1, (Jan 2006), pp. 29-33, ISSN 0147-8389

Byrd, CL.; Wilkoff, BL.; Love, CL.; Sellers, TD.; Turk, KT.; Reeves, R.; Young, R.; Crevey, B.; Kutalek, SP.; Freedman, R.; Friedman, R.; Trantham, J.; Watts, M.; Schutzman, J.; Oren, J.; Wilson, J.; Gold, F.; Fearnot, NE. & Van Zandt, HJ. (1999). Intravascular extraction of problematic or infected permanent pacemaker leads: 1994-1996. U.S. Extraction Database, MED Institute. *Pacing Clin Electrophysiol*, Vol.22, No.9, (Sept 1999), pp. 1348-1357, ISSN 0147-8389

Byrd, CL. & Wilkoff, BL. (2000). Techniques and devices for extraction of pacemaker and implantable cardioverter-defibrillator leads, In: *Clinical Cardiac Pacing and*

Defibrillation, Wilkoff, BL., 669-706, WB Saunders, ISBN 0-7216-7683-9, Philadelphia

Byrd, CL.; Wilkoff, BL.; Love, CJ.; Sellers, TD. & Reiser, C. (2002). Clinical study of the laser sheath for lead extraction: the total experience in the United States. *Pacing Clin Electrophysiol*, Vol.25, No.5, (May 2002), pp. 804-808, ISSN 0147-8389

Catanchin, A.; Murdock, CJ. & Athan, E. (2007). Pacemaker infections: a 10-year experience. *Heart Lung Circ*, Vol.16, No.6, (Dec 2007), pp.434-439, ISSN 1444-2892

Centella, T.; Oliva, E.; García-Andrade, I.; Martín-Dávila, P.; Cobo, J.; Moya, JL.; Hernández-Madrid, A. & Epeldegui, A. (2007). Percutaneous extraction of pacemaker and defibrillator leads. *Rev Esp Cardiol*, Vol.60, No.6, (Jun 2007), pp.607-615, ISSN 1885-5857

Chua, JD.; Wilkoff, BL.; Lee, I.; Juratli, N.; Longworth, DL. & Gordon, SM. (2000). Diagnosis and management of infections involving implantable electrophysiologic cardiac devices. *Ann Intern Med*, Vol.133, No.8, pp. 604-8, ISSN 0003-4819

Cosgrove, SE.; Vigliani, GA.; Fowler, VG.; Abrutyn, E.; Corey, GR.; Levine, DP.; Rupp, ME.; Chambers, HF.; Karchmer, AW. & Boucher, HW. (2009). Initial low-dose gentamicin for Staphylococcus aureus bacteremia and endocarditis is nephrotoxic. *Clin Infect Dis*, Vol.48, No.6, (March 2009), pp.713-721, ISSN 1058-4838

Da Costa, A.; Lelièvre, H.; Kirkorian, G.; Cèlard, M.; Chevalier, P.; Vandenesch, F.; Etienne, J. & Touboul, P. (1998). Role of the preaxillary flora in pacemaker infections: a prospective study. *Circulation*, Vol.97, No.18, (May 1998), pp.1791-1795, ISSN 0009-7322

Daouriche, RO. (2001). Device-associated infections: a macroproblem that starts with microadherence. *Clin Infect Dis*, Vol.33, No.9, (Nov 2001), pp.1567-1572, ISSN 1058-4838

Daouriche, RO. (2004). Treatment of infections associated with surgical implants. *N Engl J Med*, Vol.350, No.14, (Apr 2004), pp.1422-1429, ISSN 0028-4793

De Alarcón, A.; Gálvez, J.; Ruiz, J.; Miralles, F.; Reguera, JM. & Lomas, JM. on behalf of the Grupo Andaluz para el Estudio de las Enfermedades Infecciosas. (2005). Infections associated with intracardiac devices (ICD). What could be its better management?. 8th International Symposium on Modern Concepts in Endocarditis and Cardiovascular Infections. May Charleston, South Carolina. USA 2005.

Del Río, A.; Anguera, I.; Miró, JM.; Mont, L.; Fowler, V.; Azqueta, M. & Mestres, CA. (2003) Surgical treatment of pacemaker and defibrillator lead endocarditis: the impact of electrode lead extraction on outcome. *Chest*; Vol.124, No.4, (Oct 2003), pp.1451-1459, ISSN 0012-3692

Dumont, E.; Camus, C.; Victor, F.; De Place, C.; Pavin, D. ; Alonso, C.; Mabo, P. & Daubert, JC. (2003). Suspected pacemaker or defibrillator transvenous lead infection. Prospective assessment of a TEE-guided therapeutic strategy. *Eur Heart J*, Vol.24, No.19, (Oct 2003), pp.1779-1787, ISSN 0195-668X

Duval, X.; Selton-Suty, C.; Alla, F.; Salvador-Mazenq, M.; Bernard, Y.; Weber, M.; Lacassin, F.; Nazeyrolas, P.; Chidiac, C.; Hoen, B. & Leport, C. (2004). Endocarditis in patients with a permanent pacemaker: a 1-year epidemiological survey on infective endocarditis due to valvular and/or pacemaker infection. *Clin Infect Dis*, Vol.39, No.1, (Jul 2004), pp.68-74, ISSN 1058-4838

Farooqi, FM.; Talsania, S.; Hamid, S. & Rinaldi, CA. (2010). Extraction of cardiac rhythm devices: indications, techniques and outcomes for the removal of pacemaker and defibrillator leads. *Int J Clin Pract*, Vol.64, No.8, (July 2010), pp. 1140-1147, ISSN 1742-1241

Fischer, A.; Love, B.; Hansalia, R. & Mehta, D. (2009). Transfemoral snaring and stabilization of pacemaker and defibrillator leads to maintain vascular access during lead extraction. *Pacing Clin Electrophysiol*, Vol.32, No.3, (Mar 2009), pp. 336-339, ISSN 0147-8389

Fowler, VG.; Boucher, HW.; Corey, GR.; Abrutyn, E.; Karchmer, AW.; Rupp, ME.; Levine, DP.; Chambers, HF.; Tally, FP.; Vigliani, GA.; Cabell, CH.; Link, AS.; DeMeyer, I.; Filler, SG.; Zervos, M.; Cook, P.; Parsonnet, J.; Bernstein, JM.; Price, CS.; Forrest, GN.; Fätkenheuer, G.; Gareca, M.; Rehm, SJ.; Brodt, HR.; Tice, A. & Cosgrove, SE. (2006). Daptomycin versus standard therapy for bacteremia and endocarditis caused by *Staphylococcus aureus*. *New Engl J Med*, Vol.355, No.7, (Aug 2006), pp.653-665, ISSN 0028-4793

Habib, G.; Badano, L.; Tribouilloy, C.; Vilacosta, I. & Zamorano, JL.; Galderisi, M.; Voigt, JU.; Sicari, R.; Cosyns, B.; Fox, K. & Aakhus, S. (2010). Recommendations for the practice of echocardiography in infective endocarditis. *Eur J Echocardiogr*, Vol.11, No.2, (Mar 2010), pp.202-219, ISSN 1097-6795

Henrikson, CA. & Brinker, JA. (2008). How to prevent, recognize, and manage complications of lead extraction. Part III: Procedural factors. *Heart Rhythm*, Vol.5, No.9, (Sept 2008), pp. 1352-1354, ISSN 1556-3871

Hurst, LN.; Evans, HB.; Windle, B. & Klein, GJ. (1986). The salvage of infected cardiac pacemaker pockets using a closed irrigation system. *Pacing Clin Electrophysiol*, Vol.9, No.6, (Nov 1986), pp. 785-792, ISSN 0147-8389

Kennergren, C.; Schaerf, RH.; Sellers, TD.; Wilkoff, BL.; Byrd, CL.; Tyres, GF.; Coe, S.; Coates, CW. & Reiser, C. (2000). Cardiac lead extraction with a novel locking stylet. *J Interv Card Electrophysiol*, Vol.4, No.4, (Dec 2000), pp. 591-593, ISSN 1572-8595

Kerut, EK.; Hanawalt, C. & Everson, CT. (2007). Role of the echocardiography laboratory in diagnosis and management of pacemaker and implantable cardiac defibrillator infection. *Echocardiography*, Vol.24, No.9, (Oct 2007), pp.1008-1012, ISSN 0742-2822

Klug, D.; Lacroix, D.; Savoye, C.; Goullard, L.; Grandmougin, D.; Hennequin, JL.; Kacet, S. & Leckieffre, J. (1997). Systemic infection related to endocarditis on pacemaker leads: clinical presentation and management. *Circulation*, Vol.95, No.8, (Apr 1997), pp.2098-2107, ISSN 0009-7322

Klug, D.; Wallet, F.; Lacroix, D.; Marquié, C.; Kouakam, C.; Kacet, S. & Courcol, R. (2003). Local symptoms at the site of pacemaker implantation indicate latent systemic infection. *Heart*, Vol.90, No.8, (Aug 2003), pp.882-886, ISSN 1355-6037

Klug, D.; Balde, M.; Pavin, D.; Hidden-Lucet, F.; Clementy, J.; Sadoul, N.; Rey, JL.; Lande, G.; Lazarus, A.; Victor, J.; Barnay, C.; Grandbastien, B. & Kacet, S. (2007). Risk factors related to infections of implanted pacemakers and cardioverter-defibrillator: results of a large prospective study. *Circulation*, Vol.116, No.12, (Sept 2007), pp.1349-1355, ISSN 0009-7322

Kratz, JM. & Toole, JM. (2010). Pacemaker and internal cardioverter defibrillator lead extraction: a safe and effective surgical approach. *Ann Thorac Surg*, Vol.90, No.5, (Nov 2010), pp.1411-1417, ISSN 0003-4975

Lawton, JS.; Moon, MR.; Curci, JA.; Rubin, BG.; Smith, TW.; Gleva, MJ. & Damiano, RJ. (2006). Management of arterial injuries caused by laser extraction of indwelling venous pacemaker and defibrillator leads. *Pacing Clin Electrophysiol*, Vol.29, No.8, (Aug 2006), pp. 917-920, ISSN 0147-8389.

Lopez, JA. (2010). Treatment of an infected pacemaker pocket with an antimicrobial envelope. *Ann Thorac Surg*, Vol.89, No.5, (May 2010), pp. 1639-1641, ISSN 0003-4975

Mason, PK.; Dimarco, JP.; Fergunson, JD.; Mahapatram, S.; Mangrum, JM.; Bilchick, KC.; Moorman, JR.; Lake, DE. & Bergin, JD. (2011). Sonication of explanted cardiac rhythm management devices for the diagnosis of pocket infections and asymptomatic bacterial colonization. *Pacing Clin Electrophysiol*, Vol.34, No.2, (Feb 2011), pp.143-149, ISSN 0147-8389

Maussoure, PL.; Reuter, S.; Lafitte, S.; Clementy, J.; Laborderie, J.; Bordachard, P.; Clementy, J. & Roudaut, R. (2007). Pacemaker endocarditis: clinical features and management of 60 consecutive cases. *Pacing Clin Electrophysiol*; Vol.30, No.1, (Jan 2007), pp.12-19, ISSN 0147-8389

Mathur, G.; Stables, RH.; Heaven, D.; Stack, Z.; Lovegrove, A.; Ingram, A. & Sutton, R. (2003). Cardiac pacemaker lead extraction using conventional techniques: a single centre experience. *Int J Cardiol*, Vol.91, No.2-3, (Oct 2003), pp.215-219, ISSN 0167-5273

Mazetti, H.; Cichero, CF.; Tentori, MC. & Mascheroni, O. (2008). Transjugular approach for lead extraction. *Europace*, Vol.10, No.2, (Feb 2008), pp. 156-160, ISSN 1099-5129

Meier-Ewert, HK.; Gray, ME. & John, RM. (2003). Endocardial pacemaker or defibrillator leads with infected vegetations: A single-center experience and consequences of transvenous extraction. *Am Heart J*, Vol.146, No.2, (Aug 2003), pp.339-344, ISSN 0002-8703

Mermel, LA.; Allon, M.; Bouza, E.; Craven, DE.; Flynn, P.; O'Grady, NP.; Raad, II.; Rijnders, BJ.; Sherertz, RJ. & Warren, DK. (2009). Clinical practice guidelines for the diagnosis and management of intravascular catheter-related infection: 2009 Update by the Infectious Diseases Society of America. *Clin Infect Dis*, Vol.49, No.1, (Jul 2009), pp.1-45, ISSN 1058-4838

Moon, MR.; Camillo, CJ. & Gleva, MJ. (2002). Laser-assist during extraction of chronically implanted pacemaker and defibrillator leads. *Ann Thorac Surg*, Vol.73, No.6, (Jun 2002), pp.1893-1896, ISSN 0003-4975

Murdoch, DR.; Corey, CR.; Hoen, B.; Miró, JM.; Fowler, VG.; Bayer, AS.; Karchmer, AW.; Olaison, L.; Pappas, Pa.; Moreillon, P.; Chambers, ST.; Chu, VH.; Falcó, V.; Holland, DJ.; Jones, P.; Klein, JL.; Raymond, NJ.; Read, KM.; Tripodi, MF.; Utili. R.; Wang, A.;

Woods, CW. & Cabell, CH. (2009). Clinical presentation, etiology and outcome of infective endocarditis in the 21st century: the International Collaboration on Endocarditis-Prospective Cohort Study. *Arch Intern Med*, Vol.169, No.5, (Mar 2009), pp.463-473, ISSN 0003-9926

Neuzil, P.; Taborsky, M.; Rezek, Z.; Vopalka, R.; Sediva, L.; Niederle, P. & Reddy, V. (2007). Pacemaker and ICD lead extraction with electrosurgical dissection sheaths and standard transvenous extraction Systems: results of a randomized trial. *Europace*, Vol.9, No.2, (Feb 2007), pp.98-104, ISSN 1099-5129

Parra-Ruiz, J.; Vidaillac, C.; Rose, WE. & Rybak, MJ. (2010). Activities of high-dose daptomycin, vancomycin, and moxifloxacin alone or in combination with clarithromycin or rifampin in a novel in vitro modes of Staphylococcus aureus biofilm. *Antimicrob Agents Chemother*, Vol.54, No.10, (Oct 2010), pp.4329-4334, ISSN 0066-4804

Perlroth, J.; Kuo, M.; Tan, J.; Bayer, A. & Miller, LG. (2008). Adjuntive use of rifampin for the treatment of Staphylococcus aureus infections: a systematic review of the literature. *Arch Inter Med*, Vol.168, No.8, (Apr 2008), pp.805-819, ISSN 0003-9926

Rodríguez-Baño, J.; De Cueto, M.; Retamar, P. & Gálvez-Acebal, J. (2010). Current management of bloodstream infections. *Expert Rev Anti Infect Ther*, Vol.8, No.7, (Jul 2010), pp.815-829, ISSN 1478-7210

Rodríguez-Martínez, JM. & Pascual, A. (2008). Actividad de los antimicrobianos en biocapas bacterianas. *Enferm Infecc Microbiol Clin*, Vol.26, No.2, (Feb 2008), pp.107-114, ISSN 0213-005X

Rohacek, M.; Wiesser, M.; Kobza, R.; Schoenenberger, AW.; Pfyffer, GE.; Frei, R.; Erne, P. & Trampuz, A. (2010). Bacterial colonization and infection of electrophysiological cardiac devices detected with sonication and swab culture. *Circulation*, Vol.121, No.15, (Apr 2010); 1691-1697, ISSN 0009-7322

Rosenheck, S.; Weiss, A.; Leibowitz, D. & Sharon, Z. (2002). Noninstrumental pacemaker and defibrillator lead removal. The importance of the rotation forces. *Pacing Clin Electrophysiol*, Vol.25, No.7, (July 2002), pp. 1029-1036, ISSN 0147-8389

Rusanov, A. & Spotnitz, HM. (2010). A 15-year experience with permanent pacemaker and defibrillator lead and patch extractions. *Ann Thorac Surg*, Vol.89, No.1, (Jan 2010), pp.44-50, ISSN 0003-4975

Rybak, MJ.; Lomaestro, BM.; Rotschafer, JC.; Moellering, RC.; Craig, WA.; Billeter, M.; Dalovisio, JR. & Levine, DP. (2009). Vancomycin therapeutic guidelines: a summary of consensus recommendations from the infectious diseases Society of America, the American Society of Health-System Pharmacists, and the Society of Infectious Diseases Pharmacists. *Clin Infect Dis*, Vol.49, No.3, (Aug 2009), pp.325-327, ISSN 1058-4838

Satsu, T. & Onoe, M. (2010). Vacuum-assisted wound closure for pacemaker infection. *Pacing Clin Electrophysiol*, Vol.33, No.4, (April 2010), pp. 426-430, ISSN 0147-8389

Smith, HJ.; Fearnot, NE.; Byrd, CL.; Wilkoff, BL.; Love, CJ. & Sellers, TD. (1994). Five-years experience with intravascular lead extraction. U.S. Lead Extraction

Database. *Pacing Clin Electrophysiol*, Vol.17, No.11, (Nov 1994), pp. 2016-2020, ISSN 0147-8389

Sohail, MR.; Uslan, DZ.; Khan, AH.; Friedman, PA.; Hayes, DL.; Wilson, WR.; Steckelberg, JM.; Stoner, S. & Baddour, LM. (2007) Risk factor analysis of permanent pacemaker infection. *Clin Infect Dis*, Vol.45, No.2, (Jul 2007), pp.166-173, ISSN 1058-4838

Sohail, MR.; Uslan, DZ.; Khan, AH.; Friedman, PA.; Hayes, DL.; Wilson, WR.; Steckelberg, JM.; Stoner, S. & Baddour, LM. (2007). Management and outcome of permanent pacemaker and implantable cardioverter-defibrillator infections. *J Am Coll Cardiol*, Vol.49, No.18, (May 2007), pp.1851-1859, ISSN 0735-1097

Sohail, MR.; Uslan, DZ.; Khan, AH.; Friedman, PA.; Hayes, DL.; Wilson, WR.; Steckelberg, JM.; Jenkins, SM. & Baddour, LM. (2008). Infective endocarditis complicating permanent pacemaker and implantable cardioverter-defibrillator infection. *Mayo Clin Proc*; Vol.83, No.1, (Jan 2008), pp.46-53, ISSN 0025-6196

Soriano, A.; Marco, F.; Martínez, JA. Pisos, E.; Almela, M.; Dimova, VP.; Alamo, D.; Ortega, M.; Lopez, J. & Mensa, J. (2008). Influence of vancomycin minimum inhibitory concentration on the treatment of methicillin-resistant Staphylococcus aureus bacteremia. *Clin Infect Dis*, Vol.46, No.2, (Jan 2008), pp.193-200, ISSN 1058-4838

Uslan, DZ.; Sohail, MR.; St Sauver, JL.; Friedman, PA.; Hayes, DL.; Stoner, SM.; Wilson, WR.; Steckelberg, JM. & Baddour, LM. (2007). Permanent pacemaker and implantable cardioverter defibrillator infection: a population-based study. *Arch Inter Med*, Vol.167, No.7, (Apr 2007), pp.669-675, ISSN 0003-9926

Verma, A. & Wilkoff, BL. (2004). Intravascular pacemaker and defibrillator lead extraction: A state-of-the-art review. *Heart Rhythm*, Vol.1, No.6, (Dec 2004), pp. 739-744, ISSN 1556-3871

Victor, F.; De Place, C.; Camus, C.; Le Bretton, H.; Leclercq, C.; Pavin, D.; Mabo, P. & Daubert, C. (1998). Pacemaker lead infection: echocardiographic features, management, and outcome. *Heart*, Vol.81, No.1, (Jan 1998), pp.82-87, ISSN 1355-6037

Vila, J.; Soriano, A. & Mensa, J. (2008). Bases moleculares de la adherencia microbiana sobre los materiales protésicos. Papel de las biocapas en las infecciones asociadas a los materiales protésicos. *Enferm Infecc Microbiol Clin*, Vol.26, No.1, (Jan 2008), pp.48-55, ISSN 0213-005X

Voigt, A.; Shalaby, A. & Saba, S. (2009). Continued rise in rates of cardiovascular implantable electronic device infections in the United States: temporal trends and causative insights. *Pacing Clin Electrophysiol*, Vol.33, No.4, (Apr 2009), pp.414-419, ISSN 0147-8389

Wazni, O.; Epstein, LM.; Carrillo, RG.; Love, C.; Adler, SW.; Riggio, DW.; Karim, SS.; Bashir, J.; Greenspon, AJ.; DiMarco, Jp.; Cooper, JM.; Onufer, JR.; Ellenbogen, KA.; Kutalek, SP.; Dentry-Mabry, S.; Ervin, CM. & Wilkoff, BL. (2010). Lead extraction in the contemporary setting: the LExICon study. *JACC*, Vol.55, No.6, (Feb 2010), pp. 579-586, ISSN 0735-1097

Wilkoff, BL.; Byrd, CL.; Love, CJ.; Hayes, DL.; Sellers, TD.; Schaerf, R.; Parsonnet, V.; Epstein, LM.; Sorrentino, RA. & Reiser, C. (1999). Pacemaker lead extraction with the laser sheath: results of the Pacing Lead Extraction With the Excimer Sheath (PLEXES) Trial. *JACC*, Vol.33, No.6, (June 1999), pp.1671-1676, ISSN 0735-1097

8

Infections of Cardiac Implantable Electronic Devices: Etiology, Prevention and Treatment

Cosimo Chelazzi, Valentina Selmi,
Luca Vitali and Angelo Raffaele De Gaudio
Department of Medical and Surgical Critical Care,
Section of Anesthesiology and Intensive Care,
University of Florence, Azienda Ospedaliero-Universitaria Careggi
Italy

1. Introduction

Since the initial use of prosthetic heart valves, the use of cardiac prosthesis and implantable devices has revolutionized the therapeutic options available to patients (de Oliveira et al.,2009). Cardiac Permanent PaceMakers (PPMs) have been implanted since the early 1960s. Over the past 50 years there have been tremendous advances in both the design of the device and the software employed. In the mid 1960s, transvenous leads were developed that could be inserted through a vein and thence into the heart, thus preventing the need for a thoracotomy. The development of 'active fixation' leads ensured a better contact with the endocardium and the presence of a steroid eluting tip helped to reduce any inflammation that might result. The introduction of the lithium iodine battery has dramatically increased the battery life to well over ten years. Radiofrequency programming became available in the 1970s, allowing simple adjustments to be made to pacemaker's settings without the need for surgery. Today, permanent pacemakers and ICD (Implantable Cardiac Defibrillator), together with any adjustments, can be completed within minutes using a portable computer. Information regarding events such as periods of bradycardia, tachycardia or ventricular fibrillation can be stored within the memory of the device and accessed by the specialist during the routine checkup. To maintain atrio-ventricular synchrony, dual chamber pacing was then introduced. Moreover, in the late 1990s, pacemaker technology had improved to the extent that it became possible to increase the pacing rate to match the patient's activity level (Allen et al., 2007).

A wide range of cardiac implantable electronic devices (CIEDs) are now available, including ICDs and cardiac resynchronization systems. PPMs are commonly used in patients with atrioventricular conduction block, sick sinus syndrome, and symptomatic sinus bradycardia, whereas ICDs target primarily patients at risk for life-threatening ventricular arrhythmias.

Since clinical trials have consistently demonstrated the ability of the ICD to reduce mortality in selected patients with moderate-to-severe left ventricular systolic dysfunction, the indications for CIEDs have expanded dramatically and the rate of implantation has greatly rosen. A recent analysis showed that rate of implantation in US between 1997 and 2004 rose by 19% and 60% for PPMs and ICDs, respectively. Approximately 70% of device recipients were 65 years of age or older, and more than 75% of them had one or more coexisting illnesses. The rate of ICD implantation has increased in the elderly (70 to 79 years of age) and very elderly (80 years of age or older). The 2001 World Survey found that in developed countries, between 20% and 35% of CIED recipients were more than 80 years old. The National Hospital Discharge Survey found a 49% increase in the number of new CIED implantations, including both PPMs and ICDs. In 2003, although the absolute number of PPMs implantations was higher than that of ICDs (180284 versus 57436 implanted devices) most of the increase in CIED device implantation was due to ICD implantations (160% and 31% increases in ICD and PPM implantations, respectively) (Baddour et al., 2010).

Despite their unquestioned clinical importance and diffusion, CIEDs may be linked to several complications, including infections, and the consequences of them may be catastrophic. Therefore, development of strategies for the prevention of device associated infections is crucial (Borer et al., 2004).

The reported rate of infection after implantation of permanent endocardial devices ranges between 0.13% and 12.6%, depending on definition. The wide use of CIEDs and increasing age of patients set the stage for higher role of associated infections and related hospitalizations increased of about 3-fold (Baddour et al., 2010). Moreover, the cost of treating device-associated infections may be enormous, thus leading to increased healthcare expenses (Borer et al., 2004). Precise data regarding the actual healthcare burden of CIED infections are not available. The financial impact is due to multiple factors, including the costs of device removal, cost of new device (which would be required in the majority of patients) and costs related to cardiac and other medical evaluations, diagnostic procedures, surgical interventions for infected device removal, medical therapy, and increased length of stay in intensive care unit (Baddour et al., 2010).

2. Epidemiology of CIED associated infections

CIED infections have been recognized as a source of major comorbidity since the early 1970s. In earlier years, the rates of PPM infection ranged widely between 0.13% and 19.9%. Although most infections have been limited to the pocket, frank PPM endocarditis accounted for approximately 10% of PPM infections. The decreased size of ICDs allowed implantation without thoracotomy. Initially, abdominal implantation with tunneling was required. Subsequently, the entire device could be implanted prepectorally; with these less extensive operations the infection rate lowered to less than 7%. In a study on all ICD primary implantations, replacements, and revisions at a single center, there were 21 ICD-related infections (1.2%) among 1700 procedures. Among 959 patients with long-term follow-up, the infection rate was 3.2% with abdominal and 0.5% with pectoral systems respectively (Mela et al., 2001). However, globally, the rate of CIED infection has been increasing. Cabell et al. reported that the rate of cardiac device infections (PPMs, ICDs, valves, and ventricular assist devices) increased from 0.94 to 2.11 per 1000 patients between 1990 and 1999, a 124% increase during the study period. The rate of frank endocarditis was relatively unchanged (0.26 and 0.39 cases/1000 patients, respectively) (Cabell et al., 2004). These findings were similar to that analyzed in Olmsted County,

Minnesota, from 1975 to 2004. A total of 1524 patients were included with a total person-time follow-up of 7578 years. The incidence of CIED infection was 1.9/1000 device years (95% confidence interval [CI] 1.1 to 3.1), with an incidence of pocket infection alone of 1.37/1000 device-years (95% CI 0.62 to 0.75) and an incidence of pocket infection with bloodstream infection or device-related endocarditis of 1.14/1000 device-years (95% CI 0.47 to 2.74) (Uslan et al., 2007). Notably, the cumulative probability of CIED infection was higher among patients with ICDs than among those with PPMs. The National Hospital Discharge Survey similarly showed that between 1996 and 2003, the number of hospitalizations for CIED infections increased 3.1-fold (2.8-fold for PPMs and 6.0-fold for ICDs). The numbers of CIED infection–related hospitalizations increased out of proportion to rates of new device implantation. Moreover, CIED infection increased the risk of in-hospital death by more than 2-fold (Voigt et al., 2006).

3. Definition and clinical presentation

CIED pocket infection is defined on the ground of signs and symptoms of local infection associated with microbiological confirmation based on results of cultures of intraoperatively collected fluid samples, explanted CIED, or purulent discharge from the pocket site. CIED infection can present as acute or chronic syndromes that can be both early or tardive. In the early, acute form, the short time elapsed between device implantation and occurrence of infection may prompt the diagnosis. In chronic and tardive infections there is often a delay between the onset of symptoms and the diagnosis. This may be due to the fact that CIED-related infections are not routinely considered in the differential diagnosis. In other cases, possible clues to the diagnosis are ignored. Clinical manifestations of pacemaker infection are linked to the portion of the device involved. Moreover, signs and symptoms may be limited to the insertion pocket or be systemic or absent altogether (Cacoub et al,. 1998).

A CIED-related infection is considered nosocomial when occurs 48 hours after admission and is not incubating at the time of admission. Infection of CIED is regarded as health care associated if patient received intravenous therapy at home, attended an outpatient hemodialysis center in the previous 30 days, was hospitalized in an acute care hospital for 2 days in the 90 days before admission, or resided in a nursing home or long-term care facility. In contrast, CIED-related infection is recognized as community acquired if it does not fit the above definitions (Tablan et al., 2003).

3.1 Clinical presentation

In the vast majority of cases, local inflammation of the generator-pocket site is present, including erythema (34%), pain (32%), swelling (21%), warmth (11.5%), and drainage through a fistulous or poorly healed incision (25%). In most severe cases cutaneous erosion (23%) with percutaneous exposure of the generator and/or leads may be seen. All these signs can be associated or not with bacteremia (Cacoub et al,. 1998). These local changes usually prompt medical attention. Some patients present with systemic symptoms that include malaise, fatigue, anorexia, or decreased functional capacity. Sometimes isolated local symptoms occurr without fever. Chua et al. reported the presence of localized signs without systemic involvement in 69% (88 of 123) of patients, a combination of local and systemic signs and symptoms in 20% (25 of 123), and systemic signs and symptoms alone in

11% (13 of 123) of patients (Chua et al., 2000). In implanted patients with unexplained fever CIED associated endocarditis should be ruled out. In CIED recipient isolated bacteremia pro,t medical investigation to rolu out endocarditis. Pacemaker endocarditis should be considered in all patients with cardiac pacemakers and chronic fever, recurrent bronchitis, pulmonary infection, and recurrent or persistent pocket infection (Cacoub et al., 1998; Klug et al., 1997). In some patients, involvement of lungs may be evident, including pleural effusions, pneumonia, pulmonary abscess, recurrent pulmonary embolism. Recurrent bronchitis is evident in 32% to 43% of patients with pacemaker endocarditis. A serious complication of pacemaker infection is generator or lead erosion through the skin. This can be the consequence of primary infection or can be the result of pressure on the overlying tissue, resulting in erosion and subsequent contamination. Erosion has been noted to be more common after elective pacemaker replacement than initial implantation (Harcombe et al., 1998). Other rare conditions associated to CIED infections are thrombosis of a vein where leads were in place (subclavian vein or superior vena cava), symptomatic pulmonary embolism, septic arthritis, vertebral, sternal or femoral osteomyelitis, splenic, brain, liver and perinephric abscess (Sohail et al., 2007a).

4. Pathophysiology

4.1 Etiology

In patients with pacemaker infection bacterial pathogens can be found in blood or pacemaker pockets. Pacemaker's hardware can be colonized as well. The most common pathogens in pocket infections are skin flora, and, specifically, Staphylococcus aureus and coagulase-negative staphylococci, including Staphylococcus epidermidis. Rarely, enteric Gram-negative bacilli can be found. Repeated cultures and percutaneous aspirates should help make the distinction between normal skin flora and pathogenic culture isolates (Gandelman at al., 2007).

Staphylococcal species cause most of CIED infections and account for 60%-80% of cases in most reported series (Fig.1). A variety of coagulase-negative Staphylococcus (CoNS) species have been described a causative agents of CIED infections. CoNS are a common cause of microbiological specimen contamination, and thus, repeated isolation of the same species of CoNS with an identical antibiotic susceptibility pattern is advisable to be diagnostic. Polymicrobial infection sometimes involves more than one species of CoNS. The prevalence of oxacillin resistance among staphylococcal strains has varied among studies ranging from 4 to 22% (Sohail et al., 2007a; Viola et al., 2010).

Several factors are responsible for the higher propensity of Staphylococci to cause CIED infections. Staphylococci are frequent colonizer of human skin and contamination of CIED generator, electrode leads or pocket tissue at the time of implantation is the predominant mechanism for the majority of the pocket infections. Staphylococci express on their membranes several adherence factors that enable them to bind the foreign materials and establish chronic infection. In addition, these organisms are capable of producing biofilm on the device surface which helps them to evade host defences and limit antimicrobial penetration. Finally, Staphylococci are the predominant pathogens responsible for secondary catheter-related bloodstream infections as they can seed the intravenous leads during an episode of bacteremia.

Corynebacterium species, Propionibacterium acnes, Gram-negative bacilli, including Pseudomonas aeruginosa, and Candida species account for a minority of CIED infections. Fungi other than Candida and nontuberculosis mycobacteria are rarely responsible for CIED infection (Sohail et al., 2010).

The microorganisms that cause CIED infections may be acquired either endogenously from the skin of patients or exogenously from the hospital environment. An association has been found between the presence of preaxillary skin flora and the pathogens isolated from pacemaker infection. Although low concentrations of methicillin-resistant CoNS have been detected in patients with no previous healthcare contact and no recent antibiotic exposure, a CIED infection due to multidrug-resistant staphylococci suggests that a healthcare environment is the site where infection was acquired (Da Costa et al., 1998a).

Pacemaker endocarditis usually presents with bacterial growth in both blood and hardware cultures. Although there is no uniform agreement regarding the rate of positive blood cultures in pacemaker endocarditis, S. epidermidis and S. aureus occur most frequently. Other pathogens include Corynebacterium sp., Pseudomonas aeruginosa, and Aspergillus niger. In one study, polymicrobial infections were found in 18.1% (Cacoub et al., 1998).

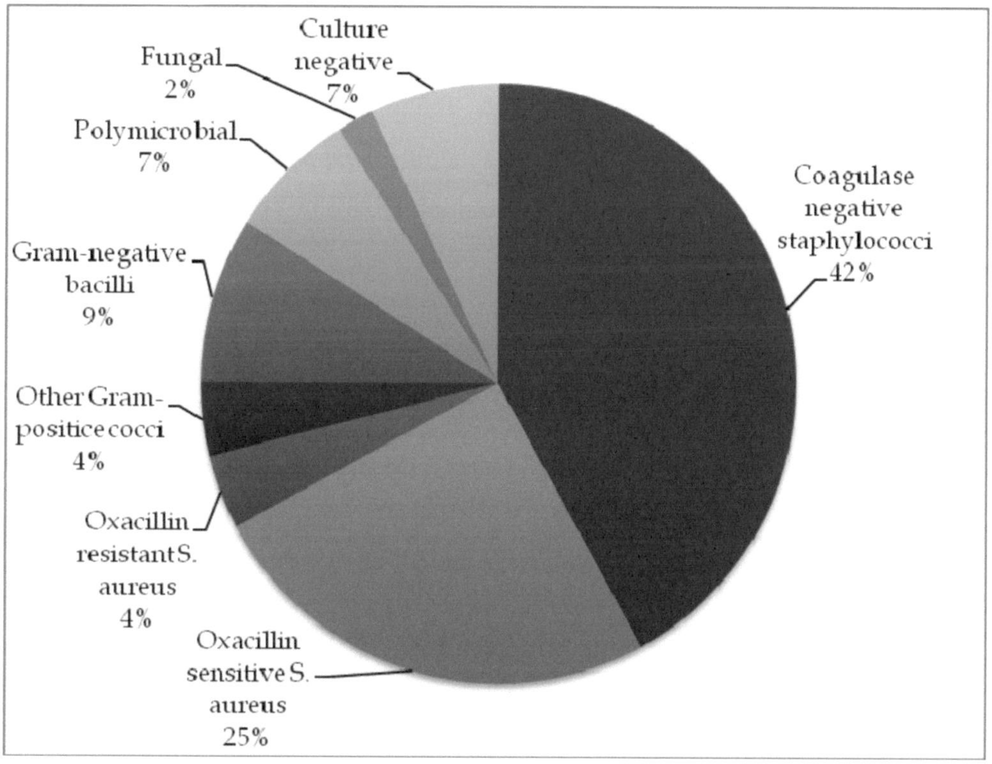

Fig. 1. Microbiology of CIED infection. Modified from Baddour et al., 2010.

4.2 Pathogenesis

The generator is placed within a surgically created space known as pocket. Electrode leads are attached to the generator and travel within the venous system to the right heart.

Pacemaker infection can be limited to the superficial portion of the pocket and leads or involve deeper intravascular and intracardiac components. The latter is known as pacemaker endocarditis. Among patients with pacemaker endocarditis, vegetations can occur on the tricuspid valve, the electrodes, and the right atrial or ventricular endocardium.

The pocket may become infected at the time of implantation, during subsequent surgical manipulation, or if the generator or subcutaneous electrodes erode the overlying skin. In this latter case, erosion can also occur as a secondary event due to underlying infection. Pacemaker endocarditis can be linked to several factors, including pacemaker lead contamination during placement, spread of the organisms along the wires from the superficial component, or hematogenous seeding of the intravascular electrodes and wires during a bacteriemic episode. While Gram-posivie bacteriamias can cause CIED infections, hematogenous seeding of a CIED is unlikely to occur in cases of Gram-negative bacteremia. The disruption of the physiologic blood flow through the tricuspid valve often caused by a pacing lead passing through the valve and associated regurgitation may contribute to pacemaker infection. Microbial adherence to endothelium has been shown to increase in areas of high shear turbulence (Baddour et al., 2010).

CIED infection is the result of the interaction between the device, the microbe, and the host.

4.2.1 Devices factors

Initial adhesion of bacteria to the device is mediated by physico-chemical properties of the plastic surface, such as hydrophobicity, surface tension, and electrostatic charge.

Factors like the nature of plastic polymer, irregularity of its surface, and its shape, can all affect bacterial adherence to the device. Plastic polymers that encase medical devices, as well as the pathogens that adhere to them, are hydrophobic. An irregularly surfaced device favours microbial adherence more than a smoothed surfaced one. When this physiochemical interaction exists, the risk of CEID infection is related to subsequent invasive manipulation of the device and may be linked to a limited experience of the physician performing the procedure (Darouiche, 2001).

4.2.2 Microbial factors

Bacteria, particularly Gram-positive cocci, can adhere to and be engulfed by endothelial cells that lie on endothelialized lead after a certain period of time. This is thought to be an important mechanism of device infection by the hematogenous route.

Microbial adherence may be linked also to interactions of bacterial surface with proteins on device's surface. CoNS may adhere directly to plastic polymers of the surface of the device via fimbria-like surface protein structures or via a capsular polysaccharide (Veenstra et al., 1996). Bacteria may also adhere to host matrix proteins that coat the surface of an implanted device. Host extracellular matrix proteins include fibrinogen, fibronectin, and collagen that are layered on implanted biomaterials. None of the major virulence factors or toxins of S Aureus have been found in CoNS, and it seems clear that the development and persistence of CoNS infections, which are so often associated with foreign materials, are due to different mechanisms, such as microbiological adherence. On the contrary, Staphylococci have a variety of surface adhesins that allow the pathogen to establish a focus of infection. Subsequent accumulation of bacteria on the device's surface requires the production of polysaccharide intercellular adhesin, which is strongly linked to with the staphylococcal cell surface and mediates cell-to-cell adhesion. The layers of bacteria on the surface of an implanted device are encased in this extracellular slime and constitute a biofilm. Biofilm is defined as a surface-associated community of one or more microbial species that are firmly attached to each other and the solid surface and are encased in an extracellular polymeric matrix that holds the biofilm together. Bacteria in a biofilm are more resistant to antibiotics and host defences, perhaps as a result of the dense extracellular matrix that protects the microbes included in the interior of the community (Lazăr & Chifiriuc, 2010). When a free-floating bacterial cell enters the biofilm, it undergoes a phenotypic shift, in which expression of large groups of genes is up-regulated. Phenotypic variation is thought to support the persistence of infection due to staphylococci in a biofilm that coats the surface of a CIED. Small colony variants are phenotypes that have caused CIED infections and harbor several characteristics that are thought to enhance the survival of staphylococci either in a biofilm or in endothelial cells covering the device, including resistance to certain antibiotics (Baddour et al., 1990; Boelens et al., 2000).

4.3 Risk factors

Several studies have identified host or procedural factors that may be associated with CIED infections.

Among the host factors, the strongest association is between renal failure and risk of CIED infection. Risk of device infection appears to be particularly high in patient with end-stage renal failure who are undergoing chronic hemodialysis via an implanted central catheter. These patients are at risk of recurrent bacteremia from their dialysis catheter and subsequent secondary seeding of the tranvenous device leads or pulse generator. Renal failure is also associated with immune dysfunction that further increases the odd of CIED infections in these patients (Bloom et al.,2006).

Anticoagulant therapy with warfarin has also been linked to a higher risk of CIED infection. Precise reasons for this association are unclear but are likely related to the increased risk of pocket hematoma, which may lead to delayed wound healing or need for surgical drainage in some cases. Reopening the pocket to drain a large hematoma increases the risk of pocket contamination with skin flora and subsequent CIED infection (Lekkerkerker et al., 2009).

Use of immunosuppressive medications, especially long term corticosteroids therapy, has also been identified as a risk factor for CIED infections (Sohail et al., 2007b).

Procedure-related factors may also play an important role in the development of CIED infections. In a prospective cohort of 6319 patients receiving CIED implantation in 44 medical centers, Klug et al. identified 42 patients who developed CIED infection during 1 year of follow-up. Factors associated with an increased risk of infection included fever within 24 hours before implantation, use of preprocedural temporary pacing, and early reintervention. Implantation of a new system compared with partial or complete system replacement and use of periprocedural antimicrobial prophylaxis were both associated with a lower risk of infection (Klug et al., 2007). There is evidence that perioperative antimicrobial prophylaxis is associated with a reduction in CIED infections (Bertaglia et al., 2006; Da Costa et al., 1998b; de Oliveira et al., 2009).

Other small studies suggest that pectoral transvenous device placement is associated with significantly lower rates of CIED infection than those implanted abdominally or by

thoracotomy. Thus, the use of a pectoral approach is not only less invasive but also appears to confer an ancillary benefit of lower infection risk (Mela et al., 2001).
Physician experience in CIED implantation may also play a role in the rate of subsequent CIED infection. In a study of Medicare administrative data, Al-Khatib et al. found a significantly higher risk of ICD infection within 90 days of device implantation in patients whose device was placed by physicians in the lowest quartile of implantation volume. Rates of mechanical complications at 90 days were also higher for lower-volume physicians (Al-Khatib et al., 2005).

5. Diagnosis

5.1 Clinical and microbiological diagnosis

In all patients with suspected CIED infection diagnosis is linked to both local and systemic signs of inflammation associated to positive microbiological culture of the skin pocket or other materials. Signs and symptoms of systemic inflammation include malaise, fever with or without chill, leucocytosis and, in most severe cases, hypotension. A new onset valvular murmur suggests CIED endocarditis. Local signs of infection include redness and oedema and pain of the skin pocket.
Definitive diagnosis of CIED infection is linked to microbiological cultures. Usually, samples are taken from the generator pocket. Alternatively, once the device has been removed, samples from lead tips may be cultured to identify the causative organism and support a diagnosis of CIED infection. Gram staining, anaerobic and aerobic bacterial cultures, should all be performed. If the initial Gram stain is negative, both tissue and the lead tip should be cultured for fungi and mycobacteria. Percutaneous aspiration of the device pocket is not recommended because of its low diagnostic accuracy and the theoretical risk of introducing microorganisms into the pocket site or spreading germ into the blood stream. Contamination of leads may also occur at the time of their extraction throught a contamined skin pocket; this may explain some of the positive lead-tip cultures found in patients without systemic manifestation and with negative blood cultures. If a CIED-related endocarditis is suspected, at least two sets of blood cultures should be obtained before starting any antimicrobial therapy. Positive blood cultures, particularly due to staphylococcal species, provide a strong clue that the clinical syndrome is due to CIED infection (Baddour et al., 2010).

5.2 Instrumental diagnosis

5.2.1 Transthoracic and transesophageal echocardiography

Endocarditis is clinically confirmed when valvular or lead neostructures consistent with vegetations are detected on echocardiography, or if the Duke criteria for infective endocarditis are met (Table 1)(Klug et al., 1997, Durak et al. 1994). Vegetation is defined as an oscillating intracardiac mass which can be seen on the electrodes, the leads or the cardiac valve leaflets. To be diagnostic, vegetation should be noted in more than one echocardiographic plane (Klug et al., 1997; Sanfilippo et al., 1991; Victor et al., 1999). Both transtoracic echocardiography (TTE) and transesophageal echocardiography (TEE) may be employed, even though TEE is more accurate and is the actual gold standard.

Definite infective endocarditis	
Pathological criteria	
Microorganisms: demonstrated by culture or histology in vegetation, in a vegetation that has embolized, or in intracardiac abscess, or demonstrated by culture of the lead	
Clinical criteria	
Two major criteria, or one major and three minor criteria, or five minor criteria	
Major criteria	
	Positive blood culture for infective endocarditis
	Typical microorganisms for infective endocarditis from two separate blood cultures
	Streptococcus viridans, *Streptococcus bovis*, HACEK group, or
	Community-acquired *Staphylococcus aureus* or enterococci, in the absence of a primary focus, or
	Persistently positive blood culture, defined as microorganism consistent with infective endocarditis from
	Blood cultures drawn >12 hours apart, or
	All of three or a majority of four or more separate blood cultures, with first and last drawn at least 1 hour apart
	Evidence of endocardial involvement:
	Positive echocardiogram for infective endocarditis:
	Oscillating intracardiac mass on PM leads or on the endocardial structure in contact with PM leads
	Abscess in contact with PM leads
Minor criteria	
	Fever >38°C
	Vascular phenomena: arterial embolism, septic pulmonary infarcts, mycotic aneurysm, intracranial hemorrhage, Janeway lesions
	Immunologic phenomena: glomerulonephritis, Osler nodes, Roth spots
	Echocardiogram: consistent with infective endocarditis but not meeting major criterion as noted previously (sleevelike appearance)
	Microbiological evidence: positive blood culture but not meeting major criterion as noted previously

Table 1. Diagnostic criteria for infective endocarditis. Modified from Durak et al., 1994.

TTE is not helpful in ruling out a diagnosis of lead-related endocarditis, particularly in adults, due to its poor sensitivity. Moreover, patients can develop both right-sided (lead-related) and left-sided endocarditis. Actually, sensitivity of TTE for left-sided and for perivalvular extension of infection is lower than TEE. On the contrary several indirect echocardiographic features of endocarditis may be better seen with TEE. They include pericardial effusion, ventricular dysfunction or dyssynchrony, and pulmonary vascular pressure estimations. TEE may be not always available and can be discomfortable for the patients. For these reasons, even if TEE rapresents the gold standard for the diagnosis of CIED infections, and is recommended for the initial diagnosis, TTE can be used during the course of patient's illness for additional studies or follow-up. It is important to underlyine that an echocardiographyc image of a mass adherent to the lead may be a sterile thrombus or infected vegetation and it is impossible to distinguish between the two with echocardiography. Masses that are detected in patients without positive blood cultures or other signs of infection are likely to sterile vegetation (thrombus). In addition, the failure to visualize a mass adherent to a lead with TEE does not exclude lead infection. Thus, even when vegetation is demonstrated, differential diagnosis may be difficult if microbiological culture are not positive. Clear guidelines for CIED infection diagnosis are lacking. Based on clinical practice and expert opinion, a summary of recommendations for diagnosis of CIED infections is provided in Table 2.

Class I
1. All patients should have at least 2 sets of blood cultures drawn at the initial evaluation before initiation of antimicrobial therapy. (Level of Evidence: C)
2. Generator-pocket tissue Gram's stain and culture and lead-tip culture should be obtained when the CIED is explanted. (Level of Evidence: C)
3. Patients with suspected CIED infection who either have positive blood cultures or who have negative blood cultures but have had recent antimicrobial therapy before blood cultures were obtained should undergo TEE for CIED infection or valvular endocarditis. (Level of Evidence: C)
4. All adults suspected of having CIED-related endocarditis should undergo TEE to evaluate the left-sided heart valves, even if transthoracic views have demonstrated lead-adherent masses. In pediatric patients with good views, transthoracic echocardiography may be sufficient. (Level of Evidence: B)
Class IIa
Patients should seek evaluation for CIED infection by cardiologists or infectious disease specialists if they develop fever or bloodstream infection for which there is no initial explanation. (Level of Evidence: C)
Class III
Percutaneous aspiration of the generator pocket should not be performed as part of the diagnostic evaluation of CIED infection. (Level of Evidence: C)

Table 2. Recommendations for Diagnosis of CIED Infection and Associated Complications. Modified from Baddour et al., 2010.

5.2.2 Positive Emission Tomography (PET)

Infection staging and identification of other septic locations may be very important in order to monitor treatment efficacy before any re-implantation. It might be useful to assess the extension of infectious disease (staging) in these patients by non-invasive whole-body imaging, and Fluoro-18 desoxyglucose (18F-FDG) PET is a potential candidate for this purpose. The use of 18F-FDG PET imaging in inflammatory processes is related to the high affinity of inflammatory cells such as neutrophils, lymphocytes and macrophage for 18F-FDG. 18F-FDG PET shows high diagnostic accuracy when infection affects the box of generator but is slightly less reliable when the leads are involved. Globally, sensitivity and specificity are optimal for box infection even if mild physiological uptake may be seen in normal cases. Physiologically, a slight 18F-FDG uptake may be observed around the box even in not infected patients, particularly in the area of the muscle interface. However, uptake around the box is much higher in case of infection. Leads infection represents a different challenge. The size of the leads and the size of the vegetation are both very small and may easily be below the theoretical resolution of the PET system. For leads, sensitivity and specificity are lower, and diagnosis is based upon visualization of mild focal uptake along the leads. Interpretation of negative cases should be cautious, particularly if patients have received prolonged antibiotherapy (Bensimhon et al., 2010).

6. Prevention

The significant morbidity and mortality associated with device infections and the need for device removal make prevention of infections extremely important. Prevention of CIED infection can be addressed before, during, and after device implantation. Before implanting intravascular devices, it is important to ensure that patients do not have clinical signs of infection. In this case definitive implantation should be posponed after the resolution of infection. Once CIEDs are implanted, both pharmacological and non pharmacological strategies can be adopted in order to reduce risk of infection.

6.1 Pharmacological strategies

A meta-analysis of 7 randomized studies on 2023 patients examining the impact of systemic antibiotics on the risk of pacemaker-related infections suggested that systemic antibiotic prophylaxis significantly reduces the incidence of serious infective complications after pacemaker implantation (Da Costa et al., 1998b). A following observational study was performed to assess the safety and long-term efficacy of a simple scheme of antibiotic prophylaxis, and to identify the predictors of long-term infective complications in patients undergoing pacemaker implantation or replacement. This study showed the efficacy of a single dose of cefazolin in preventing infective complications (Bertaglia et al., 2006). Finally a prospective, randomized, double-blinded, placebo-controlled trial was developed to determine whether prophylactic antibiotic administration reduces the incidence of infection related to device implantation was. This double blinded study included 1000 consecutive patients who presented for primary device implantation or generator replacement randomized in a 1:1 fashion to prophylactic antibiotics or placebo. Intravenous administration of 1 g of cefazolin or placebo was done immediately before the procedure. Follow-up was performed at 10 days and 1, 3, and 6 months after discharge. The primary end point was any evidence of infection at the surgical incision (pulse generator pocket), or systemic infection related to the procedure. The safety committee interrupted the trial after 649 patients were enrolled because of a significant difference in favor of the antibiotic arm and concluded that antibiotic prophylaxis significantly reduces infectious complications in patients undergoing implantation of pacemakers or cardioverter-defibrillators (de Oliveira et al., 2009). Most experts continue to advocate a first-generation cephalosporin, such as cefazolin, as prophylaxis agent. Although not generally recommended, some authors advocate the use of vancomycin, particularly in centers where oxacillin resistance among staphylococci is high. If vancomycin is used, then it should be administered 90 to 120 minutes before the procedure. Vancomycin also represents an alternative to a first-generation cephalosporin in patients who are allergic to cephalosporins (Sohail et al., 2007b). In patients who are allergic to both cephalosporins and vancomycin, daptomycin and linezolid are alternative agents for prophylaxis. Antibiotic prophylaxis is also recommended if subsequent invasive manipulation of the CIED is required. Currently, there are no data to support the administration of postoperative antibiotic therapy, and this is not recommended because of the risk of drug adverse events, selection of drug-resistant organisms, and costs (Baddour et al., 2010).

6.2 Non pharmacological strategies

Several preventive measures are recommended in combination with prophylactic antibiotics. Using a strictly aseptic technique during implantation is of paramount importance, including surgical scrubbing, use of standard operating room, facemasks, caps, and sterile gowns and gloves, and the use of sterile, dry gauze pads to cover surgical incisions (Voet et al., 1999). Other preventive strategies include to limit the duration of temporary pacing to the shortest time and to limit the number of people in the room during the procedure to those absolutely necessary. Prevention of hematoma during the procedure is important, and several interventions have been used, although there are no data to support their use (Lekkerkerker et al., 2009). This can be achieved by meticulous cauterization of bleeding sites and packing the pocket with antibiotic-soaked sponges to provide tamponade while leads are being placed. The application of topical thrombin may be helpful, particularly in anticoagulated patients. Irrigation of the pocket is useful to remove debris and may reveal persistent bleeding that could lead to a pocket hematoma. In addition, irrigation with an antimicrobial-containing solution for pocket cleansing has been used. Use of monofilament suture for closure of the subcuticular layer may avoid superficial postoperative cellulitis. A compressive dressing applied 12-24 hours after skin closure may further decrease the risk of hematoma formation. In the immediate postoperative period, recent data indicate that low-molecular-weight heparin predisposes to hematoma formation and should be avoided (Robinson et al., 2009). A hematoma should be evacuated only when there is increased tension on the skin. Needle aspiration should otherwise be avoided because of the risk of introducing skin flora into the pocket and subsequent development of infection. Finally, routine ambulatory care follow-up after CIED placement to detect early infectious complications has been performed in many centers and this is actively recommended (Deuling et al., 2009).

7. Therapy

7.1 Conservative treatment

Optimal management of CIED infection depends on the clinical presentation and causative pathogen. Conservative treatment with antibiotics alone without removal of the device may be sufficient in patients with local signs without sepsis, endocarditis or skin erosion. Seven to ten days of antibiotic therapy with an oral agent with activity against staphylococci is reasonable (Gandelman et al., 2007).

7.2 Device removal

Complete removal of all hardware is the recommended treatment for patients with established CIED infection or sepsis (Chua et al., 2000; Sohail et al., 2007a). This includes cases in which a localized pocket infection occurs in the absence of signs of systemic infection. Complete removal of hardware is needed because infection relapse rates due to retained hardware are high (Field et al., 2007). Erosion of any part of the CIED should imply contamination of the entire system, including the intravascular portion of leads, and complete device removal should be performed. Complete CIED removal should be performed when patients undergo valve replacement or repair for infective endocarditis, because the CIED could serve as a nidus for relapsing infection and subsequent seeding of the surgically treated heart valve. An epicardial system should be considered if a new CIED is required after valve surgery with initial CIED removal. Device removal is also recommended in those patients with S. aureus bacteremia with clinical or echocardiographic evidence of CEID infection, un-explained bacteremia, or relapsing bacteremia after antibiotic treatment (Chamis et al., 2001).

7.2.1 Approach to hardware removal

Two techniques for removing pacemaker systems are currently available: invasive thoracotomy and percutaneous extraction. The choice of the less invasive percutaneous technique is usually based on time elapsed from implantation, vegetation size, absence of vegetation on the tricuspid valve, and the general conditions of the patient. Percutaneous lead extraction has become the preferred method for removal of CIED hardware. However, these procedures involve significant risks, including cardiac tamponade, hemothorax, pulmonary embolism, lead migration, and death, even in experienced hands. Thus, the performance of these procedures should be limited to centers with the appropriate facilities and training, including the presence of immediate availability of cardiothoracic surgery to provide backup in the event of complications. In high-volume centers, percutaneous lead removal can be accomplished relatively safely with a high rate of success (Jones et al., 2008). A primary surgical approach to lead removal in patients with CIED infection should be limited to patients who have significant retained hardware after one attempt at percutaneous removal. Another scenario in which a preference for surgical lead removal has been advocated is in patients with lead vegetations >2 cm in diameter, because of concerns about the risk of pulmonary embolism with percutaneous lead extraction. Experience suggests, however, that percutaneous removal in patients with large vegetations can be done without precipitating a clinically apparent pulmonary embolism. Until additional data are available, decisions regarding percutaneous versus surgical removal of leads with vegetations larger than 2 cm in diameter should be individualized and based on a patient's clinical parameters and the extractor's evaluation (Field et al., 2007; Gandelman et al., 2007; Sohail et al., 2007a).

Antimicrobial therapy is adjunctive in patients with CIED infection, and complete device removal should not be delayed, regardless of timing of initiation of antimicrobial therapy. Selection of the appropriate antimicrobial agent should be based on identification and in vitro susceptibility testing results. Because most infections are due to staphylococcal species, treatment agent should be effective against those germs. In case of oxacillin resistant infections is suspected, vancomycin should be administered initially as empirical antibiotic coverage until microbiological results are known. Patients with infections due to oxacillin-susceptible staphylococcal strains can be given cefazolin or nafcillin alone with discontinuation of vancomycin. Vancomycin should be continued in patients who are not candidates for betalactam antibiotic therapy and those with infections due to oxacillin-resistant staphylococci. Compared with Gram-positive infections, Gram-negative and fungi are less frequently isolated and empiric coverage against those microorganisms is not routinely indicated; it should be started after microbiological identification has been performed.

Pathogen identification and in vitro susceptibility testing can be used to guide treatment in patients with nonstaphylococcal CIED infections. When microbiological culture are available, a de-escalation approach should be considered in order to minimize the development of antimicrobial resistances (De Gaudio et al., 2010). There are no clinical trial data to define the optimal duration of antimicrobial therapy for CIED infections, regardless of the extent of infection, or to determine when conversion to an oral agent is appropriate once complete device removal has been achieved. Factors that influence duration of therapy include the extent of device infection, the causative organism, the persistence of positive blood cultures, and associated complications such as valvular involvement, septic thrombophlebitis, or osteomyelitis. Blood cultures should be obtained from all patients after device removal. Therapy can be switched to an oral regimen once susceptibility results are known if there is an oral agent available that is active against the pathogen and the infected CIED has been removed. At least two weeks of parenteral therapy are recommended after removal of an infected device and for patients with bloodstream infection. Patients with sustained (>24 hours) positive blood cultures despite CIED removal and appropriate antimicrobial therapy should receive parenteral therapy for at least 4 weeks, even if TEE is negative for valvular vegetations.

7.2.2 Hardware reimplantation

It is important to assess the need for new device placement in any patient with an infected CIED. Based of available data, one third to one half of patients will not require new CIED placement. There are several factors, including reversal of the pathological processes that precipitated the need for CIED implantation and lack of appropriate clinical indications, that may obviate the need for new CIED placement (Sohail et al., 2007b). Adequate debridement and control of infection at all sites, both at the generator site and metastatic, if present, must be achieved before new device placement (Baddour et al., 2010). Removal of infected hardware should not be attempted until a careful assessment of a new implantation strategy has been performed, particularly in patients with pacemakers for complete heart block and resynchronization therapy devices. When implantation of a new device is necessary, it should be performed on the counterlateral side if possible to avoid relapsing device infection. If this is not possible, a transvenous lead can be tunneled to a device placed subcutaneously in the abdomen. Implantation is usually postponed to allow for resolution of infection, but patients who are CIED dependent represent a challenge, because they cannot be discharged with a temporary pacemaker. Active-fixation leads attached to pacing generators or defibrillators are now being used as a bridge until PPM implantation is deemed appropriate. Use of active-fixation leads connected to external devices permits earlier mobilization of patients dependant on cardiac stimulators and has been associated with a reduced risk of pacing-related adverse events, including lead dislocation, and local infection (Braun et al., 2006).

Optimal timing of device replacement is unknown. There have been no prospective trials that examined timing of new device replacement and risk of relapsing infection; however, several investigators recommend waiting for blood cultures to be negative before a new device is placed (Gandelman et al., 2007; Sohail et al., 2007a)

8. Conclusions

Currently, 3 million implanted cardiac pacing systems and 180000 implantable cardioverter-defibrillators exist worldwide. The rate of device implantations is increasing due to the aging of the general population and the development of new indications. Although conferring obvious benefits, the use of these implantable devices is associated with some complications. Infections must be considered as a serious and potentially fatal complication. The clinical presentation of device infection ranges from superficial wound infection to frank device-related endocarditis.

The incidence of infection related to pacemakers varies from 0.13% to 19.9% in prospective and retrospective studies. Serious complications, such as endocarditis and sepsis, may occur in 0.5% of patients. In addition, infectious complications have a significant economic impact to health care systems due to the high cost of treatment.

Data to guide treatment of patients with this condition are limited. However, the consensus from the published literature recommends prompt and complete device removal, combined with antimicrobial therapy of appropriate duration. Conservative treatment without explantation of all hardware is frequently unsuccessful. Given the progressive rise in antimicrobial-resistant bacteria in general, and gram-positive pathogens in particular, treatment of cardiovascular infections is likely to become more difficult in the future.

Finally, because a substantial number of patients may no longer require such devices, reimplantation should be done only after the continued need for such therapy has been reassessed.

9. References

Al-Khatib, SM.; Lucas, FL.; Jollis JG.; Malenka, DJ. & Wennberg, DE. (2005). The relation between patients' outcomes and the volume of cardioverter-defibrillator implantation procedures performed by physicians treating Medicare beneficiaries. *J Am Coll Cardiol*. Vol. 46, No. 8, (October 2005), pp. 1536-40, ISSN 0735-1097

Allen, M. (2006). Pacemakers and implantable cardioverter defibrillators. *Anaesthesia*. Vol. 61, No. 9, (September 2006), pp. 883-90, ISSN 0007-0912

Baddour, LM.; Barker, LP.; Christensen, GD.; Parisi, JT. & Simpson, WA. (1990). Phenotypic variation of Staphylococcus epidermidis in infection of transvenous endocardial pacemaker electrodes. *J Clin Microbiol*. Vol. 28, No. 4, (April 1990), pp. 676-9, ISSN 0095-1137

Baddour, LM.; Epstein, AE.; Erickson, CC.;, Knight, BP.; Levison, ME.; Lockhart, PB.; Masoudi, FA.; Okum EJ, Wilson, WR.; Beerman, LB.; Bolger, AF.; Estes, NA.; Gewitz, M. ; Newburger, JW. ; Schron, EB. & Taubert, KA. (2010). Update on cardiovascular implantable electronic device infections and their management: a scientific statement from the American Heart Association. *Circulation*. Vol. 121, No. 3, (January 2010), pp. 458-77, ISSN 0009-7322

Bensimhon, L.; Lavergne, T.; Hugonnet, F.; Mainardi, JL.; Latremouille, C.; Maunoury, C.; Lepillier, A.; Le Heuzey, JY. & Faraggi, M. (2010) Whole body [(18) F]fluorodeoxyglucose positron emission tomography imaging for the diagnosis of pacemaker or implantable cardioverter defibrillator infection: a preliminary prospective study. *Clin Microbiol Infec*. Epub ahead of print. ISSN 1469-0691

Bertaglia, E.; Zerbo, F.; Zardo, S.; Barzan, D.; Zoppo, F. & Pascotto P.(2006). Antibiotic prophylaxis with a single dose of cefazolin during pacemaker implantation: incidence of long-term infective complications. *Pacing Clin Electrophysiol*. Vol. 29, No. 1, (January 2006), pp. 29-33, ISSN 1540-8159

Bloom, H.;, Heeke, B.; Leon, A.; Mera, F.; Delurgio, D.; Beshai, J. & Langberg J. (2006). Renal insufficiency and the risk of infection from pacemaker or defibrillator surgery. *Pacing Clin Electrophysiol.* Vol. 29, No. 2, (February 2006), pp. 142-5, ISSN 1540-8159

Boelens, JJ.; Dankert, J.; Murk, JL.; Weening, JJ.; van der Poll, T.; Dingemans, KP.; Koole, L.; Laman, JD. & Zaat, SA. (2000). Biomaterial-associated persistence of Staphylococcus epidermidis in pericatheter macrophages. *J Infect Dis.* Vol. 181, No. 4, (April 2000), pp. 1337-49, ISSN 1537-6613

Borer, A.; Gilad, J.; Hyam, E.; Schlaeffer, F.; Schlaeffer, P.; Eskira, S.; Aloni, P.; Wagshal, A. & Katz A. (2004). Prevention of infections associated with permanent cardiac antiarrhythmic devices by implementation of a comprehensive infection control program. *Infect Control Hosp Epidemiol.* Vol. 25, No. 6, (June 2004), pp.492-7, ISSN 0899-823X

Braun, MU.; Rauwolf, T.; Bock, M.; Kappert, U.; Boscheri, A.; Schnabel, A. & Strasser, RH. (2006). Percutaneous lead implantation connected to an external device in stimulation-dependent patients with systemic infection: a prospective and controlled study. *Pacing Clin Electrophysiol.* Vol. 29, No. 8, (August 2006), pp. 875-9, ISSN 1540-8159

Cabell, CH.; Heidenreich, PA.; Chu, VH.; Moore, CM.; Stryjewski, ME.; Corey, GR. & Fowler, VG Jr. (2004). Increasing rates of cardiac device infections among Medicare beneficiaries: 1990-1999. *Am Heart J.* Vol. 147, No.4, (April 2004), pp.582-6, ISSN 1751-7168

Cacoub, P.; Leprince, P.; Nataf, P.; Hausfater, P.; Dorent, R.; Wechsler, B.; Bors, V.; Pavie, A.; Piette, JC. & Gandjbakhch, I. (1998). Pacemaker infective endocarditis. *Am J Cardiol.* Vol. 82, No. 4, (August 1998), pp. 480-4, ISSN 0002-9149

Chamis, AL.; Peterson, GE.; Cabell, CH.; Corey, GR.; Sorrentino, RA.; Greenfield, RA.; Ryan, T.; Reller, LB. & Fowler, VG Jr. (2001). Staphylococcus aureus bacteremia in patients with permanent pacemakers or implantable cardioverter-defibrillators. *Circulation.* Vol. 104, No. 9, (August 2001), pp. 1029-33, ISSN 0009-7322

Chua, JD.; Wilkoff, BL.; Lee, I.; Juratli, N.; Longworth, DL. & Gordon, SM. (2000). Diagnosis and management of infections involving implantable electrophysiologic cardiac devices. *Ann Intern Med.* Vol. 133, No. 8, (October 2000), pp. 604-8, ISSN 1539-3704

Da Costa, A.; Kirkorian, G.; Cucherat, M.; Delahaye, F.; Chevalier, P.; Cerisier, A.;Isaaz, K. & Touboul, P. (1998). Antibiotic prophylaxis for permanent pacemaker implantation: a meta-analysis. *Circulation.* Vol. 97, No. 18, (May 1998), pp. 1796-801, ISSN 0009-7322

Da Costa, A.; Lelièvre, H.; Kirkorian, G.; Célard, M.; Chevalier, P.; Vandenesch, F.; Etienne, J. & Touboul, P. (1998). Role of the preaxillary flora in pacemaker infections: a prospective study. *Circulation.* Vol. 97, No. 18,(May 1998), pp.1791-5, ISSN 0009-7322

Darouiche, RO. (2001). Device-associated infections: a macroproblem that starts with microadherence. *Clin Infect Dis.* Vol. 33, No. 9, (November 2001), pp. 1567-72, ISSN 1058-4838

De Gaudio, AR.; Selmi, V. & Chelazzi, C. (2010). Antibiotics and artificial nutrition in the cardiac intensive care unit. *G Ital Cardiol.* Vol. 11, No. 4, (April 2010), pp.274-84, ISSN 1827-6806 de Oliveira, JC.; Martinelli, M.; Nishioka, SA.; Varejão, T.; Uipe, D.; Pedrosa, AA.; Costa, R.; D'Avila, A. & Danik, SB. (2009). Efficacy of antibiotic prophylaxis before the implantation of pacemakers and cardioverter-defibrillators: results of a large, prospective, randomized, double-blinded, placebo-controlled trial. *Circ Arrhythm Electrophysiol*. Vol. 2, No. 1, (February 2009), pp. 29-34, ISSN 1941-3149

Deuling, JH.; Smit, MD.; Maass, AH.; Van den Heuvel, AF.; Nieuwland, W.; Zijlstra, F. & Van Gelder, IC. (2009). The value and limitations of a wound inspection clinic after cardiac device implantation. *Eur J Cardiovasc Nurs*. Vol. 8, No. 4, (March 2009), pp. 288-92, ISSN 1474-5151

Field, ME.; Jones, SO. & Epstein, LM. How to select patients for lead extraction. *Heart Rhythm*. Vol. 4, No. 7, (July 2007), pp. 978-85, ISSN 1556-3871

Gandelman, G.; Frishman, WH.; Wiese, C.; Green-Gastwirth, V.; Hong, S.; Aronow, WS. & Horowitz, HW. (2007). Intravascular device infections: epidemiology, diagnosis, and management. *Cardiol Rev*. Vol. 15, No. 1, (January 2007), pp.13-23, ISSN 1538-4683

Harcombe, AA.; Newell, SA.; Ludman, PF.; Wistow, TE.; Sharples, LD.; Schofield, PM.; Stone, DL.; Shapiro, LM.; Cole, T. & Petch, MC. (1998). Late complications following permanent pacemaker implantation or elective unit replacement. *Heart*. Vol. 80, No. 3, (September 1998), pp.240-4, ISSN 1355-6037

Heinle, S.; Wilderman, N.; Harrison, JK.; Waugh, R.; Bashore, T.; Nicely, LM.; Durack, D. & Kisslo, J. (1994). Value of transthoracic echocardiography in predicting embolic events in active infective endocarditis. Duke Endocarditis Service. *Am J Cardiol*. Vol. 74, No. 8, (October 1994), pp. 799-801, ISSN 0002-9149

Jones, SO.; Eckart, RE.; Albert, CM. & Epstein, LM. (2008). Large, single-center, single-operator experience with transvenous lead extraction: outcomes and changing indications. *Heart Rhythm*. Vol. 5, No. 4, (April 2008), pp. 520-5, ISSN 1556-3871

Klug, D.; Balde, M.; Pavin, D.; Hidden-Lucet, F.; Clementy, J.; Sadoul, N.; Rey, JL.; Lande, G.; Lazarus, A.; Victor, J.; Barnay, C.; Grandbastien, B. & Kacet, S. (2007). Risk factors related to infections of implanted pacemakers and cardioverter-defibrillators: results of a large prospective study. *Circulation*. Vol. 116, no. 12, (September 2007), pp. 1349-55, ISSN 0009-7322

Klug, D.; Lacroix, D.; Savoye, C.; Goullard, L.; Grandmougin, D.; Hennequin, JL.; Kacet, S. & Lekieffre, J. (1997). Systemic infection related to endocarditis on pacemaker leads: clinical presentation and management. *Circulation*. Vol. 95, No. 8, (April 1997), pp. 2098-107, ISSN 0009-7322

Lazăr, V. & Chifiriuc, MC. (2010). Architecture and physiology of microbial biofilms. Roum *Arch Microbiol Immunol*. Vol. 69, No. 2, (April 2010), pp. 95-107, ISSN 1222-3891

Lekkerkerker, JC.; van Nieuwkoop, C.; Trines, SA.; van der Bom, JG.; Bernards, A.; van de Velde, ET.; Bootsma, M.; Zeppenfeld, K.; Jukema, JW.; Borleffs, JW.; Schalij, MJ. & van Erven, L. (2009). Risk factors and time delay associated with cardiac device infections: Leiden device registry. *Heart. Vol*. 95, No. 9, (May 2009), pp. 715-20, ISSN 1355-6037

Mela, T.; McGovern, BA.; Garan, H.; Vlahakes, GJ.; Torchiana, DF.; Ruskin, J. & Galvin, JM. (2001). Long-term infection rates associated with the pectoral versus abdominal approach to cardioverter-defibrillator implants. *Am J Cardiol*. Vol. 88, No. 7, (October 2001), pp. 750-3, ISSN 0002-9149

Robinson. M.; Healey, JS.; Eikelboom, J.; Schulman, S.; Morillo, CA.; Nair, GM.; Baranchuk, A.; Ribas, S.; Evans, G.; Connolly, SJ. & Turpie, AG. (2009). Postoperative low-molecular-weight heparin bridging is associated with an increase in wound hematoma following surgery for pacemakers and implantable defibrillators. *Pacing Clin Electrophysiol*. Vol. 32, No. 3, (March 2009), pp. 378-82, ISSN 1540-8159

Sanfilippo, AJ.; Picard, MH.; Newell, JB.; Rosas, E.; Davidoff, R.; Thomas, JD. & Weyman, AE. (1991). Echocardiographic assessment of patients with infectious endocarditis: prediction of risk for complications. *J Am Coll Cardiol*. Vol.18, No. 5, (November 1991), pp. 1191-9, ISSN 0002-9149

Sohail, MR.; Sultan, OW. & Raza, SS. (2010). Contemporary management of cardiovascular implantable electronic device infections. *Expert Rev Anti Infect Ther*. Vol. 7, No. 7, (July 2010), pp. 831-9, ISSN 1478-7210

Sohail, MR.; Uslan, DZ.; Khan, AH.; Friedman, PA.; Hayes, DL.; Wilson, WR.; Steckelberg, JM.; Stoner, S. & Baddour, LM. (2007). Management and outcome of permanent pacemaker and implantable cardioverter-defibrillator infections. *J Am Coll Cardiol*. Vol. 49, No. 18, (May 2007), pp. 1851-9, ISSN 0002-9149

Sohail, MR.; Uslan, DZ.; Khan, AH.; Friedman, PA.; Hayes, DL.; Wilson, WR.; Steckelberg, JM.; Stoner, SM. & Baddour, LM. (2007). Risk factor analysis of permanent pacemaker infection. *Clin Infect Dis*. Vol. 45, No. 2, (July 2007), pp.166-73, ISSN 1058-4838

Tablan, OC.; Anderson, LJ.; Besser, R.; Bridges, C. & Hajjeh, R. (2003). Guidelines for preventing health-care-associated pneumonia, 2003: recommendations of the CDC and the Healthcare Infection Control Practices Advisory Committee. *MMWR Recomm Rep*. Vol. 53, No. 3, (March 2004), pp. 1-36, ISSN 1057-5987

Uslan, DZ.; Sohail, MR.; St Sauver, JL.; Friedman, PA.; Hayes, DL.; Stoner, SM.; Wilson, WR.; Steckelberg, JM. & Baddour, LM. (2007). Permanent pacemaker and implantable cardioverter defibrillator infection: a population-based study. *Arch Intern Med*. Vol. 167, No. 7, (April 2007), pp. 669-75, ISSN 1538-3679

Veenstra, GJ.; Cremers, FF.; van Dijk, H. & Fleer, A. (1996). Ultrastructural organization and regulation of a biomaterial adhesin of Staphylococcus epidermidis. *J Bacteriol*. Vol. 178, No. 2, (January 1996), pp. 537-41, ISSN 1098-5530

Victor, F.; De Place, C.; Camus, C.; Le Breton, H.; Leclercq, C.; Pavin, D.; Mabo, P. & Daubert, C. (1999). Pacemaker lead infection: echocardiographic features, management, and outcome. *Heart*. Vol. 81, No. 1, (January 1999), pp. 82-7, ISSN 1355-6037

Voet, JG.; Vandekerckhove, YR.; Muyldermans, LL.; Missault, LH. & Matthys, LJ. (1999). Pacemaker lead infection: report of three cases and review of the literature. *Heart*. Vol. 81, No. 1, (January 1999), pp. 88-91, ISSN 1355-6037

Voigt, A.; Shalaby, A. & Saba, S. (2010). Continued rise in rates of cardiovascular implantable electronic device infections in the United States: temporal trends and causative insights. *Pacing Clin Electrophysiol*. Vol. 33, No. 4, (April 2010), pp. 414-9, ISSN 1540-8159

9

Clinical Concerns and Strategies in Radiation Oncology

Michael S. Gossman
Regulation Directive Medical Physics^{SM}
United States

1. Introduction

The Chapter was constructed to offer the recommended tactics of clinical practice in radiation oncology, since pacemaker patients generally maintain their implanted pacemaker throughout their cancer treatment. Recent improvements to the functionality and stability of implantable pacemakers involve changes for greater battery power consumption efficiency as well as radiation hardened electrical circuits. Manufacturers have also pursued MRI-compatibility for these devices with some success. While such newer models of pacemakers are similar in construction to previously marketed devices, even for the recent MRI-compatible designs currently in clinical trials, there is increased interest now with regard to radiation therapy dose effects when a device is near or directly in the field of radiation. This manuscript provides the radiation safety precautions clinically incorporated for the management of patients having implantable pacemakers with a required need for radiation therapy. It provides guidance and current recommendations for the cardiac physician, radiation oncologist and medical physicist prior to and during radiation delivery.

The Chapter first details extensively the concepts of CT imaging, computerized treatment planning, and dose aim analysis with mock treatments. The later sections deal with current research observations from investigators concerned with the consequences of using different modalities of treatment and imaging for a patient having a pacemaker implanted. These sections include novel research on electronic device instability induced by x-rays, neutrons, and proton beams as well as radiation from radioactive material. The recent advancement of technology for magnetic resonance imaging and its limitations are also provided. This Chapter should provide a sound basis for comprehension of the complex nature of dealing with a patient having a pacemaker, while requiring continual treatment for cancer care after their implant. It is also a significant educational source for the detailed research on device interactions presented.

2. Radiation oncology methods

It is not a common occurrence for radiation oncologists to be referred a patient having a cardiac pacemaker implanted. At a clinic operating up to 60 patients per day with two radiation oncologists, only two patients may be referred to them for consultation in any calendar year. However, when faced with the dilemma of how to treat such a patient, the radiation oncologist often finds one of their greatest challenges. Not only do they have to determine the best chances of survival for the patient given their type of disease, classification, staging, and current physiological status, but they also have to be aware of the possible harm to the stationary pacemaker when the prescribed amount of radiation is directed at the patient. Treatments most commonly performed for cancer patients involve radiation originating from external beam particle accelerators. Many of these machines are capable of emitting x-ray radiation in the clinical energy range of 6-18 MV and at dose-rates[1] of 6 Gy/min. Figure 1 shows a commonly used particle accelerator found in a Radiation Oncology Department.

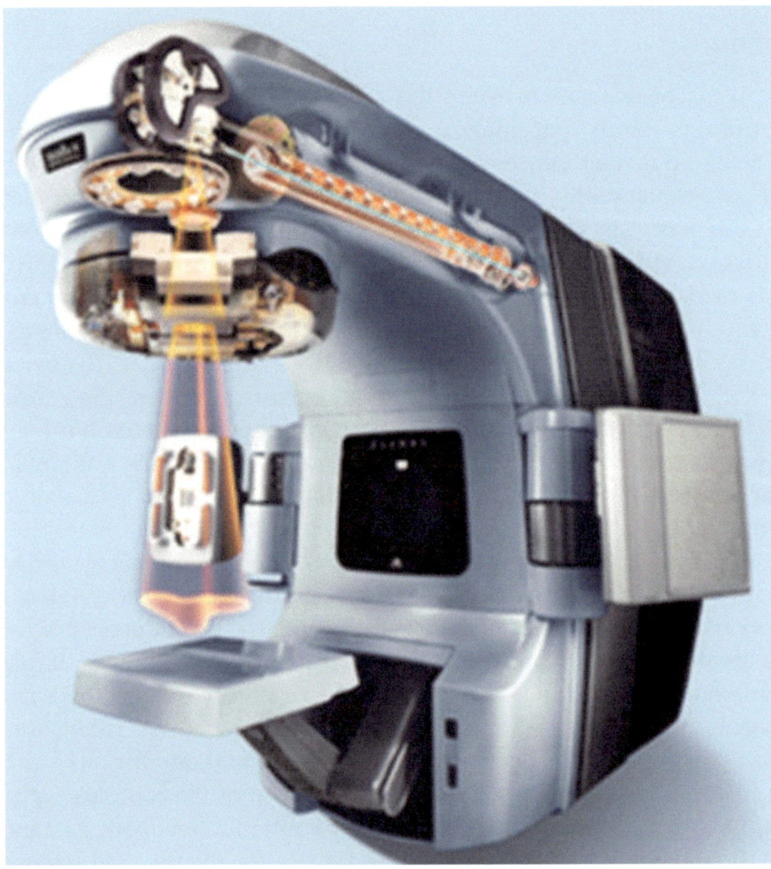

Fig. 1. Varian Medical Systems (Palo Alto, CA) Clinac® model Trilogy particle accelerator [Varian Medical Systems, Inc. - All rights reserved]

[1] The gray (Gy) is the International System of Units standard unit for absorbed dose, defined as the absorption of 1 Joule of ionizing radiation by 1 kilogram of matter (i.e. human tissue or water). It is equivalent to 100 cGy or 100 rads.

The radiation oncology community practice guidelines used when dealing with radiation safety issues for patients that have a pacemaker implanted are those published by the American Association of Physicists in Medicine (AAPM) through Task Group-45 (Marbach et al., 1994). Now seventeen years later, much of the electronics in pacemakers have been reengineered. Therefore, designs and mechanisms addressed in that literature are now outdated. While the newly formed AAPM Task Group-203[2] is actively researching to update and recreate a new guidance document, pacing specialists, radiation oncologists and medical physicists struggle to determine standards to these issues clinically. Even the effect of simple computerized tomography (CT) scanning on pacemakers is not well defined (Solan et al., 2004).

Nearly all radiation oncology treatments are performed in the accompaniment of a CT scan of the patient's anatomy. This is something that most cancer centers have within their department. Although the CT scan is not intended to diagnose the patient, the three-dimensional data may be utilized within planning computers to simulate the intended delivery of dose to the patient before they are actually treated with radiation. Such computers, referred to as treatment planning systems, contain radiation data measured by the medical physicist from the particle accelerator. By applying the radiation measurements at the various depths in water, and for the various beam aperture sizes that can be used, one may be able to visualize the distribution of dose overlay on the patient's CT scan. It is this preliminary dosimetric simulation that the radiation oncologist uses to determine the intended plan for treating the targeted cancer. The ability to predict the consequential dose distribution is important to assist in the predetermination of excessive doses to pacemakers as well.

There are two important issues concerning pacemakers in radiation oncology. First, does the treatment planning system model the dose to the pacemaker accurately? In general, incident radiation has three possible directional pathways to travel when directed at an object. It can pass directly through the device with some blocking affects (attenuation), it can bounce backward (back-scattering), or it can ricochet outward (side-scattering) from it. Research has proven that treatment planning systems underestimate all three of these interactions for metallic structures. Under the most standard geometry, the amount of radiation blocked by the pacemaker and scattered from it were determined to be less when calculated by computer then when measured with ionization detectors.

Specifically, for a selection of pacemaker generators investigated over a span of 2 years identically from Medtronic (Gossman, et al., 2010, 2011) (Adapta model ADDR01, Versa model VEDR01, Sensia model SEDR01, and Enpulse2 model E2DR01) as well as those from Boston Scientific (Gossman, 2011) (Altrua 60 EL model S606 and Altrua 60 model S603) attenuation results varied between computer and measurement up to a maximum disagreement of 5.3%. Actual measurements revealed attenuation ranges for all devices to be significant with respect to normal tissue at -6.4% to -15.9% at 6 MV and -5.2% to -9.4% at 18 MV respectively. Back-scattering and side-scattering were of the least consequence of the three. Back-scattering results were shown to range from 0.0-2.8% at 6 MV and 0.0-3.4% at 18 MV, whereas side-scattering ranged from 0.0-2.5% at 6 MV and 0.0-5.7% at 18 MV.

Electrode leads exhibit similar affects in altering the distribution of dose used therapeutically, although at less drastic levels. In these studies, marginally significant attenuation dose changes were observed only for electrode leads and connector ports, at less

[2] This author is a member of the American Association of Physicists in Medicine (AAPM) Task Group-203 on the Management of Radiotherapy Patients with Implanted Cardiac Pacemakers and Defibrillators.

than 3.1% for Boston Scientific (Gossman, 2011) devices (LD CV Acuity Spiral Up lead model 4593, Fineline II Sterox EZ lead model 4469, and Fineline II Sterox lead model 4457) and 3.8% for a Medtronic (Gossman et al., 2010, 2011) lead (Single wire lead model 5076-85CM) similarly. Scattering was determined to be negligible for either set of leads.

As a result of those publications, medical physicists have noted that the viability of computer modeling is heavily dependent upon the mathematical algorithms used. Still, the measured results forecast a concern as to the accuracy of computer approximations when electronics are included within the calculation matrix. This is true even when the pacemaker is not directly irradiated. Dose calculations compute dose throughout the anatomy of the patient regardless of whether or not the beam path projects through it. This leaves the radiation oncologist with no alternative recourse than to rely heavily on the medical physicist to best approximate treatment planning system results, while understanding from this published research that dosimetric results may be underestimated.

To enable treatment modeling on computer, the patient must first undergo a CT scan. These image data provide anatomical information specific to the patient in three dimensions. The CT is instrumental to be able to plan for the angle and size of the radiation beam prior to delivering radiation. Irradiation for imaging in this modality can result in pacemaker oversensing, although these effects are predominantly transient (McCollough et al., 2007; Yamaji et al., 2006). As explained in one group, benign problems are discovered when either there is a trigger for non-physiologic tracking that results in inappropriate rapid-paced ventricular rates, or perhaps when extra senses simulate an atrial arrhythmia that inducing a false detection and delivery of an unnecessary atrial antitachycardia pacing therapy. However, oversensing did cause inhibition of pacing in some tests. This delay is important if the heart resorts back to the same problematic functionality, putting them at risk for asystole. The researchers proved that dynamic CT scanning without table movement should not be employed. They further demonstrated that it is appropriate to consider situations in the future with other imaging modalities, in review of possible effects that may produce clinically important risks (White, 2008).

The material of the pacemaker can cause imaging limitations for the radiation oncologist using CT scans as well. Research has shown that the digitally reconstructed radiograph of a patient having a pacemaker implanted often contains artifacts which could lead to errant computer calculations if not corrected properly by a qualified medical physicist (Gossman 2010, 2011a, 2011b). These artifacts show up as non-uniform lines that obscure normal tissue anatomy. Closer analysis of these artifacts lead to marked observations that the Hounsfield units (HU) assigned by the convoluted reconstructor of the CT scanner at locations not containing the pacemaker actually have metallic values of upwards of 3000-8000 HU. At physical locations where no metallic pacemaker is present, normal tissues values in its immediate vicinity typically registers values more near to 0-250 HU. As these values are directly related to the density of the material, it is not appropriate to scan such a patient using the "normal HU range" which extends from -1000 HU (air) to 0 HU (water) and upward to +1000 HU (dense bone: 900 mg/cm^3). Rather, it is recommended to use the "extended HU range" (Coolens & Childs, 2003) to account for these very high density metals. Incorrect HU scaling for locations around the pacemaker will happen no matter what. These must be corrected in the treatment planning process. Medical physicists refer to this process as contouring with Boolean operation. Planning system software used should have the capability of permitting manual reassignment of HU values as a solution. An example of this correction is shown in Figure 2.

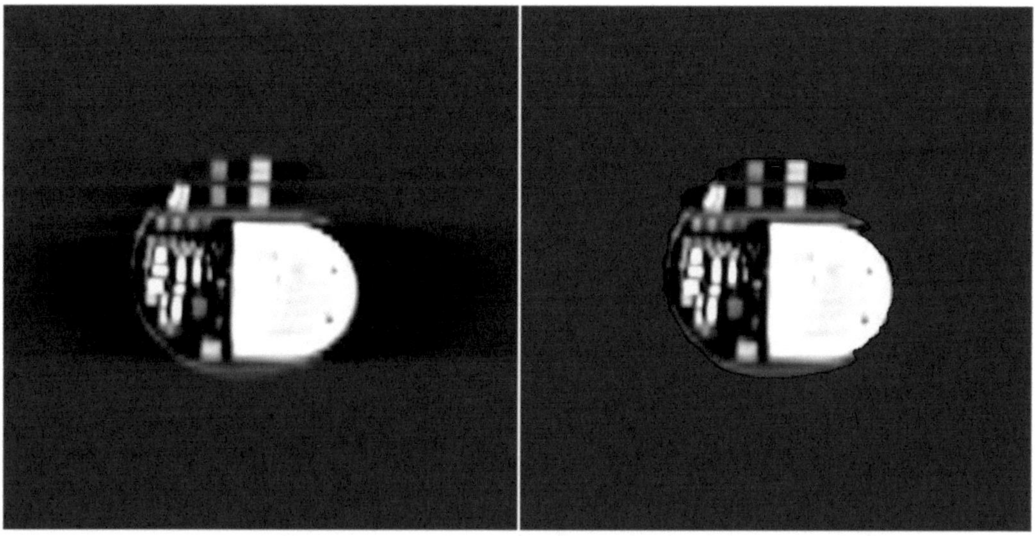

Fig. 2. General Electric (Fairfield, CT) CT scanner model LightSpeed RT® digital reconstructed radiograph in the coronal plane detailing a Medtronic ICP Adapta® model ADDR01 in water; (Left) with unavoidable artifact distortion and (Right) following appropriate manual Hounsfield unit correction

Treatment planning system dose calculations should also be conducted with care. Only the best algorithms should be employed to handle dose distributions around pacemakers and any other high density device (Gossman et al., 2009), such as electrode leads for that matter.

While some calculation algorithms provide only results assuming the entire patient is comprised of water density, this is not true for a real patient. Instead, the algorithm chosen by the medical physicist should be one which performs results with heterogeneity density correction throughout the entirety of the patient's anatomy. In this manner, as radiation passes through the body and hits the pacemaker, a more accurate depiction of dose will result from the computer having calculated consequential scattering and attenuation from it. Likewise, a more accurate dose will result when radiation passes through local organs which have their own unique density. As an aid to the radiation oncologist, where both algorithm tools are available, the medical physicist should provide results with the pacemaker's density computed as metal, and with it assigned as water as a second plan (Reft et al, 2003). Then, the differences between the two plans can illustrate for the radiation oncologist observable consequence of having the pacemaker in the calculated dose region. The treatment plan modeling described is exhibited in Figure 3.

The second issue concerning the irradiation of pacemakers in radiation oncology are the consequential malfunctions and damage that a device might incur if irradiated. In clinical practice pacemakers should be placed outside of the unshielded beam as recommended by the AAPM[3] (1). It should be well understood that even though a radiation therapy beam aperture can be adjusted in shape to not aim radiation directly at the pacemaker, radiation

[3] The AAPM is a scientific and medical organization with society membership affiliation to the American Institute of Physics. Publications include the scientific "Medical Physics Journal", technical reports, and symposium proceedings.

will also penetrate the shielding of the head of the particle accelerator that shapes the beam (transmission), resulting in imperceptible and possibly significant dose to the pacemaker.

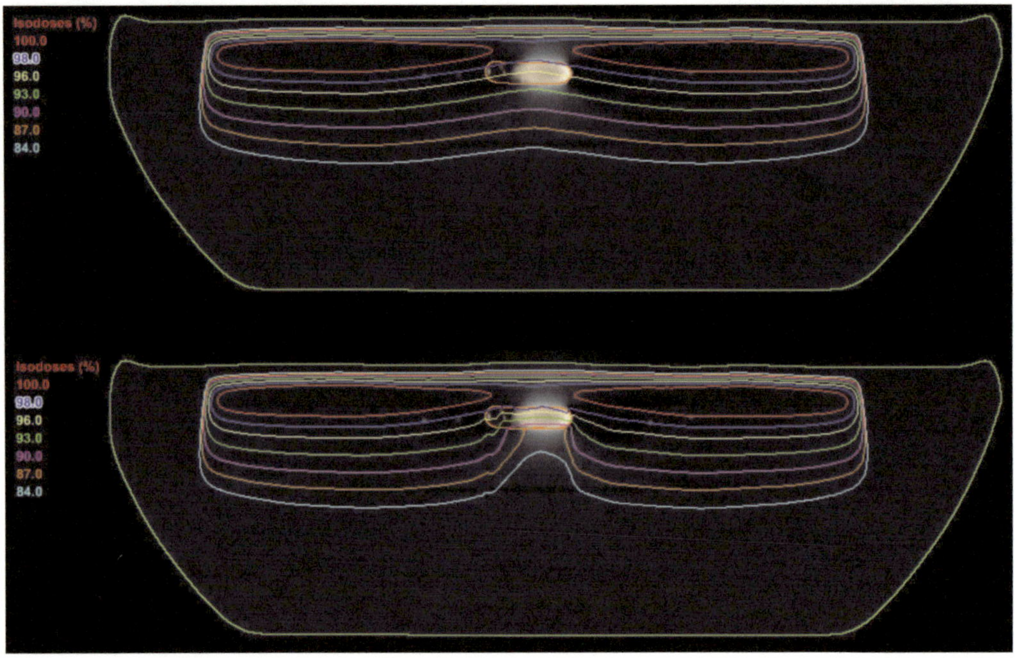

Fig. 3. Treatment plan dose distributions in the axial plane at 6 MV x-rays involving the Boston Scientific ICP Altrua® 60 EL model S606 in water; (Top) with no density correction and (Bottom) following appropriate heterogeneity correction

Some radiation will also scatter from the patient to the pacemaker as back-scatter and side-scatter. Under geometrical conditions where the pacemaker is out of the direct radiation beam although near a field edge, which is defined within the beam profile where the intensity falls-off laterally, as much as 80% of the intended dose to the target structure can be given. Even if the directed beam is adjusted to just barely keep the pacemaker out of the field, it can very easily absorb a significant amount of dose prescribed to a tumor that is not intended for the generator. The variation of dose across the irradiated field is shown in Figure 4. Inspecting the dose profile shape, one will notice that the relative dose within the beam is very symmetric in shape and flat. A closer inspection reveals that between the 80% and 20% relative dose, the intensity decreases dramatically away from the center of the radiation beam. This distal off-axis region on each side of the scan axis is called the penumbra. This is considered to be out of the ideal treatment intensity, since therapeutic dose is not well controlled in this region. Still further away from the penumbra, the dose continues to be present, although continually diminishing. This area constitutes the scattering of radiation outward, which resembles the aperture transmission as well as the scatter caused by the patient or phantom media. The plot provided is the definitive proof that a pacemaker can get a significant dose, even if it is not placed directly within the field intended to target the tumor. By definition, penumbral doses of up to 80% can be registered, while scattering doses can range of up to 20% as shown. Depending on how close the beam is to the pacemaker, there can be significant escalations in the absorbed dose to it.

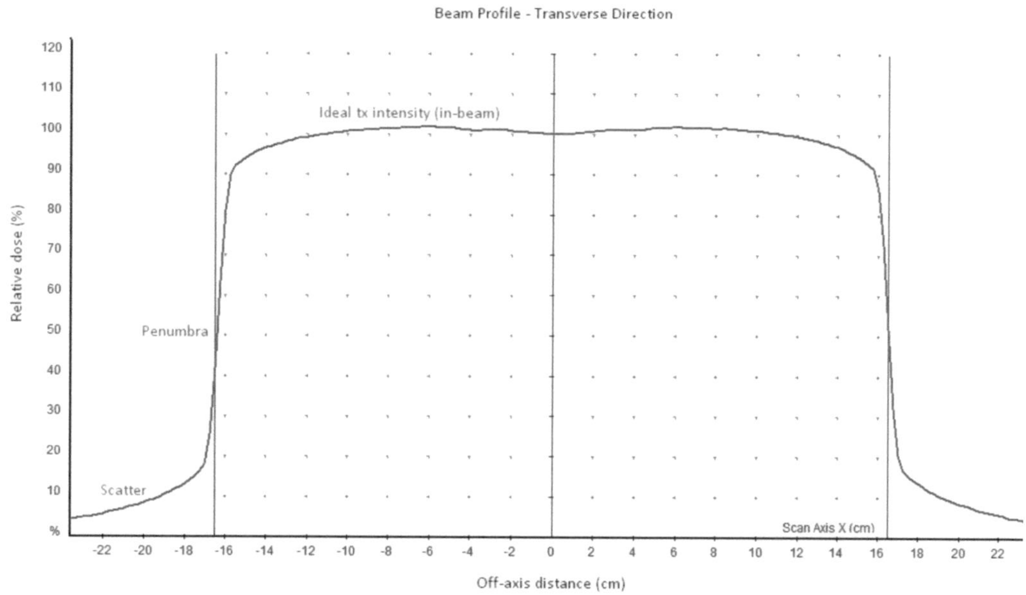

Fig. 4. Beam profile for a square aperture in water from 6 MV x-rays of the particle accelerator

With these facts, the medical physicist needs to pay close attention to the dose given to the pacemaker over the entire course of treatment.

As an example, let's consider an early stage non-small cell lung cancer prescribed to receive a low dose boost of 20 Gy over 10 fractional days of treatment. If we assume the pacemaker can only tolerate 2 Gy of radiation from the particle accelerator in accordance with the current guidelines of the AAPM (Marbach et al., 1994) and assume a single beam is assigned with a profile represented in Figure 4 with a plan for treatment such that the pacemaker is 2.0 cm away from the field, then theoretically we would see a scattered relative dose of nearly 11% possibly being absorbed by it. Each fractional dose prescribed to the tumor is scheduled to receive 2 Gy. Although 11% of this dose is small at only 0.22 Gy, the total dose after all 10 fractions yields a pacemaker total dose of 2.2 Gy. This is beyond the specified limit of 2 Gy. Therefore, the medical physicist will need to incorporate more beams with various oblique angles to avoid contribution of dose to the pacemaker.

A second example details the concern for an implantable cardioverter-defibrillator (ICD) similarly placed too close to the field as presented in Figure 5. It illustrates what is often experienced with pacemakers in this treatment planning process, similar to an ICP. Three beams are oriented at different angles to target a tumor in the example patient's right lung. The first beam is directed anterior at 180°. The second beam is directed to the tumor at a left anterior oblique angle of 250°. Then, the third beam is angled with a left posterior oblique angle of 310°. At 180° the AP beam passes through the generator. At 250° the LAO beam is directed such that the device is within the penumbra region of the beam. At 250° in this example, the LPO resulting geometry leaves the generator out of the field of radiation in the scatter region only. The beams-eye-view of each radiation field is shown in Figure 6 with the tumor and generator contoured for illustration. The proximity of the generator to the beam aperture is well observed in each example. Figure 7 provides the dosimetric results for the mock treatment in terms of a dose-volume histogram. Each scenario is analyzed in Table 1.

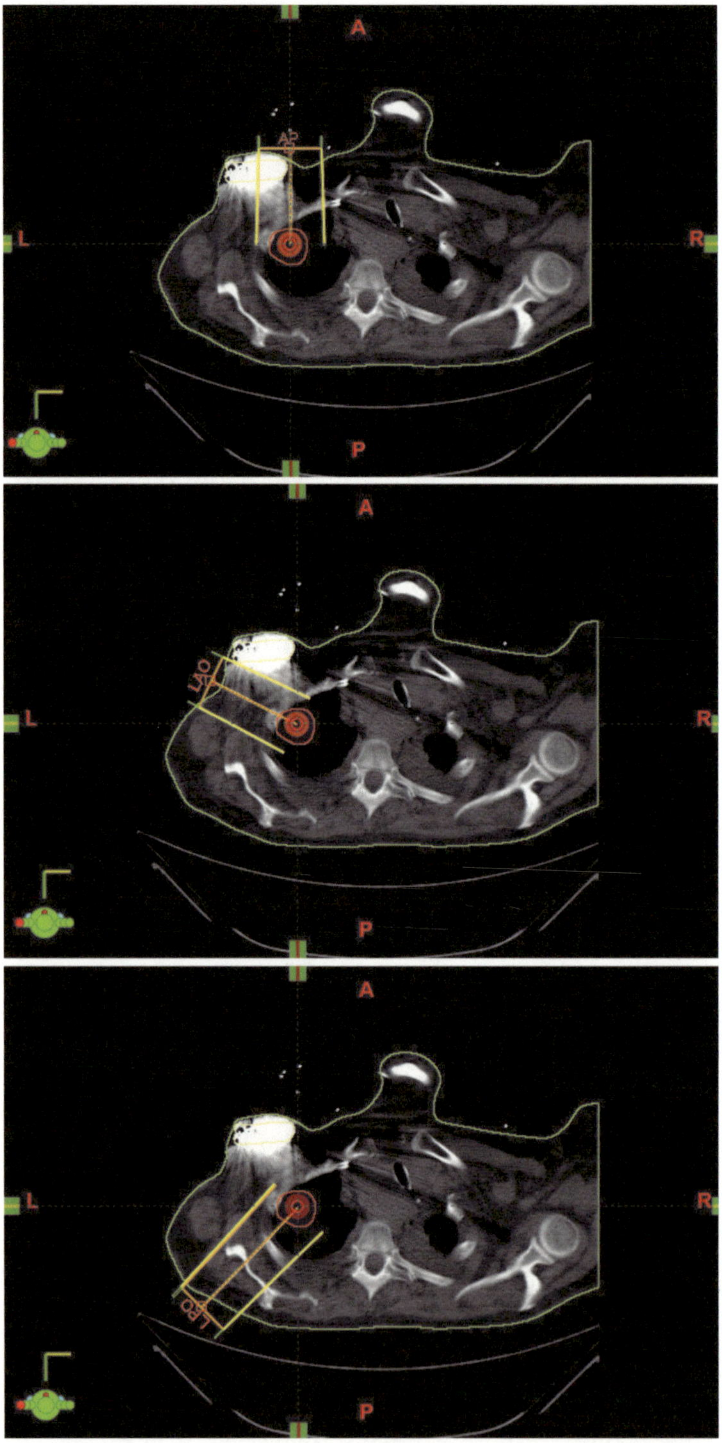

Fig. 5. Mock treatment projected beam paths in the axial view for a patient having the St. Jude Medical (St. Paul, MN) ICD Atlas® model V-242 implanted

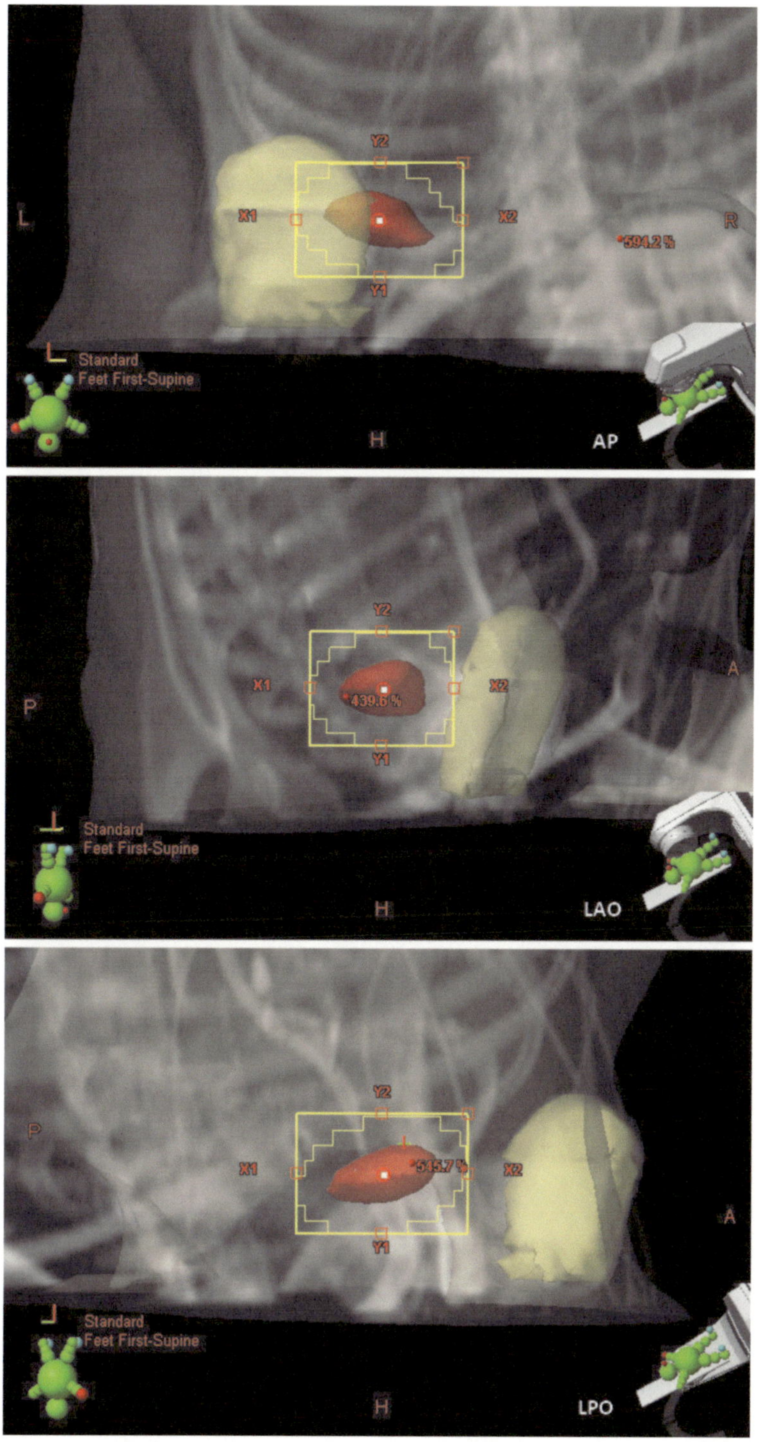

Fig. 6. Mock treatment beams-eye-views for a patient having the St. Jude Medical (St. Paul, MN) ICD Atlas® model V-242 implanted

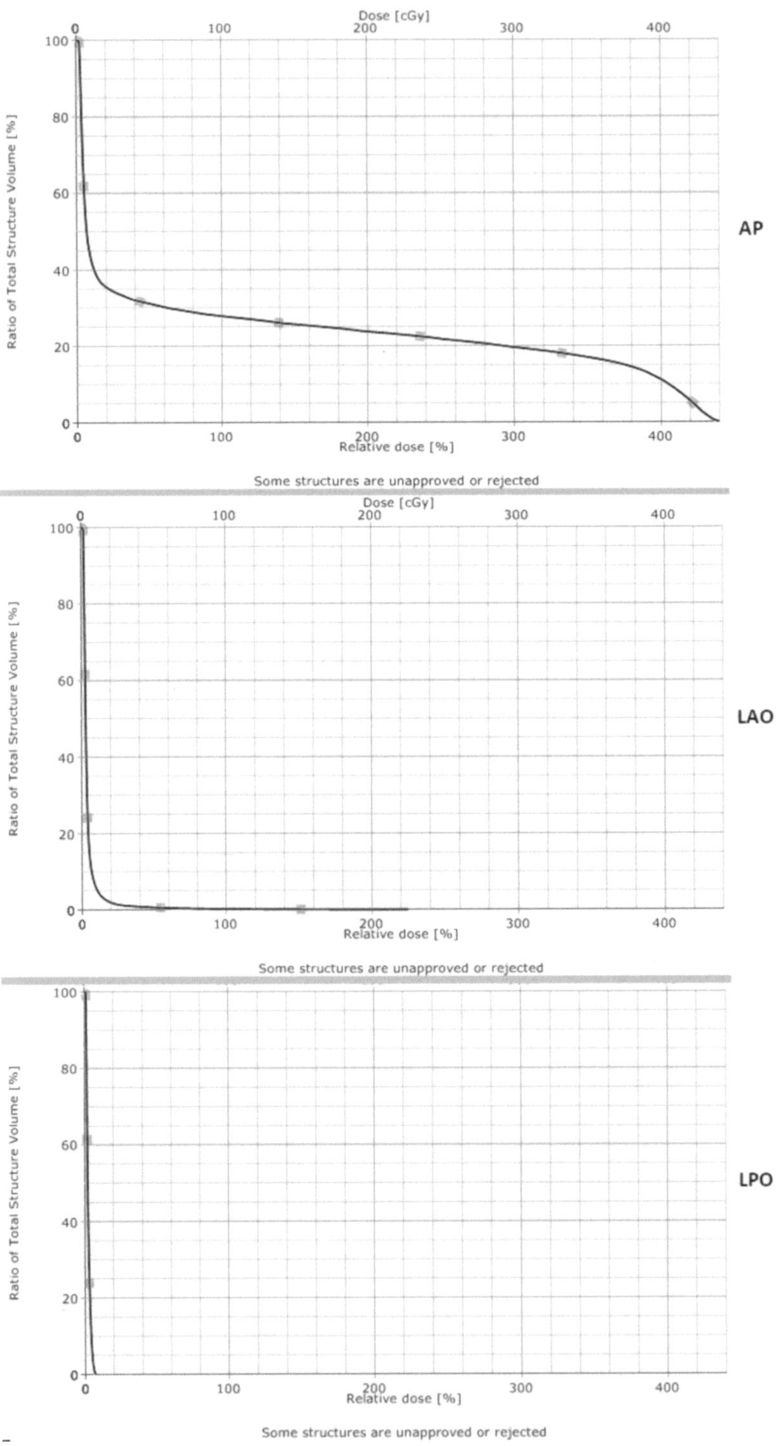

Fig. 7. Mock treatment dose-volume histogram resulting dose to the pacemaker for a patient having the St. Jude Medical (St. Paul, MN) ICD Atlas® model V-242 implanted

Beam Direction	Percentage ICD Volume	Percentage Dose Received	Maximum Percentage Dose on Entire Volume
AP	90%	3%	
	50%	7%	
	30%	60%	
	10%	405%	443%
LAO	90%	2%	
	50%	3%	
	30%	4%	
	10%	6%	225%
LPO	90%	1%	
	50%	2%	
	30%	3%	
	10%	4%	8%

Table 1. Dose-volume histogram results for the mock treatment detailing absorbed dose to the ICD from radiation

Looking at the maximum percentage dose absorbed by the generator for the example of a patient scheduled for 2 Gy in 10 fractions with an overall dose of 20 Gy, only the LPO beam yielded satisfactory results of dose to the generator, as it was in the scatter region outside of the direct radiation field and the penumbra. At a maximum dose of 8% of that 20 Gy prescription, the resulting dose to the electronics of the device is 1.6 Gy. This is the only beam arrangement that satisfies the 2 Gy recommendation. The medical physicist could benefit from the application of a variety of different beams at different angles. Using this approach, the dose absorbed to the device will be spread out over the entire surface rather than one directed device volume, resulting in less maximum percentage dose.

This is the definitive dilemma for the medical physicist and radiation oncologist. Some diseases may be best suited for a simple 2-field technique. An anterior-posterior opposed field technique is the likely tactic approached for a small lung tumor medially located. In this example with a patient lying supine on the treatment couch, an anterior-to-posterior beam aimed from the patient's chest to their back, and a posterior-to-anterior beam aimed through their back up through their chest may only be assigned. With the pacemaker having been implanted in the anterior chest wall of the patient, it then resides not only in the field of the entering anterior beam, but also in the field of the posterior field about to exit upward through the chest. These APPA beams are likely of little use now given the radiation tolerance limitations of the pacemaker as shown in the example.

Instead, oblique angles should be considered (Riley et al., 2004) as shown. The radiation oncologist will now have to concentrate their awareness of the limitations of dose to the pacemaker as well as the elevated doses that will now be incurred by all these other organs resultantly (Gullane, 1991), while insuring the pacemaker is considerably away from the radiation field edge.

The practice of irradiating pacemakers beyond levels recommended by society-based entities and manufacturers is discouraged. Many researchers have sought out to investigate the consequences of extensive irradiation to pacemakers in order to test their susceptibility to induced operation changes that is unwanted. For such testing, researchers often place the devices directly in the path of the beam. However, the approach is safely conducted when the generator is implanted into a phantom environment, thus removing concerns for patient radiation safety as well as needs for clinical trials. Further, with devices tested directly in the path of the beam, the total time for irradiation is much less than if it were placed out of the field, to arrive at the same cumulative dose for testing. Numerous issues were discovered by researchers. These will now be summarized here.

3. X-ray radiation

A large pacemaker study was performed (Mouton et al., 2002) incorporating a batch of 96 used pacemakers to test the influence of radiotherapy and the electromagnetic field. Several dose-rates (from 0.05 to 8 Gy/min) where used to yield pacemaker cumulative doses ranging from 6.2 Gy to 120 Gy. According to this group, approximately 15% of the irradiated pacemakers showed an important failure under 5 Gy. Below 2 Gy, the results indicated failure occurrences to drop by 9% although still present. There maintained the observance of important defects noted at cumulative doses of merely 0.15 Gy.

Later, a smaller study (Hurkmans et al., 2005) was initiated involving 19 new pacemakers having radiation delivered directly to each in fractional increments up to doses of 120 Gy while being monitored. Results for pacing pulse tests included 25% amplitude deviations in 5 devices, a complete loss of signal in 7 devices, and 30-50% pulse duration decreases. Pacing frequency tests revealed inhibitions during irradiation for 8 devices. Sensing thresholds changed more than 25% for 2 devices with no recovery. Telemetry capability was lost entirely for 3 devices. Battery problems were exhibited in 5 devices. Lead impedance changes were seen in nearly all devices. Finally, although 5 devices did not show any error, 7 lost output completely. With the exception of one device, which showed its point of failure at 20 Gy, all other devices could withstand a dose of 90 Gy or more before it reached a point of failure.

Devices differ in their susceptibility to radiation interference and damage (Yerra & Reddy, 2007). The effect on the device is cumulative, depending on the total dose to the device. There was no safe threshold observed in either study, validating the concerns of the AAPM (Marbach et al., 1994).

4. Electromagnetic interference

Forty-five irradiated patients implanted with a heart rhythm device was prospectively investigated in an 8 years span (Ferrara, 2010) to identify any relationship between the various types of devices with the electric and magnetic fields produced near the linear accelerator. An analysis of radiation damage to pacemakers, depending on the geometric and dosimetric characteristics of the radiation beams was carried out. There were no discovered problems with the devices due to the interaction with the electromagnetic fields. Acute (3 cases) and late (2 cases) cardiac events were observed only in 5 patients who underwent treatment, but with no dysfunction observed in any pacemaker for electromagnetic interference (EMI).

5. Neutron radiation

Neutrons are created in interactions involving high energy x-rays or high energy protons. Most proton beams can produce a knock-out neutron. However, neutrons can only be produced by x-ray beams operating above 8.04 MV. The flux of thermal neutrons created by an 18 MV x-ray beam of a radiotherapy linear accelerator has been observed to have caused a high rate of soft errors in integrated circuits that contain ^{10}B compounds (Wilkinson et al., 2005). These memory-loss effects can be removed entirely if 6 MV x-rays are used alternatively.

6. Proton radiation

Investigations on proton beam radiation therapy with implanted cardiac pacemaker function have been studied in at least one group (Oshiro et al., 2008). After a phantom study confirmed the safety of proton therapy in patients with cardiac pacemakers, 8 patients were treated using proton therapy to a total tumor dose of 33-77 Gy in dose fractions of 2.2–6.6 Gy. Although all pulse generators remained outside the treatment field, 4 patients had pacing leads in the radiation field. All patients were monitored by means of electrocardiogram during treatment, and pacemakers were routinely examined before and after proton therapy. The phantom study could not distinguish between proton dose and neutron scatter dose contributions on pacemaker generators. However, device functionality observances were well documented. In the study, changes in heart rate occurred in 2 patients. Proton therapy can result in pacemaker malfunctions that manifest as changes in pulse rate and pulse patterns. Minor malfunctions of implanted cardiac pacemakers occurred in 25% of patients receiving relatively high dose-rate proton therapy. Therefore, it was recommended that patients with cardiac pacemakers should be monitored by means of electrocardiogram during proton therapy.

7. Brachytherapy

Limited research can be found with regard to radiation induced effects on pacemakers from sealed source radioactive material. This is mainly due to the large variety of types and energies of radiation that is emitted by all the different radionuclides available. Heavier emissions, such as alpha particles, beta particles and electrons each have mass. Therefore, they have no ability to penetrate the metal casing of the pacemaker. However, gamma radiation may pass through the device entirely, depending on the energy of the photon being considered. Some brachytherapy sources emit kilovoltage photons, whereas others emit megavoltage energies. In general for electronics, the greater the mass and energy of the incident radiation, the greater the likelihood for it to interact with metallic components that affect pacemaker functionality.

The limited research involving brachytherapy sources are also due to their intensity of emission. The radioactivity of a source is dependent on the stability of the atom and the quantity of emissions per unit time increment when it decays.. Most radiation oncology sources have relatively low activity concentrations. Consequently, radioactive material for human use generally does not deliver as high a dose-rate as a particle accelerator. Still, one such investigation was found (Abner et al., 2002). Intravascular brachytherapy has been used for more than 10 years to treat restenosis within the heart. The doses imparted to a pacemaker from intraluminal brachytherapy sources was calculated to be less than 0.01 Gy for ^{89}Sr as compared to 0.74 Gy for ^{192}Ir, maximally. Both were deemed non-consequential by the investigators, since no patient induced side effects were noted in the clinical study.

8. Magnetic resonance imaging

The presence of a cardiac pacemaker had been a strict FDA (Ahmed & Shellock, 2001; U.S. FDA, 1988) contraindication for patients undergoing a magnetic resonance imaging (MRI) procedure for pacemaker dependent patients since 2000. According to estimates, 50-75 percent of patients worldwide with implanted cardiac devices are expected to need an MRI scan during the lifetime of their devices (Kalin & Stanton, 2005). Consequences with the use of non-FDA approved devices as determined in computer modeling, in vitro testing, animal in vivo studies and clinical trials include a considerable list of concerns (Kalin & Stanton, 2005; Bassen & Mendoza, 2009; Roguin et al, 2004). These include: thermal injury to the myocardium and endocardium from electrode radiofrequency absorption heating of the electrode tip causing thermal tissue damage locally. Other consequences include induced voltage in leads that couple with pacing electrodes to trigger unwanted stimulation or sustained tachycardia, electrical in-operation, conductivity of the pacemaker case, vibration of the device, and a static magnetic field forcing of translation or rotation of the device or lead.

Recently, the U.S. FDA (U.S. FDA, 2011) relaxed their position with the advancement of an MRI compatible pacemaker; the Medtronic model Revo MRI™. The device may only be used with the associated CapSureFix MRI™ SureScan leads that are FDA approved for use in the MRI environment. The pacemaker may only be prescribed for certain patients under specific conditions. This comes after a few years of experience with a similar device outside of the United States. The Medtronic model EnRhythm had been approved since 2009 in Europe and is the first pacing system approved for MRI acquisition anywhere (Kalin & Stanton, 2005).

9. Summary

The following are a summary of the recommendations for medical physicists and radiation oncologists to consider for implantable pacemakers and cardioverter defibrillators when continuing care for a patient having a pacemaker implanted in the treatment planning process.

Recommendations for treatment planning:

i. Only conduct computed tomography scanning using the commissioned extended Hounsfield unit range when using these scans for computer modeled dose delivery simulation calculations.
ii. Incorporate known implant device outer dimension information provided by the manufacturer in assisting manual contouring of the device in simulation software.
iii. Remove all streaking artifacts local to the pacemaker implant device that may cause the resulting calculation to be inaccurate.
iv. Position reference points for computer prescriptions away from all high density areas.

v. Use algorithms for calculation that minimally have three dimensional convolution superposition capabilities for most accuracy in determining dose with high density implants.
vi. Avoid directly aiming radiation through the pacemaker through the pacemaker and provide a considerable margin away from the field edge so that it is away from the penumbra region.
vii. Facilitate both homogeneous and heterogeneous calculations while comparing the differences observed for a better understanding of the magnitude and direction of profile shifts in the isodose distribution.
viii. Review published research on treatment planning system inaccuracies involving these devices.

Recommendations for treatment & imaging:

i. Particulate radiation at low energies, such as those from brachytherapy sealed sources, generally cannot penetrate the casing of a pacemaker and will therefore likely not be of any considerable cause of device malfunction, unless they are adjacent to high dose-rate afterloader devices containing ^{192}Ir at high activity.
ii. With proven consequences resulting with higher dose-rates for x-ray radiation, the smallest clinical dose-rate should be utilized.
iii. X-ray radiations at 6 MV energy are preferred over higher energies, since lower nominal x-ray energies and those from radioactive material brachytherapy sources will avoid neutron production and their consequences.
iv. Proton and neutron radiations have indicated the ability to induce malfunctions in similar to x-rays. Proton irradiation is known to create secondary neutrons, which can interact heavily with devices containing ^{10}B compounds. All such patients should be monitored with an electrocardiogram before and after treatment.
v. EMI changes have yet to be verified in the research referenced.
vi. Cumulative dose testing has shown no real absolute threshold for a safe dose to the pacemaker. However, the least dose possible should be considered strongly as the suitable plan for treatment. This is consistent with the ALARA standard; "As low as reasonably achievable."

Finally, consultation with the implanting pacing specialist, radiation oncologist and medical physicist should always be obtained for each patient, aside of the initial preparation for such cases, in an attempt to devise an in-house quality assurance protocol addressing timelines for assessing patient and device status during all imaging and radiation therapy procedures. As a general precaution for situations that arise beyond material presented here, it is strongly recommended that the clinician contact the manufacturer about the specific model in question, while referring to the most recent investigative research and updated formal guidance from the AAPM Task Group-203, which is now pending.

10. References

Abner AL, Meskell P, Carrozza J, et al. (2002). Dose to cardiac pacemakers and implanted defibrillators from beta and gamma coronary artery brachytherapy. *International*

Journal of Radiation Oncology Biology and Physics, Vol. 54, No. 2 (Supplement 1), pp. 301, ISSN 0360-3016

Ahmed S and Shellock FG. (2001). Magnetic resonance imaging safety: implications for cardiovascular patients. *Journal of Cardiovascular Magnetic Resonance*, Vol. 3, No. 3, pp. 171-182, ISSN 1097-6647

Bassen HI, Mendoza GG. (2009). In-vitro mapping of E-fields induced near pacemaker leads by simulated MR gradient fields. *Biomedical Engineering Online*, Vol. 8, No. 1, pp. 39, ISSN 1475-925X

Coolens C, Childs PJ. (2003). Calibration of CT Hounsfield units for radiotherapy treatment planning of patients with metallic hip prostheses: the use of the extended CT-scale. *Physics in Medicine and Biology*, Vol. 48, No. 11, pp. 1591-1603, ISSN 0031-9155

Ferrara T, Baiotto B, Malinverni G, et al. (2010). Irradiation of pacemakers and cardio-defibrillators in patients submitted to radiotherapy: a clinical experience. *Tumori* Vol. 96, No. 1, pp. 76-83, ISSN 0300-8916

Gossman MS. (Mar 21, 2011). Radiation Oncology dose gradients induced by heart rhythm devices. *Diagnostic & Interventional Cardiology Magazine*, ISSN 1551-6091, 04.06.2011, Available from: http://www.dicardiology.net/node/39108/

Gossman MS, Graves-Calhoun AR and Wilkinson JD. (2010). Establishing radiation therapy treatment planning effects involving implantable pacemakers and implantable cardioverter-defibrillators. *Journal of Applied Clinical Medical Physics*, Vol. 11, No. 1, pp. 1-13, ISSN

Gossman MS, Nagra B, Graves-Calhoun AR and Wilkinson JD. (2011). Beam profile disturbances from interactions with implantable pacemakers and implantable cardioverter-defibrillators. *Medical Dosimetry Journal*, Vol. 36, No. 2, pp. In print, ISSN 0958-3947

Gossman MS, Seuntjens JP, Christian KJ, et al. (2009). Dosimetric effects near implanted vascular access ports: an examination of external photon beam dose calculations. *Journal of Applied Clinical Medical Physics*, Vol. 10, No. 3, pp. 3-15, ISSN 1526-9914

Gullane PJ. (1991). Primary mandibular reconstruction: analysis of 64 cases and evaluation of interface radiation dosimetry on bridging plates. *Laryngoscope*, Vol. 101, No. 6 Pt. 2 Suppliment 54, pp. 1–24, ISSN 1531-4995

Hurkmans C, Scheepers E, Springorum B, et al. (2005). Influence of radiotherapy on the latest generation of pacemakers. *Radiotherapy and Oncology*, Vol. 76, No. 1, pp. 93-98, ISSN 1067-8140

Kalin R, Stanton MS. (2005). Current clinical issues for MRI scanning of pacemaker and defibrillator patients. *Pacing and Clinical Electrophysiology*, Vol. 28, No. 4, pp. 326-328, ISSN 1540-8159

Marbach JR, Sontag MR, Van Dyk J, Wolbarst AB. (1994). AAPM Report No. 45 (TG-34) - Management of Radiation Oncology patients with implanted cardiac pacemakers. *Medical Physics*, Vol. 21, No. 1, pp. 85-90, ISSN 0094-2405

McCollough CH, Zhang J, Primak AN, et al. (2007). Effects of CT irradiation on implantable cardiac rhythm management devices. *Radiology*, Vol. 243, No. 3, pp. 766-774, ISSN 1527-1315

Mouton J, Haug R, Bridier A, et al. (2002). Influence of high-energy photon beam irradiation on pacemaker operation. *Physics in Medicine and Biology*, Vol. 47, No. 16, pp. 2879-93, ISSN 0031-9155

Oshiro Y, Sugahara S, Noma M, et al. (2008). Proton beam therapy interference with implanted cardiac pacemakers. *International Journal of Radiation Oncology Biology and Physics*, Vol. 72, No. 3, pp. 723-727, ISSN 0360-3016

Reft C, Alecu R, Das IJ, Gerbi BJ, et al. (2003). Dosimetric considerations for patients with HIP prosthetics undergoing pelvis irradiation - Report of the AAPM Radiation Therapy Committee Task Group 63. *Medical Physics*, Vol. 30, No. 6, pp. 1162-1182, ISSN 0094-2405

Riley B, Garcia J, and Guerrero T. (2004). The utilization of a 3-dimensional non-coplanar treatment plan to avoid pacemaker complications. *Medical Dosimetry*, Vol. 29, No. 2, pp. 92-96, ISSN 0958-3947

Roguin A, Zviman MM, Meininger GR, et al. (2004). Modern pacemaker and implantable cardioverter defibrillator systems can be magnet resonance imaging safe. *Circulation*, Vol. 110, No. 5, pp. 475-482, ISSN 0009-7322

Solan AN, Solan MJ, Bednarz G and Goodkin MB. (2004). Treatment of patients with cardiac pacemakers and implantable cardioverer-defibrillators during radiotherapy. *International Journal of Radiation Oncology Biology and Physics*, Vol. 59, No. 3, pp. 897-904, ISSN 0360-3016

U.S. Food and Drug Administration. (1988). Magnetic resonance diagnostic device: panel recommendation and report on petitions for MR reclassification. *Federal Register*, Vol. 53, pp. 7575-7579, ISSN 0097-6326

U.S. Food and Drug Administration. (Feb 8, 2011). FDA News Release: FDA approves 1st pacemaker designed to work safely during some MRI exams, 04.06.2011, Available from: http://www.fda.gov/NewsEvents/Newsroom/PressAnnouncements/ucm242651.htm

White GA. (Apr 21, 2008). AAPM response to DRAFT Preliminary Public Health Notification: Possible malfunction of electronic medical devices during computed tomography (CT) scanning, 04.06.2011, Available from: http://www.aapm.org/government_affairs/documents/AAPM_comments_FDA_notification_CT_integrated_04-21-08.pdf

Wilkinson, JD, Bounds C, Brown T, et al. (2005). Cancer-radiotherapy equipment as a cause of soft errors in electronic equipment. *Device and Materials Reliability, IEEE Transactions*, Vol. 5, No. 3, pp. 449-451, ISSN 1530-4388

Yamaji A, Imai S, Saito F, et al. (2006). Does high-power computer tomography scanning equipment affect the operation of pacemakers? *Circulation Journal*, Vol. 70, No. 2, pp. 190-197, ISSN 1347-4820

Yerra L and Reddy PC. (2007). Effects of electromagnetic interference on implanted cardiac devices and their management. *Cardiology in Review*, Vol. 15, No. 6, pp. 304-309, ISSN 1061-5377

Part 4

Non-Cardiac Pacemakers

10

Pacemakers in the Upper Urinary Tract

Antonina Di Benedetto[1], Salvatore Arena[1], Francesco Arena[2], Carmelo Romeo[2], Piero Antonio Nicòtina[3] and Carlo Magno[1]
[1]*Unit of Urology, University of Messina,*
[2]*Unit of Pediatric Surgery, University of Messina,*
[3]*Unit of Human Pathology, University of Messina,*
Italy

1. Introduction

In the upper urinary tract, the mechanisms by which urine is transported from the kidney to the bladder remain little understood. For the last 35 years, it has been thought that pyeloureteric autorhythmicity arises in specialized electrically active atypical smooth muscle cells (SMC) that have many of the morphological and electrical features of cardiac sino-atrial cells and are predominantly located in the proximal regions of the ureteropelvic junction (UPJ). However, increasing evidence indicates that ICC-like cells (ICC-LC), displaying many of the morphological features of intestinal ICC and immuno-reactivity to antibodies raised against the c-*Kit* proto-oncogene, are present in the UPJ of a number of mammals. These cells are c-Kit-positive in upper urinary tract (UUT) of mouse and Human, c-kit-negative in guinea pig (Lang JR et al 2006.) c-*Kit* immuno-reactivity also appears developmentally at the same time of coordinated unidirectional peristaltic contractions in mouse embryonic ureters in organ culture. Moreover, the development of the ureteric structure and peristaltic contractions in organ colture can be prevented upon exposure to the c-Kit antibody, ACK45 (David SG et al 2005), suggesting that ICC-LC play a crucial role in promoting pyeloureteric peristalsis.
ICCs were first described by Ramon Y Cajal in 1893 as primitive neurons in the gastrointestinal system (GIS) (Lang JR et al 2006; Cajal SR 1893). Infact, ICCs were firstly found in relation to the Auerbach plexus, but also in the submucosal plexus and between the muscle layers. Moreover, mice with spontaneous mutations of the c-kit genes, and that are deficient in ICCs, lack spontaneous slow waves in the intestine and display uncoordinated peristalsis (Streuker et al 2003). Further investigations revealed that ICCs play a role as pacemaker cells, between neurons and smooth muscle cells, are originally derived from the mesenchymal tissue, and are responsible for conduction of the slow wave electrical potential for peristaltic movements (Sanders KM 1996). Local decreases in or a lack of c-kit immunoreactivity on ICCs in the gut have been detected in Hirschsprungs's disease, infantile hypertrophic pyloric stenosis, and slow transmission constipation. Recently, mucosal ICC were reported at the human ureteropelvic junction (UPJ), the submucosal and muscolar layers of the rat vase deferents, between the stroma of smooth muscle layers and glandular layers of guinea pig prostate, between the smooth muscle fibers and neurons of guinea pig bladder and in the rabbit urethra (Solari V et al 2003). Also in the UUT, ICCs

have shown to be responsible for initiating, coordinating and producing ureteropelvic peristaltic movements at the intercaliceal area, providing the passage of urine from the caliceal system through the ureter to the bladder (Sergeant et al 2000).
Several studies have been performed in uni-calyceal mammals as mouse, dog, rat, guinea pig and rabbit as well in multi-calyceal species such as human and pig. In multi-calyceal mammals minor calyces combine to form several major calyces, which fuse together to form the renal pelvis. In the isolated pig renal pelvis, small amplitude contractile and electrical activity originates at the border of the major and minor calyces. Upon injection of saline into the upper calyx, these peristaltic waves propagate through the lower calyces to the renal pelvis and the UPJ. During periods of low urine production only a few of the muscle contractions in the renal pelvis travel through to the ureter (Morita T et al 1981). With higher rates of diuresis, transmission improves until there is a one-to-one propagation of all contractions to the ureter (Constantinou CE et al 1974, 1976). The ureter in human and pig displays spontaneous contractions *in vitro*. In contrast the ureter in dog, rabbit, pig and rat contracts spontaneously *in vitro* only in the presence of excitatory agonists (Morita T et al 1986; Patacchini R et al 1998) or if the renal pelvis is left attached (Golenhofen K et al 1973; Gosling JA et al 1971; Lang RJ et al 2001). In both uni-calyceal and multi-calyceal mammals, circumferentially cut strips of muscle wall dissected from the same region contract at the same frequency. However contraction frequency decreases with distance from the renal fornix as strips are dissected from the middle and lower calyces, renal pelvis and UPJ (Gosling JA et al 1971; Hannapel J et al 1978; Zhang Y & Lang RJ 1994). Thus researchers have located the primary pacemaker in the most proximal calyceal regions of the renal pelvis.

2. Ultrastructure of the upper urinary tract (UUT)

A compact layer of epithelial cells (mucous membrane) lines the lumen on the full length of the UUT stand, on a lamina propria of varying thickness containing collagen fibrils, myofibroblasts, as well as numerous small blood vessels and unmyelinated axon bundles. A layer of smooth muscle cells (SMC) surrounds the lamina propria. In the most proximal inter-renal regions of attachment of the UUT to the renal fornix, the pelvi-calyceal junction, cells are arranged in an open network, with large areas of intervening connective tissue. In the renal pelvis, SMC are arranged in small randomly oriented bundles, which create a plexiform layer of interconnecting bundles, separated by areas of connective tissue. In contrast the muscle wall of the ureter is arranged into an inner circular and an outer longitudinal layer of closely pace SMC. Surrounding these layers the adventitia is made up of connective tissue and fibroblasts and containing blood vessels, nerve bundles and lymphatic vessels (Notley RG 1978).

3. Atypical, typical smooth muscle and ICC-like cells in the UUT

Two types of smooth muscle cells within the muscle wall of the UUT have been identified under the light and electron microscope: 'atypical' and 'typical' SMC (Gosling JA & Dixon JS 1972,1974). A third population of electrically-active cells has been described in the UUT in human and many mammals (Lang RJ et al 2001; Gosling JA & Dixon JS 1974) which may well play a fundamental role in pyeloureteric autorythmicity.
Atypical SMCs have an irregular morphology and a non-specific cholinesterase. They have been described as long thin cells, having a small nucleus and being irregularly-shaped due to

the presence of many long branching processes. Their contractile myofilaments are arranged in bundles which are separated by large areas of cytoplasm containing Golgi cisternae, granular endoplasmic reticulum and small mitochondria occupying 3% of cell sectional area (Klemm MF et al 1999; Gosling JA & Dixon JS 1972) . They form areas of close apposition with each other and with typical SMC, these appositions being separated by long portions of naked membrane. In uni-calyceal kidneys, atypical SMC were firstly described as forming a discrete layer which begins at the pelvi-calyceal junction and continues the length of the renal pelvis to the UPJ (Dixon JS & Gosling JA 1970; Gosling JA & Dixon JS 1970,1971). In the rat and guinea pig, atypical SMC represent 22% and 80%, respectively, of the SMC present in the pelvi-calyceal junction. (Lang RJ et al 2001; Gosling JA & Dixon JS 1974)

In multi-calyceal kidneys, 'atypical' SMC alone form the muscle coat of each minor calyx. A thin sheet of loosely-arranged atypical SMC extends between the minor calyces creating an open network near the point of attachment to the kidney (Gosling JA & Dixon JS 1972,1974; Dixon JS & Gosling JA 1973,1982), the space between cells being filled with collagen-rich connective tissue and axon bundles (Lang RJ et al 2001; Klemm MF et al 1999; Dixon JS & Gosling JA 1970). A gradual thickening of the wall of the UUT of all mammals with distance from the pelvi-calyceal junction indicates the increasing presence of 'typical' SMC.

'Typical' SMC are described as long spindle-shaped cell, filled by contractile filament and surrounded by a continuous basal lamina and containing a large round/oval shaped nucleus and generally grouped into bundles. In the pig 'typical' SMC are evident in the major calyx, renal pelvis and ureter (Gosling JA & Dixon JS 1974 ; Dixon JS & Gosling JA 1970) . In the guinea pig and rat, typical SMC represent 78–83% and >98% of the SMC in the proximal renal pelvis and UPJ, respectively. The relative proportion of contractile-filament rich typical SMC and atypical SMC has been shown by immuno-staining sections of the pelvi-calyceal junction (P-CJ), renal pelvis (RP) and ureter for α smooth muscle actin, and it has been reported that the intensity of immuno-reactivity for α smooth muscle actin increases along the length of the UUT (Lang RJ et al 2001; Gosling JA & Dixon JS 1974).

ICC-like cells (ICC-LC) are the recently described population of electrically- active cells in the UUT (Lang RJ et al 2001; Gosling JA & Dixon JS 1974) and they seem to play a fundamental role in pyeloureteric autorythmicity. Under the electron microscope, these cells are stellate in appearance, the cytoplasmic area containing an oval-shaped nuclear region, numerous mitochondria (4% of cell sectional area), well-developed Golgi apparatus, but no contractile filaments or immuno-reactivity to α smooth muscle actin. The plasma membrane of these cells also displays a discontinuous basal lamina and numerous calveolae. These interstitial cells form close appositions both 20nm and adherens junctions, with themselves (80% of cells) and SMC. Thus these cells display many of the morphological features used to distinguish ICC, from fibroblasts within the wall of the intestinal tract (Huizinga JD et al 1997; Huizinga JD 2005). In the guinea-pig UUT, ICC-LC lay within in the lamina propria of the pelvi-calyceal region and the renal pelvis and do not form close associations (<30nm) with nerve bundles, nor they were identified in the ureter (Gosling JA & Dixon JS 1974). These cells are also immunoreactive to antibodies raised against c-kit proto oncogene, a member of the receptor-tyrosine kinase family. Several studies described ICC-LC in UUT. Solari *et al.* described that *c-kit* positive cells in human UPJ had a fusiform cell body with 2 distinct dendrites (Solari et al 2003), Pezzone *et al.* described *c-kit* positive cells in the mouse UUT as being stellate in appearance (Pezzone MA et al 2003). Networks of these *c-kit* positive cells were located adjacent to the inner longitudinal muscle layer and between the inner and outer SMC layers (Solari et al 2003, Pezzone MA et al 2003).

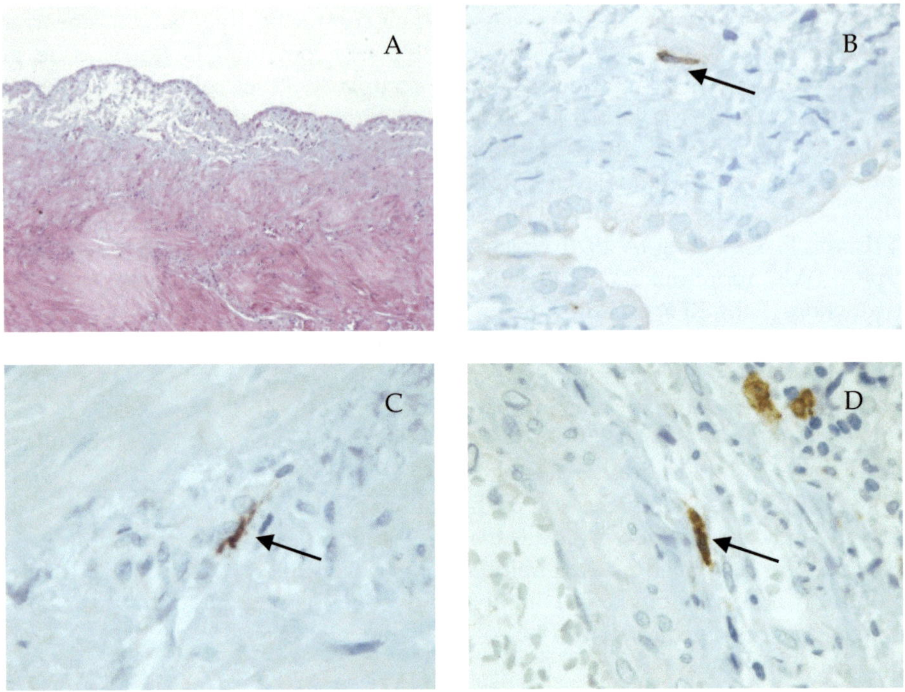

Fig. 1. Ureteral wall showing both the urothelium layer and a portion of smooth muscle layer (A) (H&H, Original magnification 125x) CD117 immunostaining displaying a cytoplasmic immunopositive Cajal cells in subepithelial (B), smooth muscle layer (C) and adventitial (D) sites (arrows), together with some mast-cells (Original magnification 250x)

There is general agreement that the number of these *c-kit* positive cells was greatest in the proximal renal pelvis and decreased with distance from the UPJ (Thompson CB 1995, Metzger R et al 2004, Pezzone MA et al 2003). Differences in technologies and antibodies used when fixing and staining preparations have been evoked to explain the variation of *c-kit* staining observed between species by different laboratories (Sleator W 1955, Pezzone MA et al 2003). Double labelling experiments have discounted the possibility that these c-kit-positive cells are mast cells, fibroblasts or macrophages (Metzger R et al 2004).

It is becoming clear that ICC and ICC-like cells in various urogenital and intestinal tissues can also be divided into a number of subpopulations on the basis of their immuno-reactivity or -negativity to c-kit, vimentin, actin filaments, ion channel populations (Lang RJ et al 2001; Gosling JA & Dixon JS 1974), receptors (Van der AaF et al 2004) and gap junction subunits. In human and less frequently pig, another population of 'vertically-orientated' *c-kit* positive spindle shape cells was present between the basal cells of the transitional epithelium (Metzger R 2004). The number of these radially arranged *c-kit* positive cells was greatest in the intermediate ureter and lowest in the renal pelvis. The role of these *c-kit* positive cells remains little unknown but it is interesting that these cells are present in an area that is richly innervated by sensory nerves suggesting that these ICC may be acting as an intermediate between the afferent innervation and the urothelium and maybe they are responsible even for initiating, coordinating and producing ureteropelvic peristaltic movements at the intercaliceal area, providing the passage of urine from the caliceal system through the ureter to the bladder.

4. Pacemaking in the UUT and electrical recordings

Pressure recordings and intracellular and extracellular electrophysiological investigations have established that every peristaltic contraction of the renal pelvis and ureter is preceded by a complex 'ureteric' or 'driven' action potential. Driven action potentials have a time course consisting of an initial slow membrane depolarization followed by a single or multiple rapidly-rising spike(s), which partially repolarize to a plateau phase (100ms to > 1s in duration) followed by a second repolarization to an afterhyperpolarization which decays back to the resting membrane potential (Sleator W et al 1955, Shuba MF 1977).

It has been also established that the probability of recording ureteric or 'driven' action potentials increased with distance from the renal fornix, from 75% of cells in the proximal renal pelvis to 89% in the distal renal pelvis and 100% of cells in the ureter. This gradient of recording action potentials with distance is due to an increasingly more negative membrane potential and a decreasing frequency of action potential discharge with distance from the renal fornix.

Atipical SMC and ICC-LC are described as pacemakers cells, essential for the induction and propagation of contractile electrical pulse.

Atypical SMC seems to be essential pacemaker cells of pelviureteric peristalsis. Investigators have envisaged that autorhythmicity within the upper urinary tract involves a 'chain of coupled linear oscillators' with the most proximal oscillator firing at the highest frequency, The decreasing presence of 'atypical' SMC with distance from the papillate base has been correlated with the decreasing frequency of contraction.

Atypical SMC have higher frequency (8-15 min-1) transient potentials of a simple waveform, those potentials are frequently (83% of cells) recorded in short "atypical" SMC (90–230μm in length) in the pelvi-calyceal junction of the guinea pig renal pelvis (Patacchini R et al 1998; Klemm MF et al 1999; Seki N et al 1990, Tsuchida S et al 1992). These transient potentials were recorded less frequently in the proximal renal pelvis (10% of recordings) and never in the ureter (Lang RJ et al 2001; Gosling JA & Dixon JS 1974). High frequency transient potentials and driven action potentials in the renal pelvis and ureter have been demonstrated by research groups, to be abolished by nifedipine, suggesting that Ca2+ entry through voltage gated L-type Ca2+ channels is essential in the initiation, maintenance or propagation of these electrical events. This model implies that the intrinsic frequency of pacemaking atypical SMC decreases with distance from the papilla base which would require morphologically similar cells having different expression profiles of voltage- and Ca2+-activated ion channels and pacemaking apparatus as their location increases with distance from the papilla.

Diuresis also has an important role in ureter peristalsis. It has been suggested that diuresis to distend the muscle wall which increases, in an unknown manner, the 'coupling' of the pacemaker regions in the longitudinal direction until the highest frequency oscillator in the proximal regions entrains the oscillators in the distal regions of the renal pelvis.

Furthermore simultaneous extracellular recordings from numerous sites on the sheep renal pelvis have revealed that only one pacemaker region on the pelvi-calyceal border is active at any one time and that the pathway of conduction might meander throughout the renal pelvis. The site of the pacemaker signal on the pelvi-calyceal border can shift spontaneously, conduction delays or block of the wave of excitation can occur at any point or time (Lammers WJ et al 1996). These observations do not support the concept of summation of subthreshold pacemaker activity. Rather it suggests that one pacemaker region in the proximal portion of the UUT dominates to drive neighbouring regions and that conduction block is a dynamic process and modulated by a number of factors such as wall stress or the hormonal/neurotransmitter/prostaglandin milieu. These mechanisms may explain the conduction block between the renal pelvis and the ureter evident *in vivo* under conditions of low urine production which is relieved during periods of increased diuresis.

ICC-LC have been described as a population of active cells which may well be responsible for additional autorythmicity. A number of investigators have demonstrated that ICC-LC form close appositions with themselves and with neighboring typical and atypical SMC, suggesting electrical connectivity and conduction.

Intracellular microelectrode impalements have been made from the serosal surface of the pelvi-calyceal junction and renal pelvis of the guinea pig and it has been that 11–17% of cells fired spontaneous action potentials with a distinctive time course consisting of a single spike followed by a quiescent plateau and a rapid repolarization. (Klemm MF et al 1999).

In the guinea pig UUT contractions occur regularly from a stable baseline at a frequency (4–7 min) essentially similar to the frequency of driven action potential discharge and lower than the frequency of discharge of transient potentials (Zhang Y et al 1994; Lang RJ et al 2002). Spontaneous transient potentials arise in atypical SMC and propagate to neighbouring typical SMC and ICC-like cells, triggering driven and intermediate action potentials, respectively.

The mechanisms involved in the generation and propagation of pacemaker potentials in SMC display considerable variation between tissues and species.

In conclusion, except for the very proximal regions of the UTT and distal ureteric regions, it looks that two populations of pacemaker cells, atypical SMC and ICC-LC, are present in any portion of UUT and that the drive of each pacemaker system on any typical SMC bundle varies with distance from the papilla base. Importantly, to the best of our knowledge, there aren't any pharmacological agents at present that selectively identify, block or activate the drive of either pacemaker system. Although c-kit antibody binding to unfixed tissues allows for the identification and selective recording from c-kit-positive ICC-LC, there are no vital stains selective for atypical SMC or c-kit-negative ICC-LC to allow a similar targeted examination of their influence on muscle wall contractility. Anyway, a complete electrophysiological and pharmacological profile of c-kit- positive/negative ICC-LC and atypical SMC at the single cell level and the establishment of any species differences or changes in properties might be crucial before the development of a complete model of UPJ autorhythmicity.

The renal pelvis and ureter represent a functional system with myogenic excitation, generation and conduction. The coordination between renal pelvis and ureteral peristalsis is an important part of the hydrodynamics of the upper urinary tract. Contraction waves arising from the upper and urinary tract, and propagation may require the direct involvement of ICCs, which are the pacemaker cells in SMC. As in gastrointestinal motility, ICCs may have a significant role in the propagation, coordination and modulation of UUT peristalsis. As in the gastrointestinal tract damage, several studies have been done to identify a possible pathogenetic factor of altered ICC in genitourinary disease as primary vesicoureteral reflux, congenital ureteropelvic junction obstruction and primary obstructive megaureter.

5. Congenital ureteropelvic junction obstruction

Congenital ureteropelvic junction (UPJ) obstruction is the most common cause of neonatal hydronephrosis with a frequency of 1/1,000 to 2,000 newborns. Previous and recent studies showed abnormal innervation patterns and abnormalities of smooth muscle or collagen in UPJ cases, including absent or deficient muscle and muscular malorientation, suggesting a basis for disordered function and obstruction (Solari V et al 2003).

The renal pelvis and ureter represent a functional system with myogenic excitation, generation and conduction. The coordination between renal pelvis and ureteral peristalsis is an important part of the hydrodynamics of the upper urinary tract. Contraction waves arising from the upper urinary tract, and propagation may require the direct involvement of ICCs, which are the pacemaker cells in smooth muscle. As described, ICCs may have a significant role in the propagation, coordination and modulation of ureteropelvic peristalsis. Decreased expression of c-kit positive ICCs in UPJ obstruction may cause the failure of transmission of peristaltic waves across the UPJ, resulting in the failure of urine to be propelled from the renal pelvis into the ureter in UPJ obstruction. Solari et al (Solari V et al 2003) examined the status of UPJ innervation using immunohistochemistry with antiperipherin antibody (type III intermediate filament, a specific marker for peripheral neurons, and nerve fibers). Peripherin immunoreactive nerve fibers were markedly decreased in obstructed UPJ samples. So in patients with UPJ obstruction there is not only defective intramuscular innervation of UPJ, but also altered distribution of ICCs, which are coordinators of peristaltic activity. The lack or deficient expression of ICCs in the UPJ may lead to defective generation of pacemaker activity, thus, causing peristaltic activity dysfunction.

The lack or absence of c-kit positive ICCs in obstructed UPJ specimens suggests that this might be responsible for motility disturbance of the upper ureter. The possible link between absent ICCs and other features reported in obstructed UPJ cases, such as neuronal depletion in the muscle layers, justify additional studies. Further investigations of ICCs are still necessary to understand better the pacemaker mechanism in the human upper urinary tract and the unknown etiology of the failure of spontaneous contractions to propel urine from the renal pelvis through the ureter in patients with UPJ obstruction.

6. Primary vesico-ureteral reflux

Primary vesico-ureteral reflux (VUR) is thought to be caused by a congenital structural deficiency of the trigonal vesico-ureteral junction (VUJ) due to maturational abnormalities. The VUJ represents the boundary line between the low-pressure upper urinary tract and the high variable pressure of the lower urinary tract. It protects the upper tract from reflux using active and passive antireflux mechanisms. The most common explanation of a competent valve mechanism is passive compression of the roof of the intravesical ureter against the underlying detrusor. The length of the intravesical ureter relative to its diameter seems to be the crucial point supporting the 'passive' reflux defence mechanism (Arena S. et al 2007). The 'active' antireflux system is due to the contraction of the longitudinal muscle coat of the VUJ. Active shortening of the longitudinal muscle layer of the transmural and submucosal ureterer areas ejects the bolus of urine into the bladder lumen.

Reductions of the total smooth muscle mass or defective configurations creating insufficient or uncoordinated contractions are accompanied by a decrease in the neuronal supply or aganglionosis. Predominantly in the upper urinary tract, coordinated peristalsis is essential to propel urine from the renal pelvis down to the bladder in a unidirectional way. Those peristaltic waves are generated in the renal pelvis and the proximal ureter by pacemaker cells. Functional and structural alterations of ureteric ends seem to impair the active valve mechanism of the VUJ, causing VUR (Schwentner C et al 2005). Several studies have shown that the reducing of the total smooth muscle fascicles or a defective configuration creating insufficient or uncoordinated contractions are accompanied by a loss of c-kit-positive ICCs at the VUJ. Manometric findings on refluxing ureteric units (RUs) showed changed manometric patterns. In fact, the pressures recorded in the VUJ in the control and patients with VUR fluctuated rhythmically from a basal pressure to a high pressure during peristalsis (Pmax). While in RUs affected by grade I to III VUR the waves were rhythmic, the manometric profile in grade IV and V VUR was an arrhythmic or 'silent' pattern, with typical bicuspid spikes in the manometric record. Moreover, the basal and maximum pressure were negatively correlated with the grade of VUR (Arena S. et al 2007).

The variable and inconsistent pressures of the peristaltic waves, and the irregular wave rhythm, are likely to result in disturbed urine transport along the distal part of RUs, while the silent ureter might represent an advanced stage of ureteric arrhythmia, suggesting a more damaged ureter resembling a ureteric arrhythmic state.

Histological and histochemical findings showed a varied extent of change in intravesical RU tracts, e.g. muscle disarrangement and atrophy, and increased interstitial fibrosis. It has been reported a significant correlation between the grades of VUR and smooth muscle lesions, in according with Gearhart *et al.* (Gosling JA 1995) who reported a degree of smooth muscle deterioration and more collagen deposition in dilated refluxing ureters than in normal ureters. Moreover, Oswald *et al.* (Oswald J et al 2004) reported a replacement of muscle bundles by connective tissue, leading to ureteric rigidity. It is patent that a defect of the longitudinal muscle coat implies an impairment of the contraction of the ureteric muscular layer, producing VUR. In fact, both the ostial valve contraction and ureteric peristalsis support an 'active' antireflux mechanism (Oswald J et al 2003). A significant decrease in c kit- positive ICCs, common tissue regulators in assisting peristalsis, has been described. It is not clear why depletion of c-kit-expressing ICCs occurs in RU ends. Interestingly, mammalian ICCs derive from smooth muscle progenitors, whose differentiation is independent of neural crest-derived cell lines (Wu JJ et al 2000). In RU there is a grade-correlated defect of muscle cells, among which c-kit-positive ICCs differentiate inside the ureteric ending, so that the loss of c-kit-positive ICCs might be a consequence of the disruption of muscle cells. Alternatively, as mesenchymal cells, surrounding the mesonephric duct, differentiate into the ureteric inner layer of smooth muscle cells, the delayed elongation of the Wolffian duct endings might be a pathogenetic event for muscular and subsequent ICC defects in VUR. Thus, the late maturation of ureteric ends is coherent with a possible spontaneous resolution of VUR, after postnatal remodelling of the VUJ, as shown for the pathogenesis of primary megaureter (Nicotina PA et al 1997). Loss of c-kit-positive ICCs could be also secondary to ureteric trauma during episodes of VUR, as reported in the proximal segment of obstructed fetal bowel (Khen N et al 2004). Consistently it is acknowledged that that mechanical stress can affect the expression of development genes, providing evidence that molecular signals are not the only forces that are involved in modelling the developing embryo.

In conclusion, RU ends share muscle disarrangement and fibrosis, dysfunction of the ostial valve and impairment of basal VUJ pressure, impairing significantly peristaltic waves. It's shown that the density of c-kit-positive ICCs in VUR negatively correlated with the grade of VUR and positively with Pmax , implying qualitative and quantitative alterations of peristaltic waves in VUR. These observations underline the assumption that VUR is related to an inadequately active mechanism, but further investigations are needed to clarify the origin of architectural lesions and the absence of c-kit- positive ICCs.

7. Congenital primary obstructive megaureter

Congenital megaureter is a term used in many cases of urinary tract dilation detected before and after birth (Shokeir AA et al 2000). In children, the ureteral diameter is usually not >5 mm, and when it is >7 mm, it could be considered a megaureter (Angerri O et al 2007).
The studies by Payabvash et al. (Payabvash S et al 2007) and Kajbafzadeh et al. (Kajbafzadeh AM et al 2006) revealed that the proportion of muscular content in the ureteral wall of an obstructed vesicoureteral junction is significantly lower than that in normal specimens. Lee et al. (Lee BR et al 1992) suggested that active and passive biomechanical wall properties, as well as morphologic parameters, such as decreased smooth muscle and increased collagen content are likely to change in various pathologic situations, including the obstructed megaureter. It has been suggested that abnormal peristalsis might have potentially contributed to the development of both obstructive and the increased collagen of the dilated ureter might be responsible for the abnormal peristalsis.

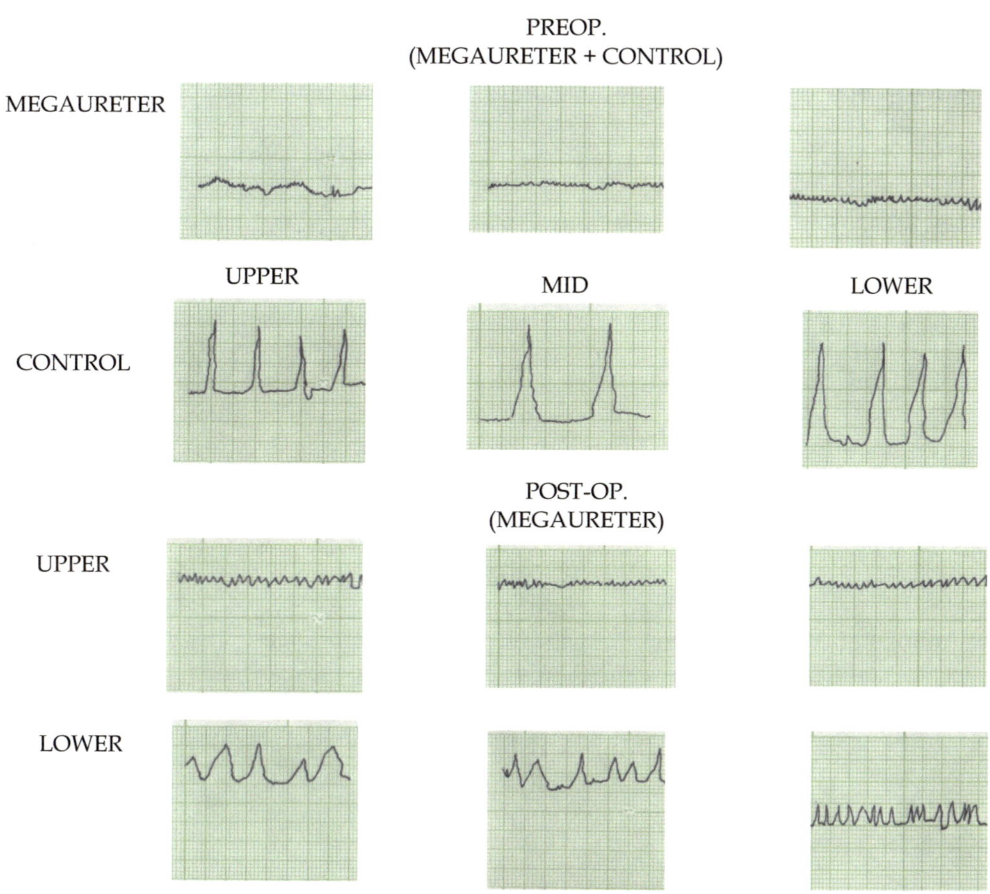

Fig. 2. Electromanometric ureteral findings in unilateral congenital megaureter: the upper track shows an impaired peristalsis in all ureteral parts as compared with contralateral ureter that has normal peristalsis . The post operative findings show only respiratory waves in the dilated upper ureter as compared with the normal peristaltic activity in the lower tract.

It was observed that apoptosis was significantly increased in the primary obstructive megaureter compared with the refluxing one. Kim et al. (Kim HG et al 2006) suggested that cell proliferation and apoptosis might play an important role in the pathogenesis of the obstructive megaureter. In fact, apoptosis of myocytes in the obstructive megaureter might affecr peristalsis. According to Kim et al. (Kim HG et al 2006) peak proliferation is noted during the early stage and apoptosis during the late stage of obstruction in animal models of obstructive ureter. We also hypothesized that the number of ICC-like cells, which are known to play an important role in peristalsis as a pacemaker of smooth muscle contraction, might be altered. As regards, it has been observed a normal distribution of ICCs in both the circular and longitudinal muscle layers of the dilated segments of patients affected by congenital primary megaureter, while a severe muscle hypoplasia and significant less of ICCs occurred in the longitudinal muscle layer of the restricted part of primary obstructive megaureter. Differently, a normal distribution of peripherin positive fibres was present in both the dilated and restricted ureteral segments (Arena F et al 2007).
Because megaureter is also a congenital disease with abnormal peristalsis, it has been hypothesized that the alterations in the number or function of ICC cells might induce discoordination between the signals of the nervous system and smooth muscle, causing abnormal peristalsis and, eventually, resulting in the development of ureteral dilation.
In contrast, a comparison between primary refluxing and obstructive magaureters showed that the number of c-kit-positive cells was clearly different between the obstructive and refluxing megaureters, with the latter having significantly fewer ICC-like cells than the former. Studies of mice with mutations leading to defects in the development of c-kit positive ICC populations have shown that without pacemakers, the coordination of smooth muscle contractions is lost.(Brading AF et al 2005).
Torihashi et al (Torihashi S et al 1999) reported that when c-kit receptors were blocked during development, the ICCs almost entirely disappeared from the small intestine. However, this loss of ICCs was not accounted for using assays for cell death, and closer examination revealed that the remaining ICCs developed ultrastructural features similar to those of smooth muscle cells. According to Burns (Burns AJ 2007) an inherent plasticity between ICCs and smooth muscle cells is regulated by c-kit signaling. c-kit signaling might be necessary for the maintenance and further development of ICC-like cells before and after birth, accounting for the spontaneous improvement of such conditions with time in some cases. According to the study by Mei et al (Mei F et al 2009) the ICC number is reduced after intestinal ischemic injury but makes a dramatic recovery. However, ischemic injury can lead to apoptosis of the ICCs, smooth muscle cells, and enteric neurons. Therefore, the higher c-kit expression in obstructive megaureters as compared to refluxing ureter might have been preceded by a reduction in ICC-like cells after ischemic injury, such as in the intestines, and the remaining increased apoptosis of smooth muscle cells might be the cause of the ureteral dysfunction.

8. Conclusions

ICC-LC are present in the UUT of a number of mammals and they have a crucial role in promoting pyeloureteric peristalsis. Studies showed that ICC-LC are responsible for initiating, coordinating and producing ureteropelvic peristaltic movements at the intercaliceal area, providing the passage of urine from the caliceal system through the ureter to the bladder. In conclusion, as well as in some gastrointestinal diseases (Hirschsprungs's disease, infantile hypertrophic pyloric stenosis, slow transmission constipation), a local decrease or a lack of c-kit immunoreactivity ICCs-LC may be involved in dysfunctional disease of urinary tract as primary vesicoureteral reflux, congenital ureteropelvic junction obstruction and primary obstructive megaureter.

9. Abbreviations

ACK:	c-kit antibodies
GIS:	gastrointestinal system
ICC:	interstitial cajal cells
ICC-LC:	ICC-like cells
P-CJ:	pelvi-calyceal junction
RP:	renal pelvis
RUs:	refluxing ureteric units
SMC:	smooth muscle cell
UPJ:	ureteropelvic junction
UTT:	upper urinary tract
VUR:	Primary vesico-ureteral reflux
VUJ:	trigonal vesico-ureteral junction

10. References

Arena F, Nicòtina PA, Arena S, Romeo C, Zuccarello B, Romeo G. C-kit positive interstitial cells of Cajal network in primary obstructive megaureter. Minerva Pediatr. 2007 Feb;59(1):7-11.

Arena S et al. Altered 'active' antireflux mechanism in primary vesico-ureteric reflux: a morphological and manometric study. BJU International (2007) 100, 407-412.

Angerri O, Caffaratti J, Garat JM, et al. Primary obstructive megaureter: initial experience with endoscopic dilatation. *J Endourol.* 2007;21:999-1004.

Brading AF, McCloskey KD. Mechanisms of disease: specialized interstitial cells of the urinary tract—an assessment of current knowledge. *Nat Clin Pract Urol.* 2005;2:546-554.

Burns AJ. Disorders of interstitial cells of Cajal. *J Pediatr Gastroenterol Nutr.* 2007;45(suppl 2):S103-S106.

Cajal SR. Sur le ganglions et plexus nerveux d' intestine. CR Soc Biol 1893; 5:217-23 (abstract).

Constantinou CE. Renal pelvic pacemaker control of ureteral peristaltic rate. *Am J Physiol.* 1974; 226: 1413–9.

Constantinou CE, Hrynczuk JR. Urodynamics of the upper urinary tract. *Invest Urol.* 1976; 14: 233–40.

David SG, Cebrian C, Vaughan ED & Herzlinger D (2005). C-kit and ureteral peristalsis. *J Urol* 173, 292–295.

Dixon JS, Gosling JA. Fine structural observations on the attachment of the calix to the renal parenchyma in the rat. *J Anat.* 1970; 106: 181–2.

Dixon JS, Gosling JA. The fine structure of pacemaker cells in the pig renal calices. *Anat Res.* 1973; 175: 139–53.

Dixon JS, Gosling JA. The musculature of the human renal calices, pelvis and upper ureter. *J Anat.* 1982; 135: 129–37.

Golenhofen K, Hannappel J. Normal spontaneous activity of the pyeloureteral system in the guinea-pig. *Pflügers Archiv - Eur J Physiol.* 1973; 341; 257–70.

Gosling JA. A quantitative histological evaluation of the dilated ureter of childhood. II. Ectopia, posterior urethral valves and the prune belly syndrome. *J Urol* 1995; 153: 172–6.

Gosling JA, Waas AN. The behaviour of the isolated rabbit calix and pelvis compared with that of the ureter. *Eur JPharmacol.* 1971; 16: 100–4.

Gosling JA, Dixon JS. Structural evidence in support of an urinary tract pacemaker. *Brit J Urol.* 1972; 44: 550–60.

Gosling JA, Dixon JS. Species variation in the location of upper urinary tract pacemaker cells. *Invest Urol.*1974; 11: 418–23.

Gosling JA, Dixon JS. Further observations on upper urinary tract smooth muscle. A light and electron microscope study. *Z Zellforsch Mikrosk Anat.* 1970; 108: 127–34.

Hannappel J, Lutzeyer W. Pacemaker localization in the renal pelvis of the unicalyceal kidney. *In vitro* study in the rabbit. *Europ Urol.* 1978; 4: 192–4.

Huizinga JD, Thuneberg L, Vanderwinden JM, Rumessen JJ. Interstitial cells of Cajal as targets for pharmacological intervention in gastrointestinal motor disorders. *Trends Pharmacol Sci.* 1997; 18: 393–403.

Huizinga JD. Frontiers in research into interstitial cells of Cajal. *J Cell Mol Med.* 2005; 9: 230–1.

Kajbafzadeh AM, Payabvash S, Salmasi AH, et al. Smooth muscle cell apoptosis and defective neural development in congenital ureteropelvic junction obstruction. *J Urol.* 2006;176:718-723.

Khen N, Jaubert F, Sauvat F *et al.*; Group for Study of Intestinal Atresia. Fetal intestinal obstruction induces alteration of enteric nervous system development in human intestinal atresia. *Pediatr Res* 2004; 56: 975–80.

Kim HG, Paick SH, Kwak C, et al. Serial microscopic changes in cell proliferation and apoptosis in obstructed ureter of rat. *J Endourol.* 2006;20:590-597.

Klemm MF, Exintaris B, Lang RJ. Identification of the cells underlying pacemaker activity in the guinea-pig upper urinary tract. *J Physiol.* 1999; 519: 867–84.

Lammers WJ, Ahmad HR, Arafat K. Spatial and temporal variations in pacemaking and conduction in the isolated renal pelvis. *Am J Physiol.* 1996; 270: F567–74.

Lang RJ, Takano H, Davidson M E, Suzuki H, Klemm MF. Characterization of the spontaneous electrical and contractile activity of smooth muscle cells in the rat upper urinary tract. *J Urol.* 2001; 166: 329–34.

Lang RJ, Hashitani H, Keller S, Takano H, Mulholland EL, Fukuta H, Suzuki H. Modulators of internal Ca2+ stores and the spontaneous electrical and contractile activity of the guinea-pig renal pelvis. *Brit J Pharmacol.* 2002; 135: 1363–74.

Lee BR, Partin AW, Epstein JI, et al. A quantitative histological analysis of the dilated ureter of childhood. *J Urol.* 1992;148:1482-1486.

Mei F, Guo S, He YT, et al. Apoptosis of interstitial cells of Cajal, smooth muscle cells, and enteric neurons induced by intestinal ischemia and reperfusion injury in adult guinea pigs. *Virchows Arch.* 2009;454:401-409

Metzger R, Schuster T, Till H, Stehr M, Franke FE, Dietz HG. Cajal-like cells in the human upper urinary tract. *J Urol.* 2004; 172: 769-772.

Morita T, Ishizuka G, Tsuchida S. Initiation and propagation of stimulus from the renal pelvic pacemaker in pig kidney. *Invest Urol.* 1981; 19: 157–60.

Morita T, Kondo S, Suzuki T, Tsuchida S. Effect of calyceal resection on pelviureteral peristalsis in isolated pig kidney. *J Urol.* 1986; 135: 151–4.

Nicòtina PA, Romeo C, Arena F, Romeo G. Segmental up-regulation of transforming growth factor-β in the pathogenesis of primary megaureter. An immunocytochemical study. *Br J Urol* 1997; 80: 946–9

Patacchini R, Santicioli P, Zagorodnyuk V, Lazzeri M, Turini D, Maggi CA. Excitatory motor and electrical effects produced in the human and guinea-pig isolated ureter and guinea-pig renal pelvis. *Brit J Pharmacol* 1998; 125: 987–96.

Payabvash S, Kajbafzadeh AM, Tavangar SM, et al. Myocyte apoptosis in primary obstructive megaureters: the role of decreased vascular and neural supply. *J Urol.* 2007;178:259-264.

Pezzone MA, Watkins SC, Albe SM, King WE, de Groat W C, Chancellor MB, Fraser MO. Identification of c-kitpositive cells in the mouse ureter: the interstitial cells of Cajal of the urinary tract. *Am J Physiol.* 2003; 284: F925–9.

Oswald J, Schwentner C, Brenner E *et al.* Extracellular matrix degradation and reduced nerve supply in refluxing ureteral endings. *J Urol* 2004; 172: 1099–102

Oswald J, Brenner E, Schwentner C *et al.* The intravesical ureter in children with vesicoureteral reflux: a morphological and immunohistochemical characterization. *J Urol* 2003; 170: 2423–7.

Richard J. Lang et al Pyeloureteric peristalsis: role of atypical smooth muscle cells and interstitial cells of Cajal-like cells as pacemakers *Physiol* 576.3 (2006) pp 695–705

Sanders KM. A case for interstitial cells of Cajal as pacemakers and mediuators of neurotransmission in the gastrointestinal tract. Gastroenterology.1996; 111: 492-515.

Schwentner C. et al. Loss of interstitial cells of Cajal and gap junction protein connexin 43 at the vesicoureteral junction in children with vesicoure. *The Journal of Urology*. Vol 174, 1981-1986, November 2005.

Seki N, Suzuki H. Electrical properties of smooth muscle cell membrane in renal pelvis of rabbits. *Am J Physiol.* 1990; 259: F888 94

Sergeant GP et al Specialized pacemaking cells in the rabbit uretra. J phisiol 2000; 526:539.

Shokeir AA, Nijman RJ. Primary megaureter: current trends in diagnosis and treatment. *BJU Int.* 2000;86:861-868.

Shuba MF. The effect of sodium-free and potassium-free solutions, ionic current inhibitors and ouabain on electrophysiological properties of smooth muscle of guinea-pig ureter. *J Physiol.* 1977; 264: 837–51.

Sleator W, Butcher HR. Action potentials and pressure changes in ureteral peristaltic waves. *Am J Physiol.* 1955; 180: 261–76.

Solari V et al. Altered expression of interstitial cells of Cajal in congenital ureteropelvic obstruction. J Urol 2003; 170:2420-2.

Streutker et al: Loss of CD117 (c-kit) and CD34-positive ICC and associated CD34-positive fibroblasts defines a subpopulation of chronic intestinal pseudo-obstruction. Am J Surg Pathol, 27: 228,2003.

Thompson CB. Apoptosis in the pathogenesis and treatment of disease. *Science.* 1995;267:1456-1462.

Torihashi S, Nishi K, Tokutomi Y, et al. Blockade of kit signaling induces transdifferentiation of interstitial cells of Cajal to a smooth muscle phenotype. *Gastroenterology.* 1999;117:140-148.

Tsuchida S, Suzuki T. Pacemaker activity of the pelvicalyceal border recorded by an intracellular glass microelectrode. *Urol Int.* 1992; 48: 121–4.

Van der Aa F, Roskams T, Blyweert W, Ost D, Bogaer G, De Ridder D. Identification of kit positive cells in the human urinary tract. *J Urol.* 2004:171: 2492–6.

Wu JJ, Rothman TP, Gershon MD. Development of the interstitial cell of Cajal: origin, kit dependence and neuronal and nonneuronal sources of kit ligand. *J Neurosci Res* 2000; 59: 384–401.

Zhang Y, Lang RJ. Effects of intrinsic prostaglandins on the spontaneous contractile and electrical activity of the proximal renal pelvis of the guinea-pig. *Br J Pharmacol.* 1994; 113: 431–8.

11

Role of Pacing in Neurally Mediated Syncope

Vikas Kuriachan and Robert Sheldon
Libin Cardiovascular Institute of Alberta, University of Calgary, Calgary, Alberta, Canada

1. Introduction

Neurally mediated syncope syndromes involve autonomic reflexes causing bradycardia and/or hypotension resulting in a transient loss of consciousness(Brignole et al., 2004). These episodes can result in injuries and emotional stress. Recurrent vasovagal syncope can have a significant detrimental effect on the quality of life comparable to chronic disease patients with chronic back pain or rheumatoid arthritis(Linzer et al., 1991; Rose, Koshman, Spreng, & Sheldon, 2000). Hence management strategies have targeted vasodepression and bradycardia. Pacing has been a tempting solution that treats the cardioinhibitory response.

2. Vasovagal syncope

Vasovagal syncope is one of the common causes of syncope and a common reason for emergency room encounters(Savage, Corwin, McGee, Kannel, & Wolf, 1985). Vasovagal syncope is seen in younger patients and the reflex may have triggers such as sight of blood, venipuncture, or prolonged standing(Brignole et al., 2004). Some patients may have a prodrome of nausea and diaphoresis prior to loss of consciousness due to hypotension and/or bradycardia. Usually the syncopal episode last less than a minute but accompanying nausea, diaphoresis, and pallor can last longer. Many patients do not have a prodrome sufficiently long upon which to act, and therefore are unable to use preventive techniques such as counterpressure maneuvers or sitting/lying down to avoid or minimize a full episode. Unlike patients with cardiac or neurologic cause for syncope, patients with vasovagal syncope have no increased risk of cardiovascular morbidity or mortality (Soteriades et al., 2002). Hence in patients with vasovagal syncope preventing injury and maintaining a good quality of life are the primary goals for management(Kuriachan & Sheldon, 2008).

3. Initial pacing studies for vasovagal syncope

Bradycardia has long been recognized as a component of vasovagal syncope(Sharpey-Schafer, 1956). In recent years, bradycardia was seen during tilt table test studies in patients with vasovagal syncope during the induced episodes(Mosqueda-Garcia et al., 1997). Bradycardic problems have also been detected by pacemaker and implantable loop recorders during clinic episodes of vasovagal syncope(Krahn, Klein, & Yee, 1997). This suggested that pacing could prevent vasovagal syncope by treating the bradycardia component. This was initially looked at in patients with tilt table induced syncope associated with bradycardia(Fitzpatrick, Theodorakis, Ahmed, Williams, & Sutton, 1991). These patients underwent repeat tilt table test with temporary pacing. This prevented syncope in over half the patients although they still experienced vasovagal symptoms and presyncope. The results of this study should also be interpreted with caution since repeated tilt table testing can have a training effect and may reduce syncopal episodes(Reybrouck, Heidbuchel, Van De Werf, & Ector, 2002). Also the hemodynamic changes seen on tilt table induced syncopal episodes may not correlate with clinical episodes(Menozzi et al., 1993).

Initial observational studies seemed to show benefit with pacing as a treatment for vasovagal syncope(Sheldon, Koshman, Wilson, Kieser, & Rose, 1998; Petersen et al., 1994; Benditt et al., 1997). These initial studies were mainly a sequential design, with no placebo group, and included highly symptomatic patients, who received a pacemaker. Open label studies then followed which also showed impressive results with pacing. The North American Vasovagal Pacemaker Study (VPS) randomized 54 vasovagal syncope patients to a pacemaker or optimal medical treatment(Connolly, Sheldon, Roberts, & Gent, 1999a). Impressive results, as shown in Figure 1, were seen with 19/27 in the medical treatment group and only 6/27 in the pacemaker arm having one or more recurrences of syncope. The Vasovagal Syncope International Study (VASIS) randomized 42 syncope patients with cardioinhibitory responses on tilt table testing to pacemaker or medical therapy(Sutton et al., 2000). Again, an impressive reduction in syncope was seen, with only 5% in the pacemaker group and 61% in the medical therapy having syncope recurrence. Another open label study, Syncope Diagnosis and Treatment Study (SYDAT), randomized 93 syncope patients to a pacemaker or atenolol(Ammirati, Colivicchi, & Santini, 2001). This also showed a significant reduction in syncope with pacing (4.3%) versus atenolol (26%). Hence initial observational and open-label studies suggest a significant reduction in syncope recurrence with pacing with up to 87% relative risk reduction(Sud et al., 2007a; Connolly, Sheldon, Roberts, & Gent, 1999b). Summaries of the observational and randomized open-label pacing studies in vasovagal syncope are shown in Table 1.

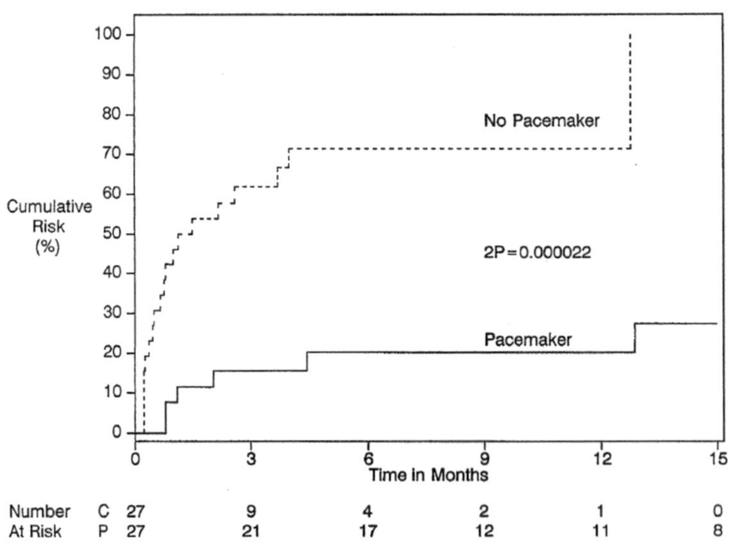

Fig. 1. Kaplan-Meier plot of time to first recurrence in VPS I of the 27 patients with pacemaker and the 27 patients without a pacemaker by intention-to-treat analysis. Figure from (Connolly et al., 1999a)

Study (year)	Type of Study	Tilt Testing part of inclusion	Study Arms	Results
Sheldon et al. (1998)	Observational	Yes	12 patients with VVS. Rate drop pacing in all patients	No syncope in 50%
Peterson et al. (1994)	Observational	Yes	37 patients with VVS. 35 had DDD and 2 had VVI	No syncope in 62%
Benditt et al (1997)	Observational	No	31 patients with VVS or CSS. Rate drop pacing in all patients	No syncope in 80%
VPS I (1999)	Open-label randomized	Yes	54 patients with VVS randomized to rate drop pacing or no implant	85% relative risk reduction
SYDAT (2001)	Open-label randomized	Yes	93 patients with VVS randomized to ppm with rate drop response or to atenolol	83 % reduction of syncope with pacing
VASIS (2000)	Open-label randomized	Yes	42 patients with VVS randomized to ppm with hysteresis and 23 with no implant	90% reduction of syncope with pacing

VVS = vasovagal syncope, CSS = carotid sinus syncope, ppm = pacemaker

Table 1. Summary of major open-label and observational studies for pacing in vasovagal syncope

4. Pacemaker programming

Various pacemaker settings have been tried in patients with vasovagal syncope. In general dual chamber (AV sequential) pacing is preferred, since both sinus and atrioventricular nodal function can be affected during a vasovagal episode. DDD pacing was compared to VVI and to sensing only (ODO) in 12 children with vasovagal syncope and found both modes of pacing to prevent syncope(McLeod, Wilson, Hewitt, Norrie, & Stephenson, 1999). All 12 were implanted with dual chamber pacemakers. Then programmed to ODO, VVI, and DDD with rate drop response for four month periods. Parents and patients were blinded to the pacemaker mode. Physician analyzing the results were blinded to patient and pacemaker mode. Even though both pacing modes prevented syncope, DDD was better than VVI for reducing presyncopal events.

Rate-changing programming has also been examined including rate hysteresis, rate smoothing, and rate drop response. The goals of these programming strategies are to treat the bradycardia and also to compensate for the hypotensive/vasodepressive response. Rate hysteresis triggers pacing at a higher rate when the intrinsic heart rate falls below a preset rate. Rate smoothing prevents sudden changes in heart rate by pacing when there is an abrupt drop in intrinsic heart rate even in just 1-2 beats. (This is also used in patients with atrial fibrillation.) Rate drop response, the most sophisticated of the three, results in high rate pacing for a few minutes when a drop in native heart rate is detected. This hopes to achieve pacing support that can overcome bradycardia and hypotension. Rate response programming has been used in many syncope studies including VPS and VPS II. One study compared DDD with rate drop response to DDI with rate hysteresis in vasovagal syncope(Ammirati et al., 1998). This study randomized 20 vasovagal syncope patients with cardioinhibitory response during tilt testing to rate drop response or rate hysteresis. During the 17 month follow up, no patients with rate drop response had syncope but 3 of 8 in the rate hysteresis group had recurrence of syncope.

Hence rate drop response was found to be more effective. Recent studies have also looked at closed loop stimulation (CLS). In closed loop stimulation variation of intracardiac impedance is tracked every beat, so that contractility changes can be detected in the early phase (prior to changes in heart rate) of a vasovagal episode and dual chamber pacing is activated(Occhetta, Bortnik, Audoglio, & Vassanelli, 2004a), as shown in Figure 2. This early initiation of pacing is believed to not only treat the bradycardic response that may follow but also overcome the transient hypotension. The INVASY trial randomized 55 patients with vasovagal syncope and positive tilt test to a CLS pacemaker or DDI and found CLS to be effective in preventing syncope over two-year follow-up period(Occhetta et al., 2004a). None of the patients had recurrences of syncope while in a CLS mode. However both groups had a reduction in syncope, likely due to a placebo effect. The recently completed, but not published, SCANSYNC study also used CLS pacing, described below. A preceding single blind cross-over study of 23 patients used a microaccelerator-equipped ventricular pace/sense leads (Sorin Biomedica, Saluggia, Italy) with a sensor at the tip that measures peak endocardial acceleration that correlates with measurements of left ventricular contractility(Deharo et al., 2003). This study compared standard DDI pacing to a rate adaptive (DDDR) specialized pacing system with a microaccelerometer in the right ventricular lead to detect myocardial contractivity. Both modalities were found to decrease syncopal episodes; in addition, the contractility-driven DDDR might have an additive benefit to conventional DDI pacing (Deharo et al., 2003).

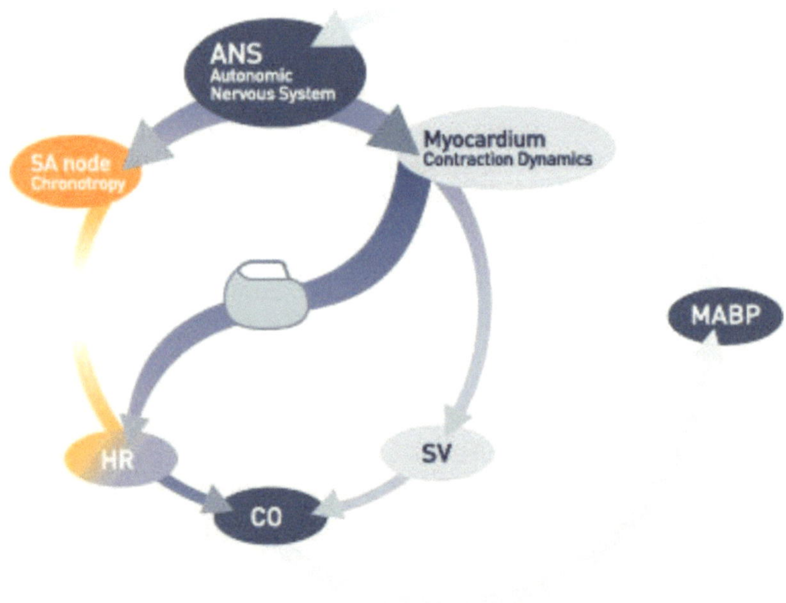

Fig. 2. Autonomic nervous system (ANS) monitors cardiac output (CO) via the mean arterial blood pressure (MABP). Cardiac output is a product of heart rate (HR) and stroke volume (SV). Myocardial contraction dynamics are monitored and changes detected early on by the closed loop stimulation pacemaker. Which enables the CLS pacemaker to provide heart rate changes help improve cardiac output. Figure taken from http://www.biotronik.com/en/in/1088 (c) Biotronik. Reproduced with permission from BIOTRONIK

5. Randomized, double blind studies comparing active pacing to sensing only

The great success of the initial studies raised the possibility a placebo effect with implant of a pacemaker for treatment of vasovagal syncope. Hence the first randomized, multicenter, double blinded study was designed and completed. VPS II, in which all 100 patients received pacemakers but were randomized to dual chamber pacing with rate drop sensing or sensing only(Connolly et al., 2003). After six months of follow up, there was no significant benefit with pacing and showed a 40% cumulative risk of syncope in the sensing group and 31% in the pacing group. This was also confirmed in a smaller study that included 29 patients with recurrent tilt-induced vasovagal syncope and one relapse after tilt testing (SYNPACE)(Raviele et al., 2004). In this study, patients all received a pacemaker and then were randomized to pacing or no pacing. Results of the first interim analysis and VPS II stopped this trial prematurely. They were unable to show a benefit with active pacing in preventing syncope.

A recent meta-analysis examined the role of pacing in vasovagal syncope(Sud et al., 2007b). Nine randomized trials were looked at in the meta-analysis, which included open label, single blind, and double blind trials. Interestingly, in contrast to open label trials, blinded trials for pacing in vasovagal syncope do not show a benefit, even in patients with marked cardioinhibitory response on tilt table testing(Sud et al., 2007a). Therefore, a cardioinhibitory response on tilt table testing probably is neither an appropriate surrogate marker for pacing studies, nor can it be used to predict patients who might respond to pacing.. The authors of the meta-analysis described that the benefits seen in open label, unblinded trials as being due to an expectation effect, by both patients and physicians. The authors of this meta-analysis synthesized a unique comparison between "inactive" pacing and no treatment and found that the expectation response alone reduces the odds of syncope by 84% (Figure 3).

Study (year)	**Number of Patients**	**Type**	**Tilt Testing part of inclusion**	**Study Arms**	**Results**
VPS II (2003)	100	Double blind randomized	No	Rate drop pacing vs ODO	Pacing did not reduce risk of syncope
SYNPACE (2004)	29	Double blind randomized	Yes	DDD rate drop vs ODO	Pacing did not reduce risk of syncope
Deharo et al. (2003)	23	Single blind randomized crossover	No	Contractility driven DDDR vs DDI	Both reduced syncope. Contractility driven may be better than DDI
INVASY (2004)	50	Single blind randomized crossover	Yes	DDD-CLS compared to DDI	Both reduced syncope. CLS pacing seems to be better than DDI.
Mcleod et al. (1999)	12	Double blind randomized	No	DDD vs VVI vs ODO	Pacing prevented syncope. DDD further reduced presyncope.

Table 2. Randomized blinded studies in pacing for Vasovagal Syncope

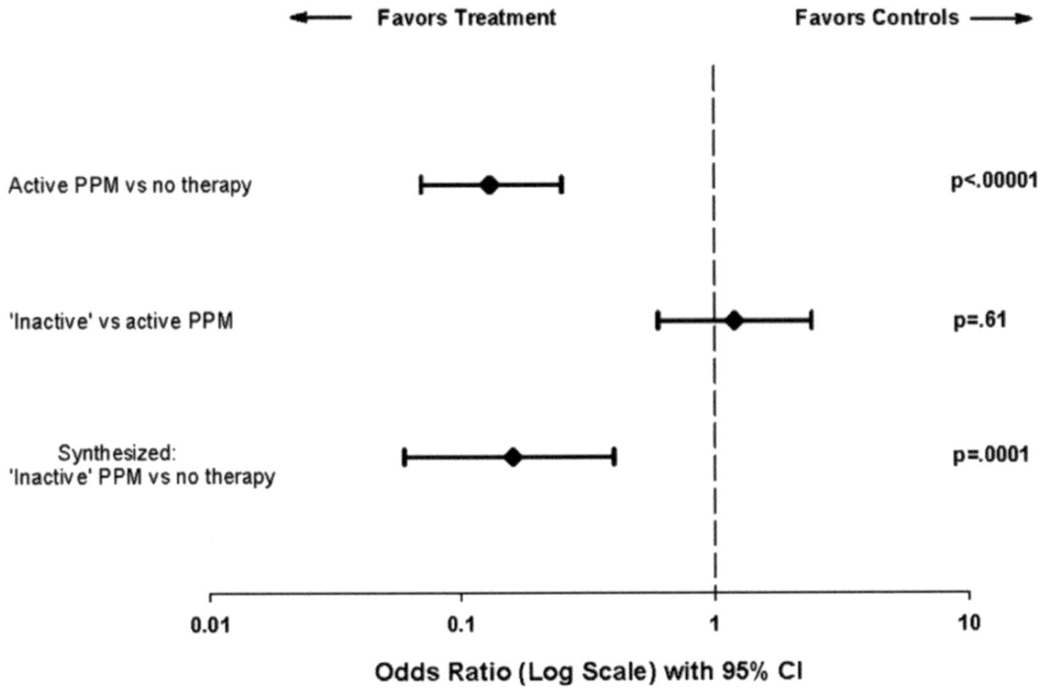

Fig. 3. Odds ratios comparing active cardiac pacing versus no therapy, "inactive" pacing versus active pacing, and a synthesized "inactive" versus no therapy. Line at OR 1.0 indicates no difference between the two groups. Estimates to the left of 1 represent treatment is better and estimates to the right represent control is better. Hence the bottom comparison represents the "expectation" effect. Figure from Sud et al 2007.

6. Placebo effect in pacing for vasovagal syncope

The placebo effect can be powerful and may be due to expectation effects of patients and health care providers, conditioning effects in patients, along with biases in patient assessment and reporting(Olshansky, 2007). Patients who receive pacemakers, due to the expense and invasive nature of the treatment, may be more willing to consider it as being a beneficial treatment for their problems. Healthcare workers who are involved in the care of these patients may not be conscious of biases they are exhibiting in assessment and reporting, and may also apparently observe a benefit from an ineffective intervention. Conversely those patients who did not receive pacemakers in studies may be disappointed and more inclined to report symptoms. Similar situations have also been encountered in the past with hypertrophic cardiomyopathy, where pacing was initially thought to improve functional status in open label studies(Nishimura et al., 1997). Similarly, atrial pacing was first reported to reduce atrial fibrillation, stroke, and death in patients with pacemakers(Gillis et al., 1999; Connolly et al., 2000). However, randomized, controlled studies did not show the benefits that were seen in the open label studies in any of these situations(Gillis et al., 1999; Connolly et al., 2000; Nishimura et al., 1997). Hence interpretation of studies in pacing that are not randomized, double blind, placebo-controlled should be done with caution since there may be important placebo effects. The vasodepressor and cardioinhibitory components may vary in each patient with different episodes and 50% to 83% of syncopal episodes may not have a cardioinhibitory component(Sheldon & Connolly, 2003). This may also explain why pacing does not seem to be of benefit in vasovagal syncope. Pacing alone may not be enough to overcome vasodepression.

7. Ongoing studies

Although the two blinded randomized trials are small (VPS II and SYNPACE), it seems pacing may not benefit most patients with vasovagal syncope. The ISSUE 2 study reported 392 patients with recurrent syncope and an implantable loop recorder (ILR)(Brignole et al., 2006). Specific treatment was then given to 53 patients based on the monitoring findings, of whom 47 received a pacemaker for asystole and 6 received anti-tachycardia treatments. A marked decrease in syncopal episodes was noted in the group that received specific treatment. In the 53 patients receiving specific treatment, the 1-year syncope recurrence rate was 10% compared to 41% in the patients without specific treatment. However the study is limited by lack of blinding and having only a minority of patients receiving specific treatment. To overcome the limitation of ISSUE 2, the ISSUE 3 study was designed (Brignole, 2007). Patients found to have asystolic pauses associated with syncope on ILR monitoring were randomized to pacemaker On or Off. This is a multicenter, randomized, placebo-controlled, prospective study of patients with a documented pause during syncope on an implantable loop recorder and then randomized to a pacemaker with pacing or only sensing. ISSUE 3 has finished recruitment and is now in the follow-up phase. The results of this study will help to clarify whether pacing may be of benefit in vasovagal syncope patients with prolonged asystolic pauses. As mentioned previously, initial studies also suggest that using a closed loop pacing (CLS) that detects contractility may be able to detect a neurocardiogenic episode early and provide pacing support better than a rate drop system(Kanjwal, Karabin, Kanjwal, & Grubb, 2010; Occhetta, Bortnik, & Vassanelli, 2003; Occhetta, Bortnik, Audoglio, & Vassanelli, 2004b). A randomized, prospective, double blind, cross over study (SCANSYNC) compared active (CLS pacing) to passive (VVI 30) pacing in patients with recurrent vasovagal syncope has been completed and is awaiting publication.

8. Other treatment options in vasovagal syncope

Other treatments for vasovagal syncope have also had similar findings with open label and observational studies showing benefit but double blind, randomized studies showing minimal benefit or no difference from placebo(Kuriachan, Sheldon, & Platonov, 2008). In patients with an identifiable prodrome there may be some benefit to using physical counterpressure maneuvers (PCM) which are safe and cost free(van et al., 2006). The maneuvers used are usually leg crossing with tensing of abdominal, buttock, and lower extremity muscles and/or gripping hands while abducting both arms. These maneuvers should be tried as first line treatments in patients with vasovagal syncope and an identifiable prodrome. Ensuring adequate volume repletion is important with salt and fluid intake. Various medications have also been studied, including beta-blockers, selective serotonin re-uptake inhibitors (SSRI), Fludrocortisone, and Midodrine. In general, no clear benefit has thus far been seen from studies with beta-blockers, SSRIs, and fludrocortisone(Kuriachan & Sheldon, 2008). The POST II study is comparing fludrocortisone to placebo in a randomized, double blind fashion and is in the follow-up phase (Raj, Rose, Ritchie, & Sheldon, 2006). Midodrine, a peripherally acting alpha-agonist, does seem to have some benefit in adults and children. Frequent dosing and some side effects, such as supine hypertension, may limits its use(Kuriachan et al., 2008). POST IV will be a double blind, randomized, placebo controlled study comparing midodrine to placebo in patients with vasovagal syncope.

The initial management approach to a patient with vasovagal syncope should include education about the condition, reassurance, and dietary intake (particularly salt and fluid). PCM should be taught to patients with a prodrome. If they still have frequent recurrent symptoms then medications attempts should be made. Pacing should be reserved as a last resort and ideally in patients documented with asystole during their syncopal episodes. A frank and open discussion should be held with the patient about the limited benefit that has been seen in studies for medications and pacing. Refer to Figure 4 for management approach for vasovagal syncope.

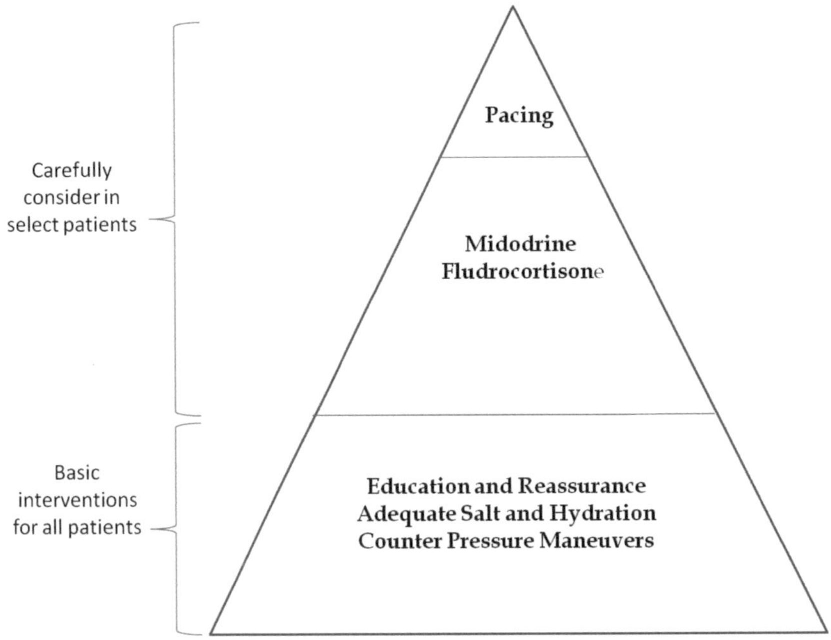

Fig. 4. Pyramid scheme of treatment for vasovagal syncope. All patients should receive the basic interventions as appropriate. Currently limited evidence for medications and pacing, hence use should be limited in very select patients who have significant, recurrent episodes after the basic interventions.

9. Carotid sinus hypersensitivity

Carotid sinus hypersensitivity and association with syncope have been known for many years. Carotid sinus hypersensitivity (CSH) is defined as a fall in systolic BP > 50mmHg and/or asystolic pause > 3 seconds with carotid sinus massage. Carotid sinus syndrome is when CSH is associated with spontaneous syncope that can be reproduced with carotid sinus massage(CSM). Carotid sinus syncope tends to happen in elderly men and the prevalence increases with cardiovascular, cerebrovascular, and neurodegenerative disease(Claesson, Kristensson, Edvardsson, & Wahrborg, 2007). A fall from syncope can result in significant injuries given the older age of this patient population. Although there is

limited evidence, carotid sinus syncope has been believed to occur in the context head turning movements that may cause pressure on the carotid, such as shoulder checking in a car with shoulder seat belt putting pressure or wearing a tight collar.
It is important to differentiate carotid sinus hypersensitivity from carotid sinus syndrome. A positive carotid sinus massage was noted in 32% of patients having an angiogram who had no history of carotid sinus syncope(Brown, Maloney, Smith, Haritzler, & Ilstrup, 1980). Asymptomatic carotid sinus hypersensitivity may be common in the elderly. Carotid sinus reflex helps with hemodynamic regulation. The vagal efferent signals increases cardiac vagal input resulting in lowering heart rate and peripheral vasodilation lowering blood pressure(LOWN & LEVINE, 1961). Hence an abnormal reflex can cause significant changes in blood pressure and heart rate which decreases brain perfusion and results in syncope.

10. Carotid sinus massage

Various protocols have been used for carotid sinus massage (Brignole et al., 2001). In one method, the carotid artery is firmly massaged at the anterior margin of the sternocleidmastoid at the cricoids cartilage level for up to 5 seconds, while the patient is in a supine position. If the first side does not yield a positive result then CSM is performed on the other side. Asystolic pause > 3 seconds (sinus pause or at times due to AV block), fall in BP > 50mmHg, and development of symptoms are necessary for a truly positive test. Abnormal responses can also be seen in patients with a history of spontaneous syncope. Some protocols use longer duration of massage to reproduce spontaneous symptoms, as well as both supine and upright positions (ensure patient safety in upright position). Heart rate changes can be readily seen on cardiac monitoring but a blood pressure drop is difficult to document without invasive monitoring (not usually practical) or noninvasive continuous digital plethysmography. CSM is contraindicated in patients with carotid bruits or history of prior stroke/TIA, due to concerns that the CSM may result in carotid plaque disruption and embolization resulting in a cerebrovascular event. Studies have looked at the safety of CSM, totaling over 5000 patients and found complication rates in the 0.1 - 0.2% range, of which most were transient neurological symptoms and full recovery was made except in two patients(Munro et al., 1994; Davies & Kenny, 1998).

11. Pacing studies in carotid sinus syncope

One of the first studies in carotid sinus syncope reported 70 patients with CSH and syncope, and found pacing to be very effective(Morley et al., 1982a). Subsequently a second study assessed 56 consecutive patients with CSH and syncope who had received no treatment (13 patients), anticholinergic medications (20), and pacemaker implant (23). In this study, pacing was effective in preventing syncope but a high rate of spontaneous remission was also observed(Sugrue et al., 1986). Another study with 21 patients, in which 13 received pacemakers, found only minimal benefit with pacing(Huang, Ezri, Hauser, & Denes, 1988). However, none of the patients with pacemakers had recurrences of syncope and only one patient had recurrence in the no pacemaker group of eight patients, demonstrating a very low recurrence rate even without receiving treatment. Other observational studies also found benefits from pacing and are listed in Table 3(Brignole et al., 1991; Brignole, Menozzi, Lolli, Sartore, & Barra, 1988).Hence some benefit was observed with pacing in CSH and syncope in the initial studies, but there were high rates of spontaneous remission.

Since many elderly patients who have syncope may not remember the details of the event and prodrome, they may present with a non-accidental fall. Hence it was thought that in many elderly patients, carotid sinus syncope might be responsible for non-accidental falls. This was first examined in the SAFE-PACE trial(Kenny et al., 2001). This open-label study included 175 consecutive patients over the age of 50 with non-accidental falls attending an accident and emergency facility. Those with carotid sinus hypersensitivity were randomized to rate drop dual chamber pacemaker or standard treatment. Paced patients were significantly less likely to fall (odds ratio 0.42) and reduced injurious event by 70%. SAFE-PACE 2 was a double blind, randomized study done to assess this(Daniel, Steen, Seifer, & Kenny, 2010). 141 patients with unexplained falls and cardioinhibitory carotid sinus hypersensitivity were randomized to a rate responsive pacemaker or implantable loop recorder. No significant reduction was seen in the pacemaker group, but this small sample size led to an underpowered study. Again, due to concerns of the open-label nature of the initial SAFE-PACE, a randomized study was conducted in which 25 patients received pacemakers but was randomized to pacemaker On (DDD) or Off (ODO)(Parry, Steen, Bexton, Tynan, & Kenny, 2009). This was a double blind study with a cross over design. There was a mean of 3.48 falls in the ODO mode and 4.04 in the DDD mode. Survival analysis showed no significant differences in time to first fall between the two groups (Figure 5). Hence no benefit was seen with pacing in this group for fall reduction. Further supporting the placebo effect in this study was the fall reduction that was seen in both groups, pacemaker On or Off, in the first six months after implant. However, this study was underpowered and should be interpreted with caution. Hence the initial impressive benefits seen in SAFE-PACE may be due to a placebo effect similar to the open-label vasovagal pacing studies.

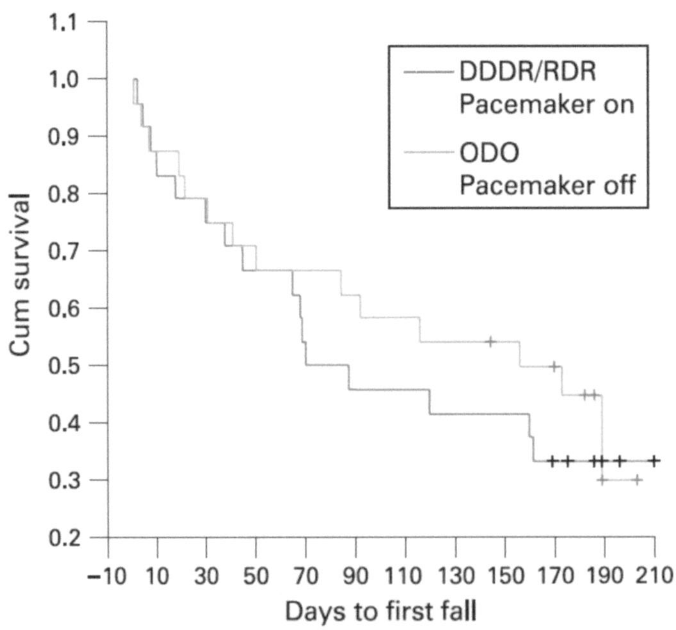

Fig. 5. Survival analysis (treating each group as independent samples) showed no significant differences in time to first fall between DDD and ODO modes. P=0.57. Figure from Parry et al. 2009.

Study (year)	Number of Patients	Methodology	Study Arms	Results
Sugrue et al. (1986)	56	Observational	13 no treatment 23 pacemaker 20 anticholinergics	Pacing was effective but high rate of spontaneous remission
Morley et al. (1982)	70	Observational	54 patients VVI 13 patients DVI 18 patients DDD	89% asymptomatic with pacing
Huang et al. (1988)	21	Observational	13 with pacemaker 8 with no implant	Pacing found to be beneficial. However only one patient had recurrence (in no pacer group)
Brignole et al. (1991)	60	Observational Crossover	26 with DDD 34 with VVI	DDD found to have less symptoms overall
Brignole et al.(1988)	35	Observational	19 no implant 11 with VVI 5 with DDD	Pacing prevented syncope recurrence
SAFEPACE 1 (2001)	175	Open label	87 with pacemaker 88 no implant	Pacing reduced falls and minimal reduction of syncope
SAFEPACE 2 (2010)	141	Double blind	71 with pacemaker 70 with loop recorder	No significant reduction in falls seen
Parry et al. (2009)	25	Double blind Crossover	25 DDD and crossover to ODO	Pacing had no effect of falls

Table 3. Pacing studies in context of Carotid Sinus Hypersensitivity, Syncope, and Falls.

Although only a few small studies have shown benefit, pacing has generally been felt to be beneficial in this condition, especially in elderly patients with a predominantly cardioinhibitory response to CSM and present with symptoms suggestive of carotid sinus syncope(Brignole, Menozzi, Lolli, Bottoni, & Gaggioli, 1992; Morley et al., 1982b; Claesson et al., 2007; Moya et al., 2009). Management should also include volume repletion and recommendations on avoiding situations that may cause syncope, such as tight collars and ties. Volume expanders and vasopressors may also be helpful but usually are limited due to problems with heart failure and hypertension that is common in the elderly population.

12. Conclusion

Initial steps in the management of vasovagal syncope should include education about the diagnosis and reassurance. Patients should be instructed on liberal intake of salt and fluid. Counterpressure maneuvers should be taught to patients with a prodrome. If they still have frequent recurrent symptoms, then medications attempts should be made. Pacing should be reserved as a last resort and ideally in patients documented with asystole during their syncopal episodes. For patients with carotid sinus syncope, pacing should be considered. Additional management should also include volume repletion and recommendations on avoiding situations that may cause syncope.

13. References

Ammirati, F., Colivicchi, F., & Santini, M. (2001). Permanent cardiac pacing versus medical treatment for the prevention of recurrent vasovagal syncope: a multicenter, randomized, controlled trial. *Circulation, 104,* 52-57.

Ammirati, F., Colivicchi, F., Toscano, S., Pandozi, C., Laudadio, M. T., De, S. F. et al. (1998). DDD pacing with rate drop response function versus DDI with rate hysteresis pacing for cardioinhibitory vasovagal syncope. *Pacing Clin.Electrophysiol., 21,* 2178-2181.

Benditt, D. G., Sutton, R., Gammage, M. D., Markowitz, T., Gorski, J., Nygaard, G. A. et al. (1997). Clinical experience with Thera DR rate-drop response pacing algorithm in carotid sinus syndrome and vasovagal syncope. The International Rate-Drop Investigators Group. *Pacing Clin.Electrophysiol., 20,* 832-839.

Brignole, M. (2007). International study on syncope of uncertain aetiology 3 (ISSUE 3): pacemaker therapy for patients with asystolic neurally-mediated syncope: rationale and study design. *Europace., 9,* 25-30.

Brignole, M., Alboni, P., Benditt, D., Bergfeldt, L., Blanc, J. J., Bloch Thomsen, P. E. et al. (2001). Guidelines on management (diagnosis and treatment) of syncope. *Eur.Heart J., 22,* 1256-1306.

Brignole, M., Alboni, P., Benditt, D. G., Bergfeldt, L., Blanc, J. J., Thomsen, P. E. et al. (2004). Guidelines on management (diagnosis and treatment) of syncope-update 2004. Executive Summary. *Eur.Heart J., 25,* 2054-2072.

Brignole, M., Menozzi, C., Lolli, G., Bottoni, N., & Gaggioli, G. (1992). Long-term outcome of paced and nonpaced patients with severe carotid sinus syndrome. *Am.J.Cardiol., 69,* 1039-1043.

Brignole, M., Menozzi, C., Lolli, G., Oddone, D., Gianfranchi, L., & Bertulla, A. (1991). Validation of a method for choice of pacing mode in carotid sinus syndrome with or without sinus bradycardia. *Pacing Clin.Electrophysiol., 14,* 196-203.

Brignole, M., Menozzi, C., Lolli, G., Sartore, B., & Barra, M. (1988). Natural and unnatural history of patients with severe carotid sinus hypersensitivity: a preliminary study. *Pacing Clin.Electrophysiol., 11,* 1628-1635.

Brignole, M., Sutton, R., Menozzi, C., Garcia-Civera, R., Moya, A., Wieling, W. et al. (2006). Early application of an implantable loop recorder allows effective specific therapy in patients with recurrent suspected neurally mediated syncope. *Eur.Heart J., 27,* 1085-1092.

Brown, K. A., Maloney, J. D., Smith, C. H., Haritzler, G. O., & Ilstrup, D. M. (1980). Carotid sinus reflex in patients undergoing coronary angiography: relationship of degree and location of coronary artery disease to response to carotid sinus massage. *Circulation, 62,* 697-703.

Claesson, J. E., Kristensson, B. E., Edvardsson, N., & Wahrborg, P. (2007). Less syncope and milder symptoms in patients treated with pacing for induced cardioinhibitory carotid sinus syndrome: a randomized study. *Europace., 9,* 932-936.

Connolly, S. J., Kerr, C. R., Gent, M., Roberts, R. S., Yusuf, S., Gillis, A. M. et al. (2000). Effects of physiologic pacing versus ventricular pacing on the risk of stroke and death due to cardiovascular causes. Canadian Trial of Physiologic Pacing Investigators. *N.Engl.J.Med., 342,* 1385-1391.

Connolly, S. J., Sheldon, R., Roberts, R. S., & Gent, M. (1999a). The North American Vasovagal Pacemaker Study (VPS). A randomized trial of permanent cardiac pacing for the prevention of vasovagal syncope. *J.Am.Coll.Cardiol., 33,* 16-20.

Connolly, S. J., Sheldon, R., Roberts, R. S., & Gent, M. (1999b). The North American Vasovagal Pacemaker Study (VPS). A randomized trial of permanent cardiac pacing for the prevention of vasovagal syncope. *J.Am.Coll.Cardiol., 33,* 16-20.

Connolly, S. J., Sheldon, R., Thorpe, K. E., Roberts, R. S., Ellenbogen, K. A., Wilkoff, B. L. et al. (2003). Pacemaker therapy for prevention of syncope in patients with recurrent severe vasovagal syncope: Second Vasovagal Pacemaker Study (VPS II): a randomized trial. *JAMA, 289,* 2224-2229.

Daniel, J. R., Steen, N., Seifer, M. C., & Kenny, R. (2010). Carotid sinus syndrome, should we pace? A multicentre, randomised control trial (Safepace 2). *Heart, 96,* 347-351.

Davies, A. J. & Kenny, R. A. (1998). Frequency of neurologic complications following carotid sinus massage. *Am.J.Cardiol., 81,* 1256-1257.

Deharo, J. C., Brunetto, A. B., Bellocci, F., Barbonaglia, L., Occhetta, E., Fasciolo, L. et al. (2003). DDDR pacing driven by contractility versus DDI pacing in vasovagal syncope: a multicenter, randomized study. *Pacing Clin.Electrophysiol., 26,* 447-450.

Fitzpatrick, A., Theodorakis, G., Ahmed, R., Williams, T., & Sutton, R. (1991). Dual chamber pacing aborts vasovagal syncope induced by head-up 60 degrees tilt. *Pacing Clin.Electrophysiol., 14,* 13-19.

Gillis, A. M., Wyse, D. G., Connolly, S. J., Dubuc, M., Philippon, F., Yee, R. et al. (1999). Atrial pacing periablation for prevention of paroxysmal atrial fibrillation. *Circulation, 99,* 2553-2558.

Huang, S. K., Ezri, M. D., Hauser, R. G., & Denes, P. (1988). Carotid sinus hypersensitivity in patients with unexplained syncope: clinical, electrophysiologic, and long-term follow-up observations. *Am.Heart J., 116,* 989-996.

Kanjwal, K., Karabin, B., Kanjwal, Y., & Grubb, B. P. (2010). Preliminary observations on the use of closed-loop cardiac pacing in patients with refractory neurocardiogenic syncope. *J.Interv.Card Electrophysiol., 27,* 69-73.

Kenny, R. A., Richardson, D. A., Steen, N., Bexton, R. S., Shaw, F. E., & Bond, J. (2001). Carotid sinus syndrome: a modifiable risk factor for nonaccidental falls in older adults (SAFE PACE). *J.Am.Coll.Cardiol., 38,* 1491-1496.

Krahn, A. D., Klein, G. J., & Yee, R. (1997). Recurrent syncope. Experience with an implantable loop recorder. *Cardiol.Clin., 15,* 313-326.

Kuriachan, V. & Sheldon, R. S. (2008). Current concepts in the evaluation and management of syncope. *Curr.Cardiol.Rep., 10,* 384-390.

Kuriachan, V., Sheldon, R. S., & Platonov, M. (2008). Evidence-based treatment for vasovagal syncope. *Heart Rhythm., 5,* 1609-1614.

Linzer, M., Pontinen, M., Gold, D. T., Divine, G. W., Felder, A., & Brooks, W. B. (1991). Impairment of physical and psychosocial function in recurrent syncope. *J.Clin.Epidemiol., 44,* 1037-1043.

LOWN, B. & LEVINE, S. A. (1961). The carotid sinus. Clinical value of its stimulation. *Circulation, 23,* 766-789.

McLeod, K. A., Wilson, N., Hewitt, J., Norrie, J., & Stephenson, J. B. (1999). Cardiac pacing for severe childhood neurally mediated syncope with reflex anoxic seizures. *Heart, 82,* 721-725.

Menozzi, C., Brignole, M., Lolli, G., Bottoni, N., Oddone, D., Gianfranchi, L. et al. (1993). Follow-up of asystolic episodes in patients with cardioinhibitory, neurally mediated syncope and VVI pacemaker. *Am.J.Cardiol., 72,* 1152-1155.

Morley, C. A., Perrins, E. J., Grant, P., Chan, S. L., McBrien, D. J., & Sutton, R. (1982a). Carotid sinus syncope treated by pacing. Analysis of persistent symptoms and role of atrioventricular sequential pacing. *Br.Heart J., 47,* 411-418.

Morley, C. A., Perrins, E. J., Grant, P., Chan, S. L., McBrien, D. J., & Sutton, R. (1982b). Carotid sinus syncope treated by pacing. Analysis of persistent symptoms and role of atrioventricular sequential pacing. *Br.Heart J., 47,* 411-418.

Mosqueda-Garcia, R., Furlan, R., Fernandez-Violante, R., Desai, T., Snell, M., Jarai, Z. et al. (1997). Sympathetic and baroreceptor reflex function in neurally mediated syncope evoked by tilt. *J.Clin.Invest, 99,* 2736-2744.

Moya, A., Sutton, R., Ammirati, F., Blanc, J. J., Brignole, M., Dahm, J. B. et al. (2009). Guidelines for the diagnosis and management of syncope (version 2009): the Task Force for the Diagnosis and Management of Syncope of the European Society of Cardiology (ESC). *Eur.Heart J., 30,* 2631-2671.

Munro, N. C., McIntosh, S., Lawson, J., Morley, C. A., Sutton, R., & Kenny, R. A. (1994). Incidence of complications after carotid sinus massage in older patients with syncope. *J.Am.Geriatr.Soc., 42,* 1248-1251.

Nishimura, R. A., Trusty, J. M., Hayes, D. L., Ilstrup, D. M., Larson, D. R., Hayes, S. N. et al. (1997). Dual-chamber pacing for hypertrophic cardiomyopathy: a randomized, double-blind, crossover trial. *J.Am.Coll.Cardiol., 29,* 435-441.

Occhetta, E., Bortnik, M., Audoglio, R., & Vassanelli, C. (2004a). Closed loop stimulation in prevention of vasovagal syncope. Inotropy Controlled Pacing in Vasovagal Syncope (INVASY): a multicentre randomized, single blind, controlled study. *Europace., 6,* 538-547.

Occhetta, E., Bortnik, M., Audoglio, R., & Vassanelli, C. (2004b). Closed loop stimulation in prevention of vasovagal syncope. Inotropy Controlled Pacing in Vasovagal Syncope (INVASY): a multicentre randomized, single blind, controlled study. *Europace., 6,* 538-547.

Occhetta, E., Bortnik, M., & Vassanelli, C. (2003). The DDDR closed loop stimulation for the prevention of vasovagal syncope: results from the INVASY prospective feasibility registry. *Europace., 5,* 153-162.

Olshansky, B. (2007). Placebo and nocebo in cardiovascular health: implications for healthcare, research, and the doctor-patient relationship. *J.Am.Coll.Cardiol., 49,* 415-421.

Parry, S. W., Steen, N., Bexton, R. S., Tynan, M., & Kenny, R. A. (2009). Pacing in elderly recurrent fallers with carotid sinus hypersensitivity: a randomised, double-blind, placebo controlled crossover trial. *Heart, 95,* 405-409.

Petersen, M. E., Chamberlain-Webber, R., Fitzpatrick, A. P., Ingram, A., Williams, T., & Sutton, R. (1994). Permanent pacing for cardioinhibitory malignant vasovagal syndrome. *Br.Heart J., 71,* 274-281.

Raj, S. R., Rose, S., Ritchie, D., & Sheldon, R. S. (2006). The Second Prevention of Syncope Trial (POST II)--a randomized clinical trial of fludrocortisone for the prevention of neurally mediated syncope: rationale and study design. *Am.Heart J., 151,* 1186-1187.

Raviele, A., Giada, F., Menozzi, C., Speca, G., Orazi, S., Gasparini, G. et al. (2004). A randomized, double-blind, placebo-controlled study of permanent cardiac pacing for the treatment of recurrent tilt-induced vasovagal syncope. The vasovagal syncope and pacing trial (SYNPACE). *Eur.Heart J., 25,* 1741-1748.

Reybrouck, T., Heidbuchel, H., Van De Werf, F., & Ector, H. (2002). Long-term follow-up results of tilt training therapy in patients with recurrent neurocardiogenic syncope. *Pacing Clin.Electrophysiol., 25,* 1441-1446.

Rose, M. S., Koshman, M. L., Spreng, S., & Sheldon, R. (2000). The relationship between health-related quality of life and frequency of spells in patients with syncope. *J.Clin.Epidemiol., 53,* 1209-1216.

Savage, D. D., Corwin, L., McGee, D. L., Kannel, W. B., & Wolf, P. A. (1985). Epidemiologic features of isolated syncope: the Framingham Study. *Stroke, 16,* 626-629.

Sharpey-Schafer, E. P. (1956). *British Medical Journal, 1,* 506-509.

Sheldon, R. & Connolly, S. (2003). Second Vasovagal Pacemaker Study (VPS II): rationale, design, results, and implications for practice and future clinical trials. *Card Electrophysiol.Rev., 7,* 411-415.

Sheldon, R., Koshman, M. L., Wilson, W., Kieser, T., & Rose, S. (1998). Effect of dual-chamber pacing with automatic rate-drop sensing on recurrent neurally mediated syncope. *Am.J.Cardiol., 81,* 158-162.

Soteriades, E. S., Evans, J. C., Larson, M. G., Chen, M. H., Chen, L., Benjamin, E. J. et al. (2002). Incidence and prognosis of syncope. *N.Engl.J.Med., 347,* 878-885.

Sud, S., Massel, D., Klein, G. J., Leong-Sit, P., Yee, R., Skanes, A. C. et al. (2007a). The expectation effect and cardiac pacing for refractory vasovagal syncope. *Am.J.Med., 120,* 54-62.

Sud, S., Massel, D., Klein, G. J., Leong-Sit, P., Yee, R., Skanes, A. C. et al. (2007b). The expectation effect and cardiac pacing for refractory vasovagal syncope. *Am.J.Med., 120,* 54-62.

Sugrue, D. D., Gersh, B. J., Holmes, D. R., Jr., Wood, D. L., Osborn, M. J., & Hammill, S. C. (1986). Symptomatic "isolated" carotid sinus hypersensitivity: natural history and results of treatment with anticholinergic drugs or pacemaker. *J.Am.Coll.Cardiol., 7,* 158-162.

Sutton, R., Brignole, M., Menozzi, C., Raviele, A., Alboni, P., Giani, P. et al. (2000). Dual-chamber pacing in the treatment of neurally mediated tilt-positive cardioinhibitory syncope : pacemaker versus no therapy: a multicenter randomized study. The Vasovagal Syncope International Study (VASIS) Investigators. *Circulation, 102,* 294-299.

van, D. N., Quartieri, F., Blanc, J. J., Garcia-Civera, R., Brignole, M., Moya, A. et al. (2006). Effectiveness of physical counterpressure maneuvers in preventing vasovagal syncope: the Physical Counterpressure Manoeuvres Trial (PC-Trial). *J.Am.Coll.Cardiol.*, *48*, 1652-1657.